Melanomas: Basic Properties and Clinical Behavior

# Pigment Cell

Vol. 2

Series Editor: V. RILEY, Seattle, Wash.

S. Karger · Basel · München · Paris · London · New York · Sydney

Proceedings of the 9th International Pigment Cell Conference
Houston, Tex., January 13–17, 1975 (Part I)

# Melanomas:
# Basic Properties and
# Clinical Behavior

Editor: V. RILEY, Seattle, Wash.

165 figures and 92 tables, 1976

S. Karger · Basel · München · Paris · London · New York · Sydney

# Pigment Cell

Vol. 1: Mechanisms in Pigmentation. Proceedings of the 8th International Pigment Cell Conference, Sydney, 1972. Editors: V. J. McGovern and P. Russell (Sydney) XIV + 414 p., 166 fig., 89 tab., 1973. ISBN 3–8055–1480–8

Vol. 3: Unique Properties of Melanocytes. Proceedings of the 9th International Pigment Cell Conference, Houston, Tex., 1975 (Part II). Editor: V. Riley (Seattle, Wash.) XVI + 430 p., 224 fig., 52 tab., 1 cpl., 1976. ISBN 3–8055–2371–8

Cataloging in Publication
International Pigment Cell Conference, 9th, Houston, Tex., 1975
Proceedings of the 9th International Pigment Cell Conference, Houston, Tex., January 13–17, 1975
Editor, V. Riley. – Basel, New York: Karger, 1976
(Pigment cell; v. 2–3)
Contents: pt. 1. Melanomas: basic properties and clinical behavior. – pt. 2. Unique properties of melanocytes.
1. Melanoma – congresses   2. Melanocytes – congresses   3. Melanin – congresses
I. Riley, Vernon, 1914– ed.   II. Melanomas: basic properties and clinical behavior
III. Unique properties of melanocytes   IV. Title   V. Series
W1 PI24 v. 2–3/QZ 200 I6094 1975p
ISBN 3–8055–2369–6

# Melanomas: Basic Properties and Clinical Behavior

Part I of the Proceedings of the 9th International Pigment Cell Conference, Houston, Tex., 1975.
For the contributions published in Part II of the Proceedings, appearing as Pigment Cell, Vol. 3, under the title 'Unique Properties of Melanocytes', see table of contents on page IX of this volume.

## Contents

### Biochemical Properties of Melanoma

### Genetics

Contents

## Cell Culture of Malignant Melanocytes

## Immunology of Experimental Melanoma

## Immunology of Human Melanoma

## Diagnosis and Physiological Influences of Melanoma

## Experimental Therapy of Melanoma

## Therapy of Melanoma

## Epidemiology of Melanoma

# Unique Properties of Melanocytes

Part II of the Proceedings of the 9th International Pigment Cell Conference,
Houston, Tex., 1975.
Published as Pigment Cell, Vol. 3.

## Contents

### Ultrastructure and Biochemical Organization of the Pigmentary System

### Structure and Unique Properties of Melanoproteins

### Enzymology of Melanin Formation and Transfer

Contents X

## Pigment Cell Genetics

## Hormone and Prostaglandin Influences on Pigment Cells

Contents

## Pigment Cell Photobiology and Control Mechanisms

## Cell Culture of Melanocytes

# Editorial

For the past thirty years the International Pigment Cell Conferences have convened periodically without the benefit of formal organization. The unstructured character of this interdisciplinary group was part of its special flavor and stimulating qualities. However, because of the increased interest in research on the pigment cell, and its application to the problems of biology including cancer, as represented by the malignant melanocyte, there is accumulating evidence that research in these areas might benefit by the establishment of an appropriate vehicle for the orderly perpetuation of the conferences, and by providing a stable literary means for publishing the proceedings of the conferences as well as interim papers of investigators working on the pigment cell.

As a consequence, the conference organizer undertook a mail survey to objectively assess the opinion of individuals who participated in previous conferences, or were otherwise identified with an interest in the field. Their views were specifically solicited concerning the formation of a pigment cell society, and whether a society journal would be desirable. The following responses were received from 143 scientists and physicians involved with pigment cell research or related clinical problems: approval was expressed by 86 percent for the formation of a Pigment Cell Society, while 11 % felt that the present informal arrangements were satisfactory and should not be changed. Three percent were undecided. In respect to the question of a society journal, 65 percent were in favor of this additional means for publishing the diverse interdisciplinary papers bearing upon pigmentation chemistry and pigment cell problems. Twenty-eight percent were against adding another journal to the world's crowded literature.

Based on the personal experiences of the editor and conference organizer, the practical accomplishment of these expressed preferences depends largely upon the availability of a physician or investigator who is not only familiar with the pigment cell field but also has available the extensive time required, as well as the interest and skills necessary to produce a journal of high quality. Special circumstances are essential to carry out the time-consuming requirements of organizing conferences and managing the business needs of such a society. Further discussion would be welcome from individuals in the field concerning practical solutions to the transformation of an organization that has served a valuable purpose in the scientific community, and deserves to be perpetuated in an appropriate manner. It would be particularly relevant to receive information about individuals whose limited teaching load, or other circumstances such as forthcoming retirement, would provide a long-term candidate to carry out the organization of such a society, and to assume primary responsibility for the organization of future International Pigment Cell Conferences.

VERNON RILEY, Series Editor
Chairman, Department of Microbiology
Pacific Northwest Research Foundation
Member, Fred Hutchinson Cancer Research Center
1102 Columbia Street, *Seattle, WA 98014* (USA)

# Preface

These proceedings contain a broad spectrum of papers dealing with the properties and behavior of malignant melanocytes. Both *in vitro* and *in vivo* studies are represented, with the investigations involving both experimental animals and man. The scope of these papers, which were delivered at the 9th International Pigment Cell Conference, encompassed a wide variety of disciplines, scientific aims, and experimental approaches. However, there was a clear division into two major research categories consisting of: (1) studies on problems concerning the malignant melanocyte, and (2), the experimental utilization of non-neoplastic melanocytes as superb, color-tagged, biological tools.

As a consequence, two separate companion volumes have been published, the first (Pigment Cell, vol. 2) containing all of the papers dealing with melanoma, while the other (Pigment Cell, vol. 3) deals with the basic research studies which utilized either normal or abnormal, nonmalignant melanocytes, or defined the subtle process associated with pigment structure, formation, and organization.

This melanoma volume will be of special interest to the oncologists, the experimental or clinical chemotherapists, and those other investigators who employ tumors as useful devices for solving basic biological problems.

The companion volume provides the most recent authoritative information on a broad spectrum of scientific investigations on natural pigment-forming processes and on the intriguing behavior of normal and abnormal, nonmalignant melanocytes. The two volumes thus complement each other, since both deal with the genetic, biochemical, or biological states of pigmented cells.

In terms of the application of such knowledge to urgent health problems of man, it is generally acknowledged that the eventual conquest of cancer requires a fuller understanding of normal life processes; and that further comprehension of the fundamental nature of life can be promoted by a careful study of pathological and neoplastic phenomena. The normal, abnormal, and transformed malignant melanocytes, all provide valuable cellular models for such studies, as exemplified by the scholarly papers contained in these two volumes.

VERNON RILEY

# The Myron Gordon Award: History and Citations

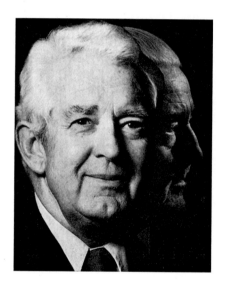

Composite portrait of VERNON TODD RILEY, recipient of the sixth Myron Gordon Award, and his father, FRANCIS VERNON RILEY. Although Dr. Riley's father was an attorney and a civil engineer by profession, he was a naturalist by avocation and inclination. Long before the advent of penicillin, he intuitively predicted from his observations of the antagonistic growth of mold and bacteria that these organisms should be a potential source of therapeutic materials. It was his enthusiastic and contagious interest in biological phenoma that was ultimately responsible for Vernon Riley's pursuit of biological research, which led to his basic studies on melanoma cells, to his discovery of the LDH-virus, and receipt of the Myron Gordon Award.

The International Pigment Cell Conferences are a continuing tribute to the scholarly pioneers who visualized their potential value to biology and medicine. The primary initiators were Dr. GEORGE MILTON SMITH of Yale, Dr. ROSS F. NIGRELLI, biologist of New York, and Dr. MYRON GORDON, internationally respected specialist in fish genetics.

During an informal gathering in Dr. SMITH's home in Pine Orchard, Conn., in 1946, these men decided to invite workers in the biological, medical, physical, and chemical sciences to meet together and to jointly analyze the nature and behavior of pigment cells, with special emphasis on the relationships to melanoma development, a formidable, early metastasizing malignancy. The formation of an integrated group of specialists was visualized, that would establish a developing pool of interdisciplinary information which would be accessible to all interested scientists and physicans. This proposal was a timely and tangible expression of the urgent need for a concerted attack upon the nature of melanomas and the overall cancer process. The first program was prepared in consultation with WALTER HESTON, VICTOR TWITTY, CORNELIUS P. RHOADS, and ROSCOE R. SPENCER. Further details on the development of this initial conference may be found in MYRON GORDON's introduction to the *Biology of Melanomas*, which was the title given to the Proceedings of the first conference. The meeting itself had the broad designation of *The Biology of Normal and Atypical Pigment Cell Growth*.

From the first, MYRON GORDON was the continuity figure, and in his intelligent and gently persuasive way he nurtured the pigment cell conferences through their sensitive formative phases. He was largely responsible for the production of the first three monographs reflecting the proceedings and discussions of those stimulating conferences.

Dr. M. J. (MIKE) KOPAC, President of the New York Academy of Science, and Professor and Chairman of the Department of Biology of New York University, had worked closely with Dr. GORDON in planning the conferences. Dr. GORDON, in turn, had solicited VERNON RILEY's assistance in editing the fourth volume of the pigment cell series. Following Dr. GORDON's sudden death in 1959, MIKE KOPAC, and others associated with the conferences, specifically asked VERNON RILEY to assume responsibility for organizing the 5th Conference. To make this invitation persuasive, MIKE KOPAC offered to make available the financial, scientific, and physical resources of the Academy in support of the Conference. In order to encourage participation by physicians and surgeons concerned with the melanoma problem, Dr. RILEY asked Dr. JOSEPH G. FORTNER, surgeon at Memorial Center, to serve as co-chairman and to promote the clinical aspects of the 5th Conference.

It was at that International Pigment Cell Conference that the Myron Gordon Award, in the form of a citation and a silver medallion, was established for outstanding contributions in the pigment cell field. The participants concurred that this was an appropriate memorial to MYRON GORDON, and would symbolize the continuity which he had anticipated.

Starting with the 5th Conference, the following individuals have been recipients of the Myron Gordon Award: GEORGE A. SWAN, Department of Chemistry, King's College, University of Durham, Newcastle upon Tyne

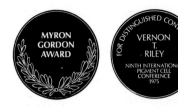

(5th Conference, New York, N.Y.); THOMAS B. FITZPATRICK, Department of Dermatology, Harvard Medical School, Massachusetts General Hospital, Boston, Mass. (6th Conference, Sofia); AARON B. LERNER, Department of Dermatology, Yale University School of Medicine, New Haven, Conn. (7th Conference, Seattle, Wash.); ELEANOR J. MACDONALD, Department of Epidemiology, M. D. Anderson Hospital and Tumor Institute, University of Texas, Houston, Tex. (8th Conference, Sydney), and VINCENT J. McGOVERN, Fairfax Institute of Pathology, Royal Prince Alfred Hospital, Sydney (8th Conference, Sydney).

Dr. VERNON RILEY, the 9th Conference recipient, has been a consistent contributor to melanoma research, involving not only the pigment cell, but has also made contributions to the field of tumor virology. He discovered and characterized a unique and important infectious entity, the Lactate Dehydrogenase-Elevating Virus (LDH-Virus), frequently called the 'Riley Virus', and has published a series of studies on the broad biological activities of this inconspicuous, non-oncogenic agent. Of special relevance to cancer was the demonstration of a correlation between the presence of this benign virus infection and an increased susceptibility of the host to the development of tumors induced by classical oncogenic viruses; and, in contrast, the ability of this virus to potentiate and enhance asparaginase therapy against cancer.

In the field of the pigment cell, Dr. RILEY was the first to adapt chromatography to the isolation and purification of melanosomes from various melanoma tissues. However, his special contribution has been the development, through carefully conducted basic research, of a variety of biochemical and biological observations that have become the building blocks upon which many subsequent investigations have depended. He has discovered or demonstrated the following basic phenomena utilizing melanomas:

The influence of various salt concentrations in altering the absorption properties of melanosomes, and other cellular components, on silica, which provided the theoretical basis for the chromatographic separation and purification of specific melanoma components.

The dual enhancement and inhibitory effects on melanoma enzyme systems of various physiological salt solutions that are conventionally employed in studying the enzymic activities of melanoma extracts and isolated cellular components, such as melanosomes.

An inhibitor, uniquely present in mouse melanoma extract, that is active against cytochrome oxidase, a fundamental cellular enzyme present in all melanomas and in all mammalian cells.

Other relevant contributions include: elucidation of the puzzling synergistic, enzyme-like reaction between *p*-phenylenediamine and melanoma extracts. He showed that identical, nonenzymic reactions could be produced by substituting dopa and related compounds for the melanoma extract.

A rational approach to the therapy of melanomas, and other malignancies, through the exploitation of toxic chemical reactions induced in the malignant cell between specific natural tumor components and known active exogenous compounds. The experimental success of this concept was demonstrated by treating mouse melanomas with various phenylenediamines to obtain tumor regressions and long-term cures. Related to these studies, was the demonstration of the antitumor properties of orthophenylenediamine.

The establishment of the biochemical ability of melanomas and other tumors to function as 'auxillary' metabolic organs in the specific detoxification or modification of various therapeutic or toxic compounds administered to the host.

The characterization, in conjunction with Dr. DARREL SPACKMAN, of alterations that occur in the concentrations of various free amino acids in the plasma and urine of melanoma patients, as well as in mice bearing melanomas.

A contribution of heroic amounts of his research time in organizing the 5th, 7th, and 8th International Pigment Cell Conferences, and in editing the proceedings of the 4th, 5th, 7th, and 8th Conferences (the 8th in conjunction with VINCENT MCGOVERN).

By virtue of these valued contributions to the understanding of the pigment cell, as well as for the manner in which he has personified the essentials of leadership by producing a friendly and stimulating spirit permeating these conferences, as envisioned by MYRON GORDON, VERNON TODD RILEY has been selected as the recipient of the sixth Myron Gordon Award, at this the Ninth International Pigment Cell Conference.

ELEANOR J. MACDONALD, Chairman
Myron Gordon Award Committee

# Acknowledgements

The following physicians and investigators reviewed the glossary terms for accuracy and relevance to pigment cell studies: PHILLIP BANDA, MARSDEN BLOIS, JAMES BOWMAN, JOHN BRUMBAUGH, GARY ELMER, M. A. FITZMAURICE, BERNARD GOFFE, JOYCE HAWKS, FUNAN HU, GEORGE ODLAND, GEORGE SANTISTEBAN, and CARL WITKOP. Editorial assistance was provided by M. A. FITZMAURICE, who also compiled the subject index and glossary. Administrative assistance by HEATHER McCLANAHAN greatly lessened the burden for the Editor. Without the organizational skills of Professor ELEANOR J. MACDONALD, and her associates in Houston, the Ninth International Pigment Cell Conference could not have taken place, and thus this monograph is a product of their activities. Thanks go to these individuals and the other unnamed contributors who made this monograph possible.

# Biochemical Properties of Melanoma

Pigment Cell, vol. 2, pp. 1–12 (Karger, Basel 1976)

# Unique Melanosomal Proteins in Murine Melanoma

W. G. KLINGLER, P. M. MONTAGUE and V. J. HEARING

Dermatology Branch, National Cancer Institute, National Institutes of Health, Bethesda, Md.

## Introduction

Melanin granules in the malignant melanocyte have many ultra-structural [22, 24, 33] and biochemical distinctions from those in the normal state. In addition, as a tumor known for occasional spontaneous regression [2], malignant melanoma has served as a model system for a broad range of immunological investigations into host antitumor defenses [14, 19, 34], and many studies have suggested the feasibility of immunotherapy for malignant melanoma [12, 15, 19, 32]. Our laboratory has been investigating these differences in melanosomes not only to further the understanding of neoplastic transformation, but also to eastablish a more specific approach to the successful immunotherapy for melanoma. This report contrasts the physical parameters of melanosomal proteins from normal and malignant murine systems, utilizing techniques which preserve protein integrity and permit subsequent immunological investigation.

## Materials and Methods

### Preparation of Fractions

The following sources of murine melanocytes were used: (1) 5- to 7-day-old normal black (C57Bl) mouse eyes; (2) 7-day-old normal black (C57Bl) mouse dorsal skin; (3) an actively growing S-91 murine melanoma (passed in $CDF_1$ mice); and (4) an actively growing B16 murine melanoma (passed in C57Bl mice). Following sacrifice of the animals, melanosomes were purified as follows (with all steps performed at 4 °C) [18]. Tissues were dissected into 0.1 M phosphate buffer (pH

7.4) and homogenized in a Tenbroeck (glass/glass) homogenizer. The homogenates were centrifuged at 1,000 $g$ for 5 min; the supernatants were recovered and centrifuged at 10,000 $g$ for 10 min. The resulting crude melanosomal pellet was resuspended in 0.1 M phosphate buffer, layered on a continuous sucrose gradient (0.3–2.0 M) and centrifuged at 80,000 $g$ for 90 min – yielding the purified melanosomal pellet. Melanosomes were solubilized overnight in 1% Triton X-100, and then cleared by centrifugation at 10,000 $g$ for 10 min. Protein concentrations of the resulting supernatant were determined by the method of BRAMHALL et al. [4].

Polyacrylamide Gel Electrophoresis

Polyacrylamide gel electrophoresis (PAGE) was conducted using the Tris-glycine buffer system (system A [36] at 2 mA/tube, 20 °C, with a constant protein load of 200 $\mu$g protein per gel. Electrophoresis was terminated as the bromphenol blue tracking dye approached the bottom of the gel. Gels were stained with Coomassie brilliant blue G [9]. Relative mobilities (Rms) of each protein band (migration calculated against the tracking dye) were determined over a range of seven different acrylamide concentrations (%T[1]): 7.5, 9.0, 10.5, 12.0, 13.5, 15.0, 18.0.

For demonstration of tyrosinase activity, additional gels were run simultaneously at selected %Ts and were placed in 0.5 M phosphate buffer (pH 7.4) with 0.1% L-3,4-dihydroxyphenylalanine (Dopa) for 60 min. The resulting darkened (Dopa-positive) bands were measured using the migration of the tracking dye as a reference.

Further, as another aid to the determination of the molecular weights of the various protein species, the Triton X-100 solubilized proteins from each tissue were passed through Diaflo Ultrafilters (Amicon, 300,000, 100,000, 50,000, and 30,000 nominal molecular weights) and the resulting filtrates were subjected to PAGE on 7.5% acrylamide gels. The molecular weight ranges of each protein band thus determined were utilized as an adjunct in the analysis of Ferguson plot data for each band, as detailed below.

Data Processing

Measurement of Rms of each protein band over a range of acrylamide concentrations and the subsequent production of a Ferguson plot (log Rm vs. %T) allowed the calculation of physical constants (free mobility [$Y_o$] and retardation coefficient [$K_r$] for each protein [36]. These constants, when compared to standard curves for known molecular weight proteins, permit the estimation of such physical parameters as molecular weight, molecular radius, and valence.

The large number of data points obtained by the above procedures were resolved into Ferguson plots with the aid of a computer, which sorted the data points into the linear Ferguson plots. Ancillary data, such as relative mobilities of Dopa-positive bands and the data from ultra-filtrations, were cross-referenced against the computer output to confirm the plots obtained.

Physical parameters of the melanosomal proteins from the various tissues obtained as above were then compared. Ferguson plots determined by PAGE and used

1    %T refers to total acrylamide concentration, including bisacrylamide (3% C [36]).

in these calculations were based on a minimum of 23 independent observations over the range of acrylamide concentrations. Physical parameters such as molecular weight were estimated by computer programs [36] using a standard curve constructed from 20 standard proteins solubilized in 1% Triton X-100 and fractionated by PAGE as above. The use of this gel system in obtaining such data is detailed in another communication [16].

## Results and Discussion

Mammalian melanoma is an extremely good model for the study of malignant transformation, especially since the malignant melanocyte does not dedifferentiate completely, but retains the ability to carry out its specific function – the production of melanosomes. However, in contrast with the normal melanosome, which is ovoid and uniformly melanized, melanin granules in the malignant melanocyte are irregular in shape, variable in size, with sporadic melanin deposition on a disordered melanosomal matrix [22, 24, 33]. Aside from ultrastructural distinctions, there is preliminary evidence (detailed below) that melanosomes from melanoma may have immunological differences, and may engender an immune response. Therefore, a biochemical characterization of both normal and melanoma melanosomal proteins could provide a molecular basis for these ultrastructural differences, and in addition, a demonstration of tumor-specific and common proteins potentially could corroborate immunological findings.

This present study reports primarily on biochemical distinctions, resolved by PAGE, between melanosomal proteins of normal and malignant pigment cells. Unlike other membrane solubilization techniques, such as urea or sodium decyl sulfate (SDS), Triton X-100 does not denature the solubilized proteins. Thus, the use of Triton X-100 not only allows the protein species to be fractionated as a function of their molecular weight and charge, but it also preserves the structure and thus the immunologic properties of the molecules [5, 29].

A schematic diagram of the melanosomal protein-banding pattern observed on 7.5% polyacrylamide gels and a photograph of one of the corresponding gels (fig. 1) demonstrates several categories of melanosomal proteins: (1) those unique to melanosomes of murine melanoma (numbers 2, 4, 17, 24); (2) those common to the normal and malignant state (numbers 3, 5–16, 18, 19, 21, 22, 25–32), and (3) proteins found only in normal melanosomes (numbers 1, 20, 23).

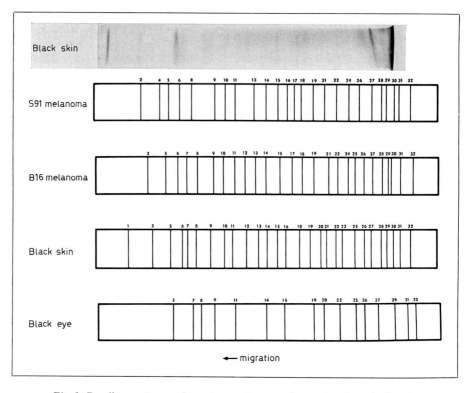

*Fig. 1.* Banding patterns of murine melanosomal proteins. Protein bands were numbered in order of decreasing mobility on 7.5% gels. Similarly migrating bands whose mobilities were within 2 standard deviations were given the same number. This manner of grouping bands was not intended to show identity among bands with the same number, but the noncorrespondence of other bands. For example, a comparison of figure 2 and table III indicates that band 14 in fact is 2 co-migrating proteins at 7.5%T: one common to all tissues, and one unique Dopa-positive protein in S-91 melanoma.

Further, the protein-banding patterns observed for comparable protein samples at many different %Ts were similarly compared and grouped. The number of protein bands found in each category is presented in table I. The variations between normal and neoplastic melanosomes are quite marked at each acrylamide concentration, even though a large number of protein species were demonstrable and the resolution of closely migrating bands is limited in the PAGE system. While fractionation of proteins at multiple %Ts allows a much more critical examina-

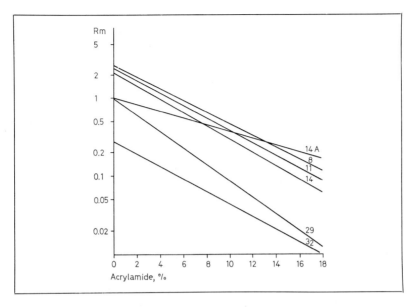

*Fig. 2.* Ferguson plots of Dopa-positive melanosomal proteins.

tion for unique protein bands, apparent discrepancies arise when numbers of unique bands at a given %T are contrasted with those at another
%T (table I). For example, at 7.5 %T, there were 3 melanosomal bands
found only in normal tissues and 4 bands unique to malignant tissue; in
contrast, at 15%T, there was one unique normal and 8 unique melanoma
melanosomal bands. Such a disparity of results arises not only from
the limitations of resolution inherent in fractionating protein bands on
gels, but is also due to overlapping slopes of Ferguson plots as shown in
figure 2. These plots demonstrate the electrophoretic migration patterns
of 6 Dopa-positive bands (characterized in table III). Note, because of a
relatively flat slope, band number 14A crosses the plot of proteins number 8, 11, and 14 at various points. Following PAGE at the appropriate
%T at or near one of these 'overlap points' only one band would be resolved; this problem of coincident bands is multiplied greatly when dealing with around 30 protein species, and accounts for the variability in
the numbers of types of bands. It should also be noted in table III that
the Dopa-positive bands also fall into the 3 general classes of proteins
found in figure 1 and table II, i.e. those common to both types of tissue,
and those unique to either.

*Table I.* Classes of murine melanosomal proteins demonstrable at various acrylamide concentrations

| %T | Normal[1] | Malignant | Common | Total |
|---|---|---|---|---|
| 7.5 | 3 | 4 | 25 | 32 |
| 9.0 | 1 | 7 | 17 | 25 |
| 10.5 | 2 | 5 | 18 | 25 |
| 12.0 | 1 | 8 | 17 | 26 |
| 13.5 | 1 | 5 | 19 | 25 |
| 15.0 | 1 | 8 | 17 | 26 |
| 18.0 | 0 | 5 | 17 | 22 |

1 Numbers of bands reported are those which were found only in *normal* (C57Bl) melanosomes, only in *malignant* (S-91 and B16) melanin granules, or those *common* to both.

As detailed in Materials and Methods, the determination of Ferguson plots (as in figure 2) permits the calculation of the approximate molecular size and charge of individual proteins. Such physical characteristics, calculated for the unique normal and unique malignant melanosomal protein bands, are presented in table II; similar data for Dopa-positive bands are listed in table III.

Analogous proteins in normal melanosomes of various species have been described [10, 17]; however, at least one of the melanosomal protein species in murine melanoma was shown to have a noncorresponding relative mobility and molecular weight [17]. In the present study, which employed Triton X-100 for solubilization, many more melanosomal proteins were resolved, presumably because the charge of the protein was also a factor affecting mobility in addition to the molecular size. In table III, for example, had SDS solubilization been used, not only would the enzymatic function of the enzyme have been lost, but protein numbers 11, 14, 32 and possibly number 8 would have been indistinguishable due to the similarity of their sizes. The melanosomal protein fraction, which contains only the T-1 isomer [31], can be shown to yield several Dopa-positive bands. The relationship between these enzymes is being studied to determine if they are truly isomers, multiple forms of the enzyme, a combination of structural protein and enzyme [23] or might reflect the presence or absence of prosthetic groups (the possible involvement of phospholipids with the enzyme has been noted [17, 30].

*Table II.* Physical characteristics of unique melanosomal proteins

| Band | Tissue | Rm 7.5% | $Y_0$[1] | $K_r$ | MW | RAD | VAL |
|------|--------|---------|----------|-------|-----|-----|-----|
| 2 | S-91 | 0.860 | 3.07 | 0.073 | 61 | 2.6 | 20 |
| 4 | S-91 | 0.805 | 1.77 | 0.045 | 23 | 1.9 | 9 |
| 0[2] | B16 | 1.000 | 1.89 | 0.038 | 16 | 1.7 | 8 |
| 17 | B16 | 0.396 | 2.04 | 0.096 | 101 | 3.1 | 17 |
| 6 | S-91, B16 | 0.750 | 2.21 | 0.063 | 46 | 2.4 | 15 |
| 8 | S-91, B16 | 0.702 | 2.56 | 0.075 | 63 | 2.7 | 17 |
| 10 | S-91, B16 | 0.620 | 2.39 | 0.078 | 68 | 2.8 | 16 |
| 24 | S-91, B16 | 0.258 | 3.65 | 0.154 | 241 | 4.1 | 50 |
| 6 | C57 | 0.750 | 2.60 | 0.071 | 58 | 2.6 | 17 |
| 8 | C57 | 0.700 | 3.25 | 0.087 | 75 | 2.9 | 9 |
| 20 | C57 | 0.327 | 3.50 | 0.136 | 197 | 3.9 | 41 |
| 23 | C57 | 0.275 | 6.20 | 0.181 | 320 | 4.6 | 93 |

1 $Y_0$ = Electrophoretic free mobility (y-intercept of Ferguson plot); $K_r$ = retardation coefficient (slope of Ferguson plot); MW = molecular weight in daltons $\times 10^{-3}$; RAD = radius in nm; VAL = valence as – (net protons per molecule) $\times 10^{-1}$. 95% confidence limits on figures are $\pm 10\%$.
2 0 reflects the fact that at 7.5% acrylamide, this band runs with the front, i.e. has Rm of 1.000.

Such unique melanosomal proteins in melanoma have several possible origin(s). (1) They could be fetal proteins derepressed in the malignant cell; in fact, an antibody cross-reacting with melanoma and fetal antigens has been noted [26]. (2) These atypical proteins could be of viral origin. (3) Such divergent proteins could be the result of their malsynthesis or aberrant degradation. One aberrant murine melanoma melanosomal protein has previously been shown [17] to have a relative mobility corresponding to the normal when electrophoresed in the presence of urea (indicating similar charge density), but having a noncorresponding relative mobility in the presence of SDS (where migration is a function of molecular size). This was interpreted to indicate the presence of a protein which in the melanoma has an abbreviated polypeptide sequence, but a charge density identical to the analogous normal protein [17]. Such data suggest that at least the third mechanism noted above is functioning in the production of altered proteins.

There is some evidence that melanin granules may be of significance in the immune response to melanoma, although the unique mela-

*Table III.* Physical parameters of Dopa-positive murine melanosomal proteins

| Band | Tissue | Rm 7.5% | $Y_0$[1] | $K_r$ | MW | RAD | VAL |
|------|--------|---------|----------|-------|-----|-----|-----|
| 11   | All    | 0.593   | 2.38     | 0.081 | 74  | 2.8 | 19  |
| 14   | All    | 0.496   | 2.11     | 0.084 | 80  | 2.9 | 18  |
| 29   | All    | 0.143   | 0.99     | 0.112 | 136 | 3.4 | 10  |
| 14A[2] | S-91 | 0.496   | 0.97     | 0.039 | 17  | 1.7 | 5   |
| 8    | C57    | 0.702   | 2.55     | 0.075 | 64  | 2.7 | 20  |
| 32   | C57    | 0.070   | 0.30     | 0.082 | 76  | 2.8 | 2   |

1 For explanation of abbreviations, see footnote 1, table II.
2 14A is so labeled to distinguish it from 14 (above) which migrates similarly on 7.5% gels.

noma melanosomal proteins have yet to be shown to be immunogenic *in vivo*. Preliminary experiments in our laboratory with the B16 melanoma using the double antibody radioimmunoassay technique [5] show circulating antibodies to at least one melanoma melanosomal antigen. Further, a recent study has shown that different melanocytic lesions evoke different types of mononuclear cell infiltrates and that this may be affected by the lesion's degree of pigmentation [10a].

A spectrum of tumor-specific host humoral [7] and cellular [25] defenses against mammalian melanoma have been shown, including tumor-specific cytoplasmic antigens [3, 11, 13, 26, 27], significant macrophage migration inhibition [21, 28], and destruction of cultured melanoma cells by autologous lymphocytes [8, 20]. Evidence for antigens common to normal and malignant melanocytes include the demonstration of delayed hypersensitivity in melanoma patients to extracts of melanoma [6, 12] and, in several cases, to extracts of normal skin [1], and the fact that anticytoplasmic antibody activity may be partially removed from positive sera by prior absorption with homogenates of pigmented skin [27]. Therefore, tumor-specific antigens, and antigens common to normal and malignant tissues, have been shown in mammalian melanoma. The unique and common melanosomal proteins described herein could result in the cytoplasmic antigenicity noted in the above studies.

A search for unique proteins responsible for tumor-specific circulating antibodies in human melanoma is currently underway, and preliminary results indicate a pattern similar to the murine melanosomal proteins presented here. Once it can be determined which, if any, of these proteins are immunogenic, data such as presented in table II will aid specific isolation of very pure antigen with significant implications for immunodiagnosis and immunotherapy. Further, a specific antibody to such unique immunogenic melanoma melanosomal proteins would be a valuable therapeutic and research tool.

In addition to our study, several biochemical comparisons of proteins in normal and malignant tissues have recently shown significant molecular distinctions in the neoplastic tissue. Nuclear proteins in normal liver and in Novikoff hepatoma ascites cells were resolved into unique and analogous protein species [35, 38]. In addition, a comparison of mitochondrial proteins of mouse mammary adenocarcinoma with normal mammary glands indicated not only a unique and an absent tumor mitochondrial polypeptide, but also an alteration of the activity of certain mitochondrial enzymes [37]. The occurrence of altered proteins in 3 different organelles of 3 different tumor systems is not likely to be coincidence, but may turn out to be a common denominator in malignancy. Hopefully, studies on the mechanism of such aberrant protein synthesis will lead to a more basic understanding of neoplasia.

## Summary

Differences in the ultrastructural appearances of melanosomes in normal pigmented tissue and melanoma have been known for some time; this study was initiated to determine if any of these differences could be resolved at the biochemical level. Melanin granules, purified from normal and malignant melanocytes, were solubilized with Triton X-100 and fractionated by gel electrophoresis. Comparison of melanosomal proteins revealed the following classes of proteins: (1) those common to all tissues, (2) proteins found in normal melanosomes but which are absent in melanoma, and perhaps most significantly, (3) unique proteins in murine melanoma. These results may provide further clues to the understanding of neoplasia, and suggest new approaches for the study of immunoassay and immunotherapy of malignant melanoma.

## References

1 BLUMING, A. Z.; VOGEL, C. L.; ZIEGLER, J. L., and KIRYABWIRE, J. W. M.: Delayed cutaneous sensitivity reactions to extracts of autologous malignant melanoma. A second look. J. natn. Cancer Inst. 48: 17–24 (1972).
2 BODENHAM, D. C.: A study of 650 observed malignant melanomas in the south-west region. Ann. R. Coll. Surg. 43: 218–239 (1968).

3   BOURGOIN, J. J. and BOURGOIN, A.: Cytoplasmic antigens in human malignant melanoma cells. Pigment Cell, vol. 1, pp. 366–371 (Karger, Basel 1973).

4   BRAMHALL, S.; NOACK, N.; WU, M., and LOEWENBERG, J. R.: A simple colorimetric method for determination of protein. Analyt. Biochem. *31:* 146–148 (1969).

5   BYSTRYN, J. C.; SCHENKEIN, I., and UHR, J. W.: Double-antibody radioimmunoassay for B16 melanoma antibodies. J. natn. Cancer Inst. *52:* 911–915 (1974).

6   CHAR, D. H.; HOLLINSHEAD, A.; COGAN, D. G.; BALLINTINE, E. J.; HOGAN, M. J., and HERBERMAN, R. B.: Cutaneous delayed hypersensitivity reactions to soluble melanoma antigen in patients with ocular malignant melanoma. New Engl. J. Med. *291:* 274–277 (1974).

7   COX, I. S. and ROMSDAHL, M. M.: Immunoglobulins associated with human malignant melanoma tumors. Pigment Cell, vol. 1, pp. 372–381 (Karger, Basel 1973).

8   CURRIE, G. A. and BASHAM, C.: Serum mediated inhibition of the immunological reactions of the patient to his own tumor: a possible role for circulating antigen. Br. J. Cancer *26:* 427–438 (1972).

9   DIEZEL, W.; KOPPERSCHLAGER, G., and HOFMANN, E.: An improved procedure for protein staining in polyacrylamide gels with a new type of Coomassie brilliant blue. Analyt. Biochem. *48:* 617–620 (1972).

10  DOEZEMA, P.: Proteins from melanosomes of mouse and chick pigment cells. J. Cell Physiol. *82:* 65–74 (1973).

10a EDELSON, R. L.; HEARING, V. J.; DELLON, A. L.; FRANK, M.; EDELSON, E. K., and GREEN, I.: Differentiation between B cells, T cells, and histocytes in melanocytic lesions: primary and metastatic melanoma and halo and giant pigmented nevi. Clin. Immunol. Immunopath. *4:* 557–568 (1975).

11  ELLIOT, P. G.; THURLOW, B.; NEEDHAM, P. R. G., and LEWIS, M. G.: The specificity of the cytoplasmic antigen in human malignant melanoma. Eur. J. Cancer *9:* 607–610 (1973).

12  FASS, L.; ZIEGLER, J. L.; HERBERMAN, R. B., and KIRYABWIRE, J. W. M.: Cutaneous hypersensitivity reactions to autologous extracts of malignant melanoma cells. Lancet *i:* 116–118 (1970).

13  FEDERMAN, J. L.; LEWIS, M. G., and CLARK, W. H.: Tumor-associated antibodies to ocular and cutaneous malignant melanoma. Negative interaction with normal choroidal melanocytes. J. natn. Cancer Inst. *52:* 587–589 (1974).

14  FOSSATI, G.; COLNAGHI, M. I.; DELLA PORTA, G.; CASCINELLI, N., and VERONESI, U.: Cellular and humoral immunity against human malignant melanoma. Int. J. Cancer *8:* 344–350 (1971).

15  GUTTERMAN, J. U.; MAVLIGIT, G.; McBRIDE, C.; FREI, E., III, and HERSH, E. M.: Immunoprophylaxis of malignant melanoma with systemic BCG. Study of strain, dose, and schedule. Natn. Cancer Inst. Monogr. *39:* 205–212 (1973).

16  HEARING, V. J.; KLINGLER, W. G.; EKEL, T. M., and MONTAGUE, P. M.: Molecular weight estimation of Triton X-100 solubilized proteins by polyacrylamide gel electrophoresis. Analyt. Biochem. *72:* 113–122 (1976).

17 HEARING, V. J. and EPPIG, J. J., jr.: Electrophoretic characterization of melanosomal proteins extracted from normal and malignant tissues. Experientia 30: 1011–1012 (1974).

18 HEARING, V. J. and LUTZNER, M. A.: Mammalian melanosomal proteins: characterization by polyacrylamide gel electrophoresis. Yale J. Biol. Med. 46: 553–559 (1973).

19 HELLSTRÖM, K. E. and HELLSTRÖM, I.: Immunity to neuroblastomas and melanomas. A. Rev. Med. 23: 19–38 (1972).

20 HELLSTRÖM, I. and HELLSTRÖM, K. E.: Some recent studies on cellular immunity to human melanomas. Fed. Proc. Fed. Am. Socs exp. Biol. 32: 156–159 (1973).

21 HENDERSON, W. R.; FUKUYAMA, K.; EPSTEIN, W. L., and SPITLER, L. E.: Demonstration of cellular immunity to tumor-specific antigens of malignant melanoma in hamsters by inhibition of macrophage migration. J. invest. Derm. 58: 229–232 (1972).

22 HIRONE, T.; NAGAI, T.; MATSUBARA, T., and FUKUSHIRO, R.: Biology of normal and abnormal melanocytes (University Park Press, Baltimore 1971).

23 HOLSTEIN, T. J.; QUEVEDO, W. C., jr., and BURNETT, J. B.: Multiple forms of tyrosinase in rodents and lagomorphs with special reference to their genetic control in mice. J. exp. Zool. 177: 173–184 (1971).

24 IWAMOTO, T.; REESE, A. B., and MUND, M. L.: Tapioca melanoma of the iris. 2. Electron microscopy of the melanoma cells compared with normal iris melanocytes. Am. J. Ophthal. 74: 851–861 (1972).

25 JEHN, U. W.; NATHANSON, L.; SCHWARTZ, R. S., and SKINNER, M.: In vitro lymphocyte stimulation by a soluble antigen from malignant melanoma. New Engl. J. Med. 283: 329–333 (1970).

26 LEWIS, M. G.; AVIS, P. J. G.; PHILLIPS, T. M., and SHEIKH, K. M. A.: Tumor-associated antigens in human malignant melanoma. Yale J. Biol. Med. 46: 661–668 (1973).

27 LEWIS, M. G.; IKONOPISOV, R. L.; NAIRN, R. C.; PHILLIPS, T. M.; FAIRLEY, G. H.; BODENHAM, D. C., and ALEXANDER, P.: Tumor-specific antibodies in human malignant melanoma and their relationship to the extent of the disease. Br. med. J. iii: 547–552 (1969).

28 MACKIE, R. M.; SPILG, W. G. S.; THOMAS, C. E., and COCHRAN, A. J.: Cell-mediated immunity in patients with malignant melanoma. Br. J. Derm. 87: 523–528 (1972).

29 MAKINO, S.; REYNOLDS, J. A., and TANFORD, C.: The binding of deoxycholate and Triton X-100 to proteins. J. biol. Chem. 248: 4926–4932 (1973).

30 MENON, I. A. and HABERMAN, H. F.: Activation of tyrosinase in microsomes and melanosomes from B16 and Harding-Passay melanomas. Archs Biochem. Biophys. 137: 231–242 (1970).

31 MIYAZAKI, K. and SEIJI, M.: Tyrosinase isolated from mouse melanoma melanosome. J. invest. Derm. 57: 81–86 (1971).

32 MORTON, D. L.: Immunotherapy of human melanomas and sarcomas. Natn. Cancer Inst. Monogr. 35: 375–378 (1972).

33 MOYER, F. H.: Genetic effects on melanosome fine structure and ontogeny in normal and malignant cells. Ann. N.Y. Acad. Sci. 100: 584–606 (1963).

34 MUKHERJI, B.; NATHANSON, L., and CLARK, D. A.: Studies of humoral and cell-mediated immunity in human melanoma. Yale J. Biol. Med. *46:* 681–692 (1973).

35 ORRICK, L. R.; OLSON, M. O. J., and BUSCH, H.: Comparison of nucleolar proteins of normal rat liver and Novikoff hepatoma ascites cells by two-dimensional polyacrylamide gel electrophoresis. Proc. natn. Acad. Sci. USA *70:* 1316–1320 (1973).

36 RODBARD, D. and CHRAMBACH, A.: Estimation of molecular radius, free mobility, and valence using polyacrylamide gel electrophoresis. Analyt. Biochem. *40:* 95–134 (1971).

37 WHITE, M. T.: Biochemical properties of mitochondria isolated from normal and neoplastic tissues of mice. J. Cell. Biol. *63:* 370a (1974).

38 YEOMAN, L. C.; TAYLOR, C. W.; JORDAN, J. J., and BUSCH, H.: Two-dimensional polyacrylamide gel electrophoresis of chromatin proteins of normal rat liver and Novikoff hepatoma ascites cells. Biochem. biophys. Res. Commun. *53:* 1067–1076 (1973).

Dr. V. J. HEARING, Bldg 10 Rm 12 N 238, National Institutes of Health, *Bethesda, MD 20014* (USA)

Pigment Cell, vol. 2, pp. 13–21 (Karger, Basel 1976)

# Studies on Oxidation and Reduction of Cytochrome $b_5$ in Microsomes of Mouse Melanoma

M. Hiraga, K. Abe, K. Morimoto, K. Nakajima and F. K. Anan[1]

Department of Internal Medicine and Clinical Pathology, Nakano General Hospital, Tokyo, Department of Biochemistry, School of Medicine, University of Tsukuba, Ibaragi-ken, and Shiseido Laboratory, Yokohama-shi

Kinetic and spectrophotometric studies of oxidation and reduction of cytochrome $b_5$ were reported in midgut homogenates of Cecropia [1], rat liver microsomes [12, 14], and hog thyroid microsomes [11]. These studies on redox properties of the pigment have contributed much in clarifying the probable pathways between pyridine nucleotides and oxygen in the microsomal electron transfer system. As a common feature of the electron transfer system in microsomes, it is generally known that flavoprotein dehydrogenase(s) and cytochrome $b_5$ are situated as redox components between pyridine nucleotides and oxygen. In addition to these components, hepatic microsomes contain cytochrome P-450 as the terminal oxidase for certain mixed function oxidations, in which the participation of cytochrome $b_5$ as the second electron donor to the oxidase was investigated [6] on the basis of the definition for mixed function oxidase [10]. Besides the participation of cytochrome $b_5$ in the function of cytochrome P-450, a cyanide-sensitive factor has been reported to be the fatty-acyl CoA desaturation system of hepatic microsomes, to which the shunt of electron from cytochrome $b_5$ is linked [2, 13]. In general, however, neither terminal oxidase linked to cytochrome $b_5$, nor has physiological role of the pigment been elucidated, although a hydrogen peroxide-generating system has been reported with NADH-oxidase system containing cytochrome $b_5$ in thyroid microsomes [11]. Conversely, recent studies on chromaffin granule membranes from adrenal medulla

1    The authors thank Prof. Y. Ogura for his helpful discussion, and Drs. F. Hu and K. Adachi for the supply of B16 melanoma.

and from splenic nerves revealed the presence of flavoprotein(s) and cytochrome $b_{561}$ in these noradrenalin storage membranes [3]. From the observation on the NADH-linked reduction of cytochrome $b_{561}$ and its oxidation by dopamine, it has been suggested that the flavoprotein and cytochrome $b_{561}$ are linked to an electron transfer chain where the copper protein enzyme, dopamine $\beta$-hydroxylase, serves as the terminal oxidase [4]. These studies on membranous type b cytochromes are very tempting in the search for terminal oxidases and to elucidate the role of the pigment in microsomes from various sorts of cells.

In the present paper, we will report on kinetic studies of oxidation and reduction of cytochrome $b_5$ in microsomes of mouse melanoma.

## Materials and Methods

Microsomes were prepared from melanotic B16 melanoma according to the method previously described [7]. For the kinetic studies of oxidation-reduction of cytochrome $b_5$, the measurement in absorbance difference between the wavelength pair 425 nm (peak) and 410 nm (trough) was performed in a Hitachi model 356 dual wavelength spectrophotometer. Recording of difference absorption spectra was carried out in a Shimadzu MPS-50 spectrophotometer. Cuvettes of 10 mm light path were used and the cell compartments were thermostatically controlled at 25 °C. NAD(P)H (purchased from Sigma Chemical Co., Missouri) solutions were spectrophotometrically standardized with the use of the extinction coefficient of 6.22 $mM^{-1} \cdot cm^{-1}$ at 340 nm [8], and the concentration of reduced cytochrome $b_5$ was estimated using an extinction coefficient of 163 $mM^{-1} \cdot cm^{-1}$ [5] in absorbance differences between the wavelength pair 425 and 410 nm. Protein concentrations were estimated by the method of LOWRY et al. [9] using crystalline bovine serum albumin as a standard. All experiments were carried out in 0.1 M potassium phosphate buffer, pH 7.5, and 2 $\mu$M rotenone was added to the reaction system only when NADH was employed as the reductant.

## Results

Reduced cytochrome $b_5$ of mouse melanoma was re-oxidizable in the aerobic state as reported in microsomes from various tissues [1, 11, 14]. Cycles of reduction and oxidation of microsomal cytochrome $b_5$ of melanoma are shown in figure 1. The rate of reduction of cytochrome $b_5$ by NAD(P)H was rapid. The extent of reduction of cytochrome $b_5$ was elevated with the increasing reductant concentration and reached each maximal plateau level at relatively low concentration of NADH or

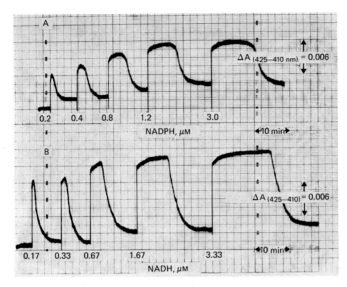

*Fig. 1.* Cycles of reduction and oxidation of cytochrome $b_5$ by NAD(P)H in aerated microsomes. Protein concentration, 10.5 mg/ml.

NADPH. The maximal plateau level of reduced cytochrome $b_5$ concentration by the use of NADH was higher than that by NADPH.

From the result shown in figure 1, kinetics similar to those reported by CHANCE and PAPPENHEIMER [1] might be applicable to the calculation of turnover number of cytochrome $b_5$ in the present study. The applicability of the kinetics is shown in figure 2. The amount of reduced cytochrome $b_5$ by the saturated concentration of NADPH or NADH reached each maximal plateau level, which did not differ by the absence or presence of cyanide. Cyanide, however, prolonged the half-time of cytochrome $b_5$ oxidation, and also increased the maximal amount of reduced cytochrome $b_5$ in the quite low concentration of NAD(P)H (not shown in fig. 2). The turnover number $k_{ox}$ of cytochrome $b_5$ was calculated (fig. 2). The value (0.0990 sec$^{-1}$) obtained by the use of NADPH was higher than that (0.0576 sec$^{-1}$) by NADH, and cyanide lowered the velocity constant for the reaction of cytochrome $b_5$ system with oxygen in both the cases by NADPH and NADH.

Conversely, the apparent first order velocity constant for the oxidation of cytochrome $b_5$ was calculated by the direct measurement of re-oxidation course of reduced cytochrome $b_5$. These results are summa-

*Table I.* Comparison of apparent first order velocity constant of cytochrome $b_5$ oxidation with turnover number calculated by the overall kinetics

| $k_{ox}$ | Reductants and inhibitor | | | |
|---|---|---|---|---|
| | NADPH | | NADH | |
| | −KCN | +1mM KCN | −KCN | +1mM KCN |
| $k_{ox} = \dfrac{2[NAD(P)H]_0}{[b_5^{2+}]_{max} \cdot t_{\frac{1}{2}off}}$, sec$^{-1}$ | 0.0990 | 0.0580 | 0.0576 | 0.0480 |
| | 41% inhibition | | 17% inhibition | |
| $k_{ox} = \dfrac{1}{t} \ln \dfrac{[b_5^{2+}]t=0}{[b_5^{2+}]t}$, sec$^{-1}$ | | | fast 0.0595 | 0.0462 |
| | | | 17% inhibition | |
| | 0.0176 | 0.0142 | slow 0.0113 | 0.0094 |
| | 19% inhibition | | 22% inhibition | |

rized in table I for comparison with the turnover number computed by the overall kinetics shown in figure 2. In the re-oxidation course of NADH-reduced cytochrome $b_5$, two consecutive first order reaction stages were observed, and 1 of the two apparent first order velocity constants was fast (0.0595 sec$^{-1}$) and consistent with the turnover number (0.0576 sec$^{-1}$) obtained by the overall kinetics. In contrast to the reduction by NADH, only one apparent first order velocity constant was obtained in the NADPH-reduced cytochrome $b_5$ system. This value was inconsistent with the turnover number (0.0990 sec$^{-1}$) calculated by the overall kinetics, and rather similar to the slow velocity constant (0.0113 sec$^{-1}$) of NADH-reduced cytochrome $b_5$ system.

Figure 3 illustrates the difference changes in the absorbance caused by NAD(P)H in aerated and anaerobic melanoma microsomes. In the NADPH-reduced system (fig. 3A), the anaerobiosis caused by the glucose-glucose oxidase system increased the change in difference absorbance from a steady state level to a second plateau level, where the successive addition of NADH and rotenone caused a slight downward deflection of the trace by the introduction of air, following upward deflection to the same plateau level before the addition of NADH. In the NADH-reduced system illustrated in figure 3B and C, the pattern similar to that shown in figure 3A was exhibited by the anaerobiosis (fig. 3C), but it was not observed in figure 3B because of the absence of glucose oxidase. The difference spectra (not presented in this paper) showed also an absorption peak at 425 nm in the Soret region.

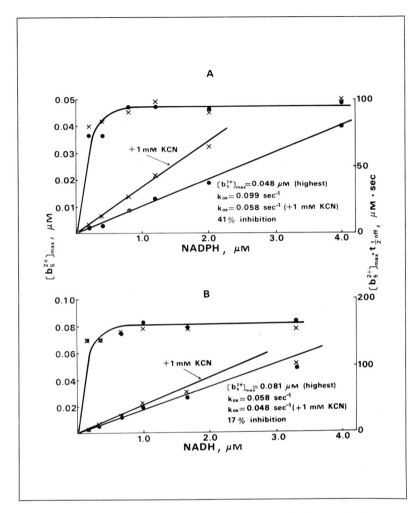

Fig. 2. Effect of initial concentration of NAD(P)H on the maximal amount of reduced cytochrome $b_5$ and the half-time of cytochrome $b_5$ oxidation. Experiments of cycling reduction and oxidation of cytochrome $b_5$ were performed in the absence (●) and presence (X) of 1 mM cyanide. The values, $k_{ox}$, expressed in the figures were calculated from the equation,

$$k_{ox} = \frac{2\,[NAD(P)H]_0}{[b_5^{2+}]_{max} \cdot t_{1/2 off}},$$

where $[NAD(P)H]_0$, the initial concentration of reductants; $[b_5^{2+}]$, the maximal amount of reduced cytochrome $b_5$; and $t_{1/2 off}$, the half-time of cytochrome $b_5$ oxidation, respectively. Protein concentration, 10.5 mg/ml.

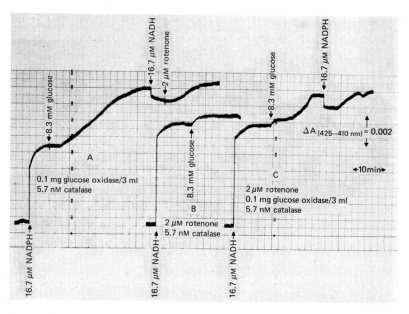

*Fig. 3.* Time courses of difference absorbance changes in aerated and anaerobic melanoma microsomes. Experimental conditions are shown as A, B, and C. Arrows indicate the addition of various reagents. Protein concentration, 2.65 mg/ml.

## Discussion

The typical time-course of reduction-oxidation of cytochrome $b_5$ by rapid recordings are schematically illustrated in figure 4. By increasing NADPH concentration, the amount of reduced cytochrome $b_5$ was elevated and reached a maximal plateau level, which was 58% reduction with respect to the anaerobic difference absorbance change. However, two consecutive reduction stages of cytochrome $b_5$ by NADH were observed, compatible with the occurrence of two consecutive oxidation stages described in table I. The fast reduction phase proceeded at an extremely rapid rate, and above a certain concentration of NADH the slow reduction phase appeared. The amount of cytochrome $b_5$ reduced in the fast phase corresponds to that reduced in the saturated concentration of NADPH. By increasing the concentration of NADH, the change in difference absorbance in the slow reduction phase gradually increased

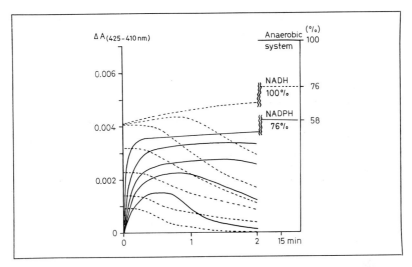

*Fig. 4.* Typical time course of reduction and oxidation of cytochrome $b_5$ by rapid recording. Solid and dotted lines indicate changes in difference absorbance caused by NADPH and NADH, respectively.

to reach a maximal plateau level of 76% reduction with respect to that in anaerobic state. Thus, the present studies suggest the following postulated pathways of electron transfer in melanoma microsomes:

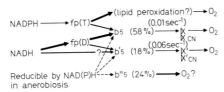

where $f_{p(T)}$ and $f_{(D)P}$ are denoted as flavoprotein dehydrogenase for NADPH and NADH; $b_5$, $b'_5$, and $b''_5$ indicate the multiple binding forms of the pigment with respect to the reductants and oxidants; X and X' are postulated factor or terminal oxidase between the pigment and oxygen; and cyanide-sensitive parts are indicated as $X_{CN}$ and $X'_{CN}$, respectively. The dotted lines do not mean the direct reduction of the pigment by NAD(P)H.

From the pathways described above, the discrepancy in the oxidation velocity constants calculated by the two different kinetic methods in the NADPH-reduced cytochrome $b_5$ system could be interpreted as the presence of a shunt, where electron leaks to oxygen through electron carriers besides cytochrome $b_5$ as observed in hog thyroid microsomes [11]. Another possibility would be referred to the contribution by the pigment having an extremely high turnover number. This possibility, however, seems unlikely because there is no discrepancy in the oxidation velocity constants obtained by the 2 different kinetic methods in the NADH-reduced pigment system. The presence of X and X' has been postulated by the results of double reciprocal plottings of $k_{ox}$ and oxygen concentration. In the plottings, $1/k_{ox}$ showed no considerable change in the range from low to infinite oxygen concentration. The cyanide inhibition of the velocity constant for the reaction of cytochrome $b_5$ system with oxygen was incomplete at 1 mM cyanide concentration, and the extent of the inhibition did not change even at 5 and 10 mM cyanide concentration.

## Summary

The oxidation and reduction of cytochrome $b_5$ was spectrophotometrically investigated by using NAD(P)H. The extent of reduction of cytochrome $b_5$ by NAD(P)H was elevated with the increasing reductant concentration, and reached each maximal plateau level at relatively low concentration of NADH or NADPH. The maximal plateau level of reduced cytochrome $b_5$ concentration by the use of NADH was higher than that by NADPH. From the turnover numbers of cytochrome $b_5$ calculated by the two different kinetic methods, and the maximal plateau levels of the reduced pigment, it has been suggested that the microsomes of mouse melanoma possess multiple binding forms of cytochrome $b_5$ with respect to the reductants (electron donor) and oxidants (electron acceptor).

## References

1   CHANCE, B. and PAPPENHEIMER, A. M., jr.: Kinetic and spectrophotometric studies of cytochrome $b_5$ in midgut homogenates of Cecropia. J. biol. Chem. 209: 931–943 (1954).
2   CORREIA, M. A. and MANNERING, G. J.: Reduced diphosphopyridine nucleotide synergism of the reduced triphosphopyridine nucleotide-dependent mixed-function oxidase system of hepatic microsomes. I. Effects of activation and inhibition of the fatty acyl coenzyme A desaturation system. Mol. Pharmacol. 9: 455–469 (1973).
3   FLATMARK, T.; LAGERCRANTZ, H.; TERLAND, O.; HELLE, K. B., and STJÄRNE, L.: Electron carriers of the noradrenaline storage vesicles from bovine splenic nerves. Biochim. biophys. Acta 245: 249–252 (1971).

4   FLATMARK, T.; TERLAND, O., and HELLE, K. B.: Electron carriers of the bovine adrenal chromaffin granules. Biochim. biophys. Acta *226:* 9–19 (1971).

5   GARFINKEL, D.: Studies on pig liver microsomes. I. Enzymic and pigment composition of different microsomal fractions. Archs Biochem. Biophys. *77:* 493–509 (1958).

6   HILDEBRANDT, A. and ESTABROOK, R. W.: Evidence for the participation of cytochrome $b_5$ in hepatic microsomal mixed-function oxidation reactions. Archs Biochem. Biophys. *143:* 66–79 (1971).

7   HIRAGA, M.; NAKAJIMA, K., and ANAN, F. K.: Microsomal electron-transfer system of mouse melanoma. Pigment Cell, vol. 1, pp. 134–141 (Karger, Basel 1973).

8   HORECKER, B. L. and KORNBERG, A.: The extinction coefficients of the reduced band of pyridine nucleotides. J. biol. Chem. *175:* 385–390 (1948).

9   LOWRY, O. H.; ROSEBROUGH, N. J.; FARR, A. L., and RANDALL, R. J.: Protein measurement with the Folin phenol reagent. J. biol. Chem. *193:* 265–275 (1951).

10   MASON, H. S.: Mechanism of oxygen metabolism. Adv. Enzymol. *19:* 79–233 (1957).

11   OHTAKI, S.; MASHIMO, K., and YAMAZAKI, I.: Hydrogen peroxide generating system in hog thyroid microsomes. Biochim. biophys. Acta *292:* 825–833 (1973).

12   OSHINO, N. and SATO, R.: Stimulation by phenols of the reoxidation microsomal bound cytochrome $b_5$ and its implication to fatty acid desaturation. J. Biochem. *69:* 169–180 (1971).

13   OSHINO, N. and SATO, R.: A function of cytochrome $b_5$ in fatty acid desaturation by rat liver microsomes. J. Biochem. *69:* 155–167 (1971).

14   MODIRZADEH, J. and KAMIN, H.: Reduction of microsomal cytochromes by pyridine nucleotides. Biochim. biophys. Acta *99:* 205–226 (1965).

M. HIRAGA, MD, Department of Internal Medicine and Department of Clinical Pathology, Nakano General Hospital, No. 59–16, 4-Chome, Chuo, Nakano-ku, *Tokyo* (Japan)

Pigment Cell, vol. 2, pp. 22–30 (Karger, Basel 1976)

# Induction of the Release of Viral Particles from Greene Hamster Melanoma Cells by Thymidine

T. W. REID, P. RUSSELL and D. M. ALBERT

Yale University School of Medicine, New Haven, Conn.

## Introduction

Previous studies have shown that addition of bromodeoxyuridine (BrdU) to certain tumor cells in tissue culture will cause the release of tumor virus particles containing reverse transcriptase activity [3, 5]. We have found that similar treatment of Greene hamster cells will result in the release of virus particles into tissue culture media [9] and that human melanomas contained reverse transcriptase type activity [8]. In examining the effect of BrdU more closely, we recently have found that the addition of low levels of thymidine to Greene hamster melanoma cells in tissue culture results in a marked increase in virus particle release [10]. This finding is of interest since it indicates that a normal constituent of the cell, when raised to higher concentrations than normal, can result in the activation of virus particle formation in tumor cells in tissue culture. In addition, this allows one to carry out experiments which may yield information concerning the actual mechanism of the induction of virus particles in tumor cells. This paper reports on the characteristics of the virus particles induced from melanoma cells and compares them with other known C-type particles released from mouse cells. A comparison is also made with virus particles released from the same cells by means of BrdU treatment.

## Experimental

The Greene transplantable hamster melanoma (Y22 Greene), a clone of mouse Balb/3T3, and a nonproducing line of clone A31 Balb/3T3 cells previously infected with Kirsten virus, were treated while in logarithmic phase of growth. Cells in 250 ml Falcon flasks were grown in culture media RPMI (1640 with 10% FCS). Following the addition of thymidine or its analogs, the cell media was not changed for 40 h. After this time, the cells were washed and fresh media was added. The culture fluid was harvested after 72–96 h. For those experiments involving labeling of the RNA, 0.1 mCi of $^3$H-uridine was added when fresh media was added to the treated culture.

After harvesting, the cell media was centrifuged at 3,000 g for 10 min and the supernatant spun at 100,000 g for 60 min. The pellet was resuspended in Tris buffer (0.05 M, pH 7.9) and layered on 20–70% linear glycerol gradient. The gradient was centrifuged for 3 h at 120,000 g. Fractions from the gradient were collected by bottom puncture; 50 $\mu$l of the fraction was added to 50 $\mu$l of 0.05 M Tris, pH 7.9, which contained 20 mM DTT, 60 mM NaCl, and 0.5% Nonident P-40. This mixture was incubated at 4 °C for 60 min. 10 $\mu$l of this solution was added to 100 $\mu$l of 0.05 M Tris (pH 7.9), 0.5 mM manganese acetate, 60 mM KCl, 20 mM DTT, 0.5% Nonident P-40, 2.25 $\mu$M ATP, 10$^{-5}$ M poly(rA) or (dA) 1.2 $\mu$mol P/ml, oligo(dT) 2.1×10$^{-6}$ M, and 0.1 $\mu$M $^3$H TTP. The reaction was allowed to incubate for 60 min at 30 °C after which a cold TCA (5% w/v) sodium pyrophosphate quench was added. The acid insoluble precipitate was collected on Whatman GF/C filter papers and counted. Any deviations from this procedure are noted in the text.

Polyribonucleotides were a product of Miles Laboratories, Elkhart, Ind.; concentrations were determined from extinction coefficients provided by the manufacturer and an assumed MW of 100,000. Oligodeoxyribonucleotides were obtained from Collaborative Research, Waltham, Mass. Chain lengths were listed at 12–18 units and their concentrations were determined from the extinction coefficient of the respective deoxyribonucleotide. The tritium-labeled thymidine triphosphate was obtained from New England Nuclear Corporation and had a specific activity of 960 cpm/pmol as used in the assay. The thymidine used came from two different lots from Sigma Chemical.

Viral pellets from cultures treated with $^3$H-uridine were prepared as described and resuspended in Tris buffer. A 20–70% linear glycerol gradient was centrifuged for 3 h at 120,000 g after the viral suspension was added. Fractions of the gradient were collected by bottom puncture and fractions were quenched with cold TCA. The acid-insoluble precipitate was collected and counted. A similar pellet was treated for 20 min with 1% SDS and 0.1 M LiCl. This solution was placed on a 10–30% linear glycerol gradient and spun for 3 h at 100,000 g. Fractions were collected by bottom puncture and the acid-insoluble precipitate collected on filter papers and counted.

## Results

In order to determine the optimum concentration of thymidine necessary for virus particle release, different concentrations of thymidine were added to the cell cultures (table I). Although 10$^{-5}$ M thymidine was

*Table I.* Viral polymerase activity released from cells with various treatments

| Cell type | Treatment | pmol $^3$H-TMP incorporated/h/10 $\mu$g protein with | |
| --- | --- | --- | --- |
| | | poly(rA) · oligo(dT) | poly(dA) · oligo(dT) |
| Y22 Greene | – | 1.2 | 0.7 |
| | $10^{-3}$ M thymidine | 8.0 | 0.6 |
| | $10^{-4}$ M thymidine | 62.0 | 0.9 |
| | $10^{-5}$ M thymidine | 130.0 | 0.8 |
| | $10^{-6}$ M thymidine | 44.0 | 0.7 |
| | $10^{-7}$ M thymidine | 10.0 | – |
| | $10^{-8}$ M thymidine | 1.2 | – |
| | $10^{-4}$ M BrdU | 104.0 | – |
| | $10^{-4}$ M BrdU + $10^{-4}$ M deoxycytidine | 125.0 | – |
| | $10^{-4}$ M thymidine | 65.0 | – |
| | $10^{-4}$ M thymidine + $10^{-4}$ M deoxycytidine | 72.0 | – |

*Table II.* Viral polymerase activity released from cells treated with thymidine, BrdU or IdU

| Cell type | Treatment | pmol $^3$H-TMP incorporated/h/10 $\mu$g protein with | |
| --- | --- | --- | --- |
| | | poly(rA) · oligo(dT) | poly(dA) · oligo (dT) |
| Y22 Greene | – | 1.2 | 0.7 |
| | $10^{-4}$ M thymidine | 60.0 | 0.9 |
| | $10^{-4}$ M BrdU | 60.0 | – |
| | $5 \times 10^{-5}$ M BrdU + $5 \times 10^{-5}$ M thymidine | 62.0 | – |
| Balb-3T3 | – | 0.4 | 0.4 |
| | $10^{-4}$ M thymidine | 0.5 | 0.9 |
| | $10^{-4}$ M BrdU | 5.0 | 0.5 |
| Balb-3T3 | – | 0.3 | 0.3 |
| Clone A31 | $10^{-4}$ M thymidine | 0.5 | 0.5 |
| Kirsten transformed | $10^{-4}$ M BrdU | 7.0 | 0.4 |
| | $10^{-4}$ M IdU | 13.0 | 0.5 |

*Table III.* Time course for virus production from Y22 cells after treatment with thymidine

| Days after treatment ($10^{-5}$ M Thy) | Polymerase activity: pmol $^3$H-TMP incorporated/h/10 $\mu$g/protein |
|---|---|
| 3 | 10.2 |
| 4 | 40.3 |
| 5 | 130.1 |
| 6 | 120.0 |
| 7 | 101.3 |
| 8 | 32.4 |

found to be the optimal concentration for virus particle release, it can be seen that $10^{-6}$ M thymidine and even $10^{-7}$ M thymidine stimulates a significant amount of virus particle release. The amount of virus is quantitated by means of the viral reverse transcriptase assay. The reverse transcriptase assay used poly(rA)·oligo(dT) as template and primer, and was significantly higher than the amount of polymerase activity found using poly(dA)·oligo(dT) as template and primer. This indicates that there are negligible amounts of cellular DNA polymerase constituent in the virus preparations. The amount of virus polymerase released by BrdU treatment and effects of adding deoxycytidine can also be seen in table I. The addition of equal amounts of deoxycytidine to the tissue culture media does not interfere with thymidine or BrdU activation of the virus particle release.

A comparison of the effects of thymidine and BrdU treatment on the Greene hamster melanoma cells and mouse 3T3 cells is seen in table II. It is seen that thymidine and BrdU cause similar increases in virus particle release from the different cell types. Also, when equal amounts of thymidine and BrdU are added to the cell media, the amount of virus released is the same as the sum of the individual effects. Thus, it would appear that BrdU and thymidine effects appear additive and there is no competition between the BrdU and thymidine.

The time course for virus production from the Y22 cells is shown in table III. Although the results vary slightly from experiment to experiment, the results in table III are representative of those generally found. The optimum day for harvesting of the virus after treatment with thymidine was usually either day 5 or 6.

*Table IV.* Viral polymerase assay for Y22 cells at various temperatures

| Temperature, °C | pmol $^3$H-TMP incorporated/h/10 $\mu$g protein | |
|---|---|---|
| | thymidine $10^{-4}$ M | BrdU $10^{-4}$ M |
| 4 | 24 | – |
| 23 | 70 | 38 |
| 30 | 60 | 39 |
| 35 | 60 | 37 |
| 41 | 42 | 30 |
| 56 | 2.7 | – |

*Table V.* Viral polymerase assay for Y22 cells at various pH values

| pH | pmol $^3$H-TMP incorporated/h/10 $\mu$g protein | |
|---|---|---|
| | $10^{-5}$ M thymidine | $10^{-5}$ M BrdU |
| 6.5 | 65.0 | – |
| 7.5 | 131.0 | 126.0 |
| 7.8 | 136.2 | 134.3 |
| 8.1 | 115.3 | 139.6 |
| 8.5 | 51.0 | – |

Further characterization of the reverse transcriptase activity associated with the virus released from the melanoma cells was carried out by assaying at various temperatures (table IV) and at different pH values (table V). These results show that the enzyme derived by thymidine activation is very similar to that derived from BrdU activation.

The cell media from the thymidine and BrdU-activated cells was spun down and the material pelleting at 100,000 $g$ was placed on a glycerol gradient. The resulting peaks of polymerase activity were determined to have densities of 1.14–1.16 g/ml (fig. 1A). This density corresponds to that of characteristic RNA tumor virus particles. Tritiated uridine was also added to the cell cultures following thymidine and BrdU treatment. Figure 1B shows that the counts from the tritiated uridine band at the same density as that of the virus particle (determined by the polymerase assay), thus indicating that the virus particle contains RNA. This RNA has been shown to have a sedimentation coefficient of 65 [10].

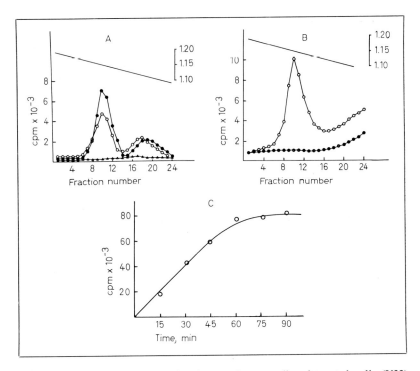

*Fig. 1. A* A virus pellet from the tissue culture media of treated cells (Y22) was resuspended in Tris buffer (0.05 M pH 7.9) and layered on a 20–70% linear glycerol gradient. The gradient was centrifuged for 3 h at 120,000 g. Thymidine treatment O; BrdU treatment ●; no treatment = ▲. *B* Virus particles obtained from thymidine-treated cells (Y22) grown in tritiated uridine were suspended in Tris buffer (0.05 M, pH 7.9) and layered on a 20–70% glycerol gradient. The gradient was centrifuged for 3 h at 120,000 g. Thymidine treatment = O; no treatment = ●. *C* Time course for the viral polymerase assay using poly(rA) · oligo(dT) as a template-primer, and tritiated thymidine triphosphate as substrate.

## Discussion

As has been pointed out by TEICH *et al.* [12], the fact that thymidine analogs such as BrdU can alter metabolism, makes attempts at understanding the basic mechanisms, while using these drugs, extremely difficult and perhaps impossible. Also, although protein synthesis inhibitors have been shown to cause the activation of virus particles [1], these compounds result in systems in which it is very hard to study mechanisms. The finding that thymidine, a normal constituent of cells, causes virus activation allows for experiments on cells which are more normal in character.

One possible complication of thymidine activation is the fact that high levels of thymidine have been shown to block cell division. This is due to the inhibition, by thymidine triphosphate (TTP), of the conversion of cytidine diphosphate to deoxycytidine diphosphate. The effects of this block can be overcome by the addition of deoxycytidine to the tissue culture media, thus allowing the formation of deoxycytidine triphosphate and its incorporation into DNA [6, 7]. However, the TTP inhibition effect is not the cause of the virus release, for when deoxycytidine is added to the tissue culture media, no decrease in virus particle release is obtained; in fact, a slight increase is seen (table I). The slight increase in virus release may be due to the fact that the small amount of thymidine added results in a slight decrease in cell growth rate, and the deoxycytidine addition brought the growth rate back to normal. This slight decrease in growth rate was not seen at lower thymidine concentrations where virus particles were also released. Thus, the side effect of decreasing deoxycytidine levels with increasing thymidine concentration seem to play no role in virus activation.

A comparison of the amount of virus released from the Y22 Greene hamster melanoma cells and Balb/3T3 mouse cells, and a nonproducing line of clone A31 Balb/3T3 cells previously infected with the Kirsten sarcoma virus (KiMSV) [4], shows that both thymidine and BrdU treatment cause a similar effect on only melanoma cell lines. In addition, it is seen that thymidine does not interfere with the addition of BrdU, thus indicating that thymidine and BrdU are probably working by the same mechanism for the release of the virus. The fact that very little activity is seen, using the poly(dA)·oligo(dT) template, indicates that the amount of contamination of cellular polymerase is very small.

The results of the temperature study seen in table IV show that the viral polymerase exhibits very little increase in activity over the temperature range from 23 to 35 °C. This is probably because the viral polymerase is unstable at higher temperatures, especially when removed from the virus particle. Thus, although it probably has more activity at a higher temperature, it also denatures more quickly. The fact that a considerable amount of activity is found at 23 °C probably is the result of this competition between the increase in polymerase activity and the rate of denaturation.

The virus particles obtained from the centrifugation study (fig. 1) were examined by electron microscopy and were found, in many cases, to inhibit a morphology similar to that descibed for hamster sarcoma virus [2]. These particles were called theta particles. We find considerable numbers of both theta and C-type particles [11]. It has been suggested by ALBINO et al. [2], that the theta particle is not a natural form of the virus, but is formed during concentration and subsequent gradient centrifugation. We also find that milder treatment does not result in the formation of theta particles. Of additional interest is the second smaller level of activity shown in figure 1A. The latter polymerase activity sedimented at 1.10 g/ml. We are presently attempting to determine whether this peak is a discrete entity or corresponds to some form of polymerase bound to membrane fragments.

## Summary

Greene hamster melanoma cells in tissue culture, when treated with low levels ($10^{-5}$ M) of thymidine, release C-type virus particles into the media. These particles are very similar to the C-type particles released from mouse cells and band at a density of 1.14–1.16 g/ml. These particles also contain reverse transcriptase activity with similar characteristics to the reverse transcriptase activity of known mouse cell C-type particles, and to reverse transcriptase released by bromodeoxyuridine treatment of the Greene hamster melanoma cells.

## Acknowledgments

We thank Drs. MICHAEL LIEBER and GEORGE TODARO for the Balb/3T3 and K31 Balb/3T3 cells and Dr. ALAN RABSON for many helpful discussions. Supported by PHS grant from the National Eye Institute NEI 00108-06 and RPB Research Professorship for T.W. REID.

## References

1   AARONSON, S. and DUNN, C.: High-frequency C-type virus induction by inhibitors of protein synthesis. Science 183: 422–423 (1974).

2   ALBINO, A.; DeHARVEN, E., and SANDERS, F.: Theta particles. A structure found in hamster sarcoma virus. J. Virol. 10: 477–483 (1972).

3   KLEMENT, V.; NICOLSON, M., and HUEBNER, R.: Rescue of the genome of focus forming virus from rat non-productive lines by 5'-bromodeoxyuridine. Nature new Biol. 234: 12–14 (1971).

4   LIEBER, M.; LIVINGSTON, D., and TODARO, G.: Superinduction of endogenous type C virus by 5-bromodeoxyuridine from transformed mouse clones. Science *181:* 443–444 (1973).

5   LOWY, D.; ROWE, W.; TEICH, N., and HARTLEY, J.: Murine leukemia virus. High-frequency activation *in vitro* by 5-iododeoxyuridine and 5-bromodeoxyuridine. Science *174:* 155–156 (1971).

6   MORRIS, N. and FISCHER, G.: Studies concerning the inhibition of cellular reproduction by deoxyribonucleosides. I. Biochim. biophys. Acta *68:* 84–92 (1963).

7   MORRIS, N.; REICHARD, P., and FISCHER, G.: Studies concerning the inhibition of cellular reproduction of deoxyribonucleosides. II. Biochim. biophys. Acta *68:* 93–99 (1963).

8   REID, T. and ALBERT, D.: RNA-Dependent DNA-polymerase activity in human tumors. Biochem. biophys. Res. Commun. *46:* 383–390 (1972).

9   REID, T.; DARLING, T.; RUSSELL, P., and ALBERT, D.: RNA-Directed DNA polymerase activity in Greene hamster melanoma. Yale J. Biol. Med. *46:* 485–491 (1973).

10   REID, T.; ALBERT, D., and RUSSELL, P.: Activation of a C-type virus from cells by treatment with low concentrations of thymidine. Cell (in press, 1975).

11   RUSSELL, P.; ALBERT, D., and REID, T.: Characteristics of virus particles released from tumor cells following treatment with low concentrations of thymidine (in preparation, 1975).

12   TEICH, N.; LOWY, D.; HARTLEY, J., and ROWE, W.: Studies of the mechanism of induction of infectious murine leukemia virus from AKR mouse embryo cell lines by 5-iododeoxyuridine and 5-bromodeoxyuridine. Virology *51:* 163–173 (1973).

Dr. T. W. REID, Departments of Ophthalmology and Visual Science, Yale University School of Medicine, *New Haven, CT 06510* (USA)

# Genetics

Pigment Cell, vol. 2, pp. 31–46 (Karger, Basel 1976)

# Melanogenesis and Tumorigenicity in Melanoma Cells and their Hybrids

F. Hu, L. M. Pasztor, R. L. White and B. J. Wilson

Oregon Regional Primate Research Center, Beaverton, Oreg.

## Introduction

The study of mammalian genetics has been given powerful assistance by the development of techniques for the *in vitro* cultivation and fusion of somatic cells. These techniques have been used to map mammalian chromosomes, including those of man, to study differentiation, and to investigate the etiology of cancer.

In the study reported here, we used these techniques to investigate the genetic control of pigmentation and tumorigenicity in somatic cell hybrids. B16 mouse melanoma cells which carry two distinct markers, pigmentation and tumor formation, were fused with mouse fibroblasts and Chinese hamster peritoneal cells, which were neither pigmented nor tumorigenic. The hybrids were then analyzed for the expression or nonexpression of pigmentation and tumorigenicity. Our aim was to determine whether these two characteristics can be expressed in the hybrid cells and what controls their expression or nonexpression.

## Materials and Methods

### Parent Cells

1) Melanoma cell line (PAZG): This 8-azaguanine-resistant line was derived from a melanoma cell line (P51) which was originally established from a B16 mouse melanoma [2]. The development of this drug-resistant line has been previously reported [16]. These cells, which were grown in Eagle's minimum essential medium (MEM) supplemented with 10% fetal calf serum (Gibco, Grand Island, New York), gentamycin (Schering, Port Reading, New Jersey) and 8-azaguanine (Sigma,

St. Louis. Mo.) at a concentration of 200 $\mu$g per ml, lack the enzyme hypoxanthine-guanine phosphoribosyl transferase (HGPRT).

2) Chinese hamster cells (CH): This is an IUdR-resistant derivative of cell line B14-150 which originated from the normal peritoneal cells of an adult Chinese hamster with a methylcholanthrene-induced fibrosarcoma (line B14 FAF 28-G3) (obtained from American Type Culture Collection CCL 14.1). These cells lack the enzyme thymidine kinase.

3) Mouse fibroblast cell line (LM[TK$^-$]): The LM(TK$^-$) cells are a thymidine-kinase-deficient derivative from the LM strain which in turn was derived from the normal subcutaneous areolar and adipose tissue of a C3H/An male mouse.

Because of their enzyme deficiency, none of the three lines could grow in medium containing hypoxanthine, aminopterin, thymidine, and glycine (HAT); in other words, when *de novo* purine and pyrimidine biosynthesis was inhibited by aminopterin, the available exogenous guanine could not be utilized by the PAZG cells nor the thymidine by the LM(TK$^-$) and CH cells.

### Cell Hybridization

Cell fusion, with Sendai virus inactivated by $\beta$-propiolactone as the fusion agent (supplied through the courtesy of Dr. H. G. COON or purchased from Connaught Laboratories, Toronto, Ont.), proceeded along the same lines as those described by COON and WEISS [4] and DAVIDSON [5].

### Karyology

The chromosome preparations were made by techniques described in another paper in this volume [17]. Both conventional Giemsa and C-band staining were used.

### Morphological and Histochemical Examination

Cells were seeded into 2-chamber slides (Lab-Tek, Miles Laboratory, Westmount, Ill.) and grown for 3–5 days until semiconfluent; they were then processed for morphological and histochemical examination. For the former, the cells were rinsed in physiological saline, fixed in methanol, and stained with May-Grünwald-Giemsa.

*Dopa reaction.* The classical dopa reaction of LAIDLAW and BLACKBERG [14] was adapted to process the monolayer culture of various cell lines. Briefly, cells in monolayers on two-chamber slides were rinsed twice with physiological saline at room temperature, fixed in phosphate-buffered 10% formalin for 15 min, and incubated in dopa reagent at pH 6.8 for 5 h. The cultures were then washed with phosphate buffer solution and again fixed in buffered formalin for at least 1 h. Finally, they were lightly stained with paracarmine, dehydrated, and coverglassed.

### Tyrosinase Assay

All of these steps, from the removal of the culture medium, and the excision of the tumors to the addition of the incubating substrate, were carried out at 0–4 °C. Cultured cells ($0.3$–$2 \times 10^6$ cells in 100 mm plastic culture dishes) were washed twice as monolayers with phosphate-buffered saline (PBS) and collected by scraping into 0.5 ml RO water (purified by reverse osmosis). Samples were homogenized in a glass tissue grinder with a motor-driven teflon pestle. Fresh tumor tissue (<0.1 g) from hamster cheek pouches was similarly homogenized in 2 ml RO water. Protein was measured by the method of LOWRY et al. [15].

Aliquots of homogenate (50 $\mu$l) were incubated for 1 h with equal volumes of substrate solution. The final concentrations of substrate constituents were L-tyrosine, 0.5 mM + 10 $\mu$Ci/ml L-[3,5-³H] tyrosine (Amersham/Searle, Arlington Heights, Ill., 30–60 Ci/mmol); L-dopa 0.2 mM; 50 mM phosphate, pH 6.8. Tritiated water was counted, after incubation, by a method modified after POMERANTZ [18].

### Test for Tumorigenicity
We used both the mouse and the hamster as host animals.

1) For PAZG × CH hybrid cells, we used the following systems:

A. C57BL/6 neonate mice. 1–2×10⁶ cells suspended in 0.1–0.2 ml of MEM were injected subcutaneously into the backs of newborn mice between 24 and 48 h after birth. At the same time, antithymocyte serum (ATS), 0.1–0.25 ml, was injected subcutaneously and again on days 1, 12, and 24 [7].

B. C57BL/6 (4- to 8-week-old male mice). Simultaneously with the injection of 5×10⁶ cells suspended in 0.1–0.2 ml of MEM, ATS (0.25 ml) was injected subcutaneously and again on days 1, 2, 4, 14, 21, and 28 after injection.

C. Cheek pouches of Syrian hamsters. Two and a half million cells suspended in 0.05 ml of MEM were inoculated into the cheek pouches of 4- to 8-week-old (50–100 g) male Syrian golden hamsters. At the same time, 0.1 ml of cortisone acetate suspension (25 mg/ml, Daylin, Los Angeles, Calif.) was injected subcutaneously and again on the second day and then twice weekly for the duration of the experiment.

2) For PAZG × LM(TK⁻) hybrid cells, we used the following systems:

A. (C57BL/6 × C3H) F₁ hybrid mice. 2.5–5×10⁶ cells suspended in 0.1–0.2 ml of PBS or MEM were injected subcutaneously into the legs of 4- to 8-week-old mice.

B. Cheek pouches of cortisone-conditioned hamsters. Same as 1.C.

### Criteria for Tumorigenicity
*Mouse system.* The tumorigenic parental cells, PAZG, were used as a standard of comparison. Within 25–30 days after injection, 10⁶ PAZG cells injected into 5- to 8-week-old C57BL/6 mice produced pigmented tumors more than 1 cm in diameter in all mice. Tumorigenicity was regarded as reduced if the appearance of the tumors was delayed for at least 30–60 days or if the tumors were noticeably smaller at the end of 60 days than 'standard' PAZG tumors.

*Hamster system.* For at least 6 weeks after cell injections, the hamsters were examined weekly, and the time of appearance, the size, and the color of the tumors were recorded. In addition, if any local tissue reactions such as inflammation, hemorrhage, necrosis, or invasion to the surrounding areas had occurred, they were recorded.

Representative tumors were examined histologically for evidence of active tumor cell proliferation.

### Criteria for Melanogenesis
Cells were considered melanogenic if they had two or more of the following characteristics: (1) if they contained brown pigment under light microscopic exami-

nation; (2) if they showed a positive dopa reaction when incubated in the dopa re-agent; (3) if tyrosinase activity was detected by our biochemical assay technique; (4) if they produced pigmented tumors when injected into appropriate host animals.

## Results

Two sets of sublines – F34-(F)-C1-4 and F34-(J) and F57-(7) and (9) – were isolated from PAZG × LM(TK⁻) and PAZG × CH fusion, respectively, and are extensively described in this discussion.

### Cytological Examination

The hybrid cells, PAZG × LM(TK⁻) (F34) and PAZG × CH (F57), differed from the parental cells, PAZG, LM(TK⁻) and CH cells in morphology and growth characteristics. The hybrid cells were generally much larger and formed colonies differently from the parental cells (fig. 1). When these cells were incubated in the dopa reagent, only the PAZG cells showed a positive reaction; the LM(TK⁻), CH, and hybrid cells were all nonreactive.

### Karyology

Mouse and hamster chromosomes were identified in metaphases by the C-banding technique. PAZG contained one large submetacentric chromosome identified by a terminal C band, 3–5 biarmed, and 49–52 acrocentric chromosomes with C bands restricted to the centromeres (fig. 2A) [16].

The parental Chinese hamster cells had 22–24 chromosomes which had only faint or practically no centromeric C bands and included an X chromosome distinguished by a totally heterochromatic long arm (fig. 2B) [8].

Fusion 57-(9) apparently arose initially from the fusion of 2 CH cells and 1 PAZG cell. PAZG chromosomes were reduced from an expected 53–57 to 22–25 (approximately 60%) (table I). In addition to the marker chromosomes contributed by PAZG, this line contained a unique marker chromosome not found in (7) (fig. 2C and E).

Six months after our initial analysis, line (9) had only 12–16 of the expected 52–57 PAZG chromosomes, i.e. an additional loss of 6–10 chromosomes, and after 10 months in culture only 10 or 11 remained (table I). Parenthetically, the submetacentric PAZG marker chromosome was lacking in every metaphase from (9) cultures analyzed after they had proliferated 6 months in vitro (fig. 2C).

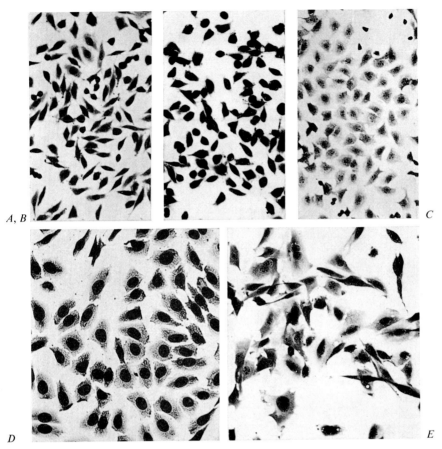

*Fig. 1.* Monolayer cell cultures. May-Grünwald-Giesma. × 240. *A* Mouse fibroblasts (LM[TK⁻]). *B* Mouse melanoma cells (PAZG). *C* Chinese hamster peritoneal cells (CH). *D* PAZG × LM(TK⁻) hybrids (F34). *E* PAZG × CH hybrids (F57).

After prolonged passage in culture (10 months), line (7) showed little loss in PAZG chromosomes, which were in the 40–45 range (table I). This line still retained the PAZG marker chromosome (the large submetacentric chromosome with a terminal C band), but did not have the unique marker chromosome seen in line (9) (fig. 2D).

Analyses revealed that the total number of Chinese hamster chromo-

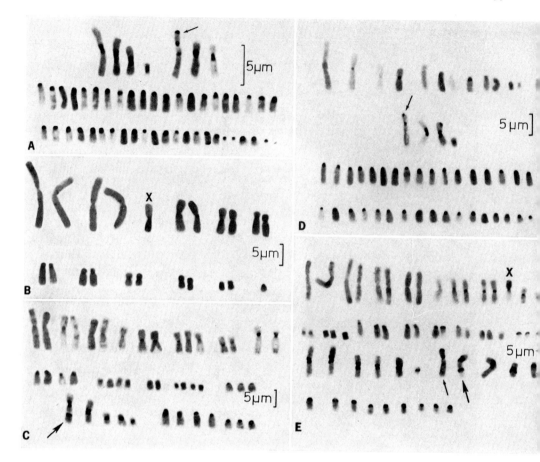

Fig. 2. Chromosomes stained to show C banding. A Karyotype of PAZG cells. Arrow indicates the marker chromosome. B Karyotype of CH cells. X chromosome as marked. C Karyotype of PAZG × CH hybrid cell F57-(9). Later cultures. Top two rows = CH chromosomes; bottom row = PAZG chromosomes. Arrow indicates a new marker chromosome unique to this line. Compare with E and note that the X chromosome, as well as the PAZG marker chromosome seen in the early cultures, is no longer present. D Karyotype of PAZG × CH hybrid cell F57-(7). Top row = CH chromosomes; bottom 3 rows = PAZG chromosomes. Arrow indicates the marker chromosome. E Karyotype of PAZG × CH hybrid cell F57-(9). Early cultures. Top 2 rows = CH chromosomes with one X chromosome as marked; bottom 2 rows = PAZG chromosomes. Thin arrow indicates the marker chromosome; thick arrow, the unique new marker.

*Table I.* Chromosome constitution and tumorigenicity of PAZG × CH hybrids

| Cell line | Date | Modal range | | Date | Tumor / animal |
|---|---|---|---|---|---|
| | | CH | PAZG | | |
| CH | | 22–24 | | | 0/3 hamster |
| PAZG | | | 53–57 | | 6/7 hamster |
| F57-(9) | 12/13/73 | 37–44 | 22–25 | | |
| | | | | 4/24/74 | 0/6 C57BL neonate (90) |
| | | | | 4/24/74 | 0/5 hamster[a] (77) |
| | 6/26/74 | 36–41 | 12–16 | | |
| | | | | 8/21/74 | 5/6 hamster |
| | | | | 10/23/74 | 1/2 hamster[b] |
| | 10/25/74 | 36–40 | 10–11 | | 9/12 |
| | | | | 11/19/74 | 3/4 hamster |
| F57-(7) | 12/12/73 | 20–22 | 40–45 | | |
| | | | | 2/28/74 | 0/14 C57BL (145) |
| | | | | 4/12/74 | 0/4 C57BL neonate (104) |
| | | | | 4/25/74 | 0/6 C57BL neonate (89) |
| | | | | 9/12/74 | 1/2 hamster |
| | 10/8/74 | 18–21 | 42–44 | 11/7/74 | 2/2 hamster   4/7 |
| | | | | 11/26/74 | 1/3 hamster |

[a] Unconditioned; all other hamsters were conditioned by cortisone injections.
[b] Only $10^6$ cells were injected in this instance; all other hamster injections were $2.5 \times 10^6$ cells.
Numbers in parentheses = total days of observation.

*Table II.* Chromosome constitution and tumorigenicity of PAZG × LM (TK⁻) hybrids

| Cell line | Modal range | | Animal host | Tumor/animal |
|---|---|---|---|---|
| | total | biarmed | | |
| PAZG | 53–57 | 3–5 | F₁ hybrid mice[a] | 8/8 (30 days) |
| | | | hamsters | 6/7 |
| LM (TK⁻) | 47–49 | 12–14 | C3H mice | 0/9 (43 days) |
| | | | F₁ hybrid mice | 0/10 (31 days) |
| | | | hamsters | 3/3 |
| F34-(F)-Cl-4 | 83–87 | 15–18 | F₁ hybrid mice | 3/7 (75 days) |
| | | | hamsters | 2/7 (small tumors) |
| F34-(J) | 80–84 | 15–18 | F₁ hybrid mice | 1/3 (62 days) |

[a] C57BL/6 × C3H.

*Table III.* Chromosome constitution of PAZG × LM (TK⁻) hybrid cells and tumors

| Parents | Date | Number of metaphases | Modal range | |
|---|---|---|---|---|
| | | | total | biarmed |
| PAZG | | 50 | 53–57 | 3–5 |
| LM (TK⁻) | | 35 | 47–49 | 12–14 |
| F34-(F)-Cl-4 continuous *in vitro* | | | | |
| | 8/15/73 | 22 | 90–98 | 11–17 |
| | 4/18/74 | 59 | 85–91 | 15–18 |
| | 5/22/74 | 56 | 80–84 | 15–18 |
| From tumor: | | | | |
| No. 1 | 7/31/74 | 34 | 80–84 | 13–17 |
| No. 2 | 8/6/74 | 64 | 80–84 | 16–18 |
| No. 3 | 8/9/74 | 50 | 80–84 | 15–17 |
| F34-(J) continuous *in vitro* | | | | |
| | 5/20/74 | 40 | 80–84 | 15–18 |
| From tumor: | 8/7/74 | 48 | 70–80 | 13–18 |

*Table IV.* Expression of melanogenic activity in different cell lines

| Cell lines | Melano-somes | Dopa oxidase histochemical | Tyrosinase assay |
|---|---|---|---|
| PAZG | + | + | + |
| CH | − | − | − |
| F57 | − | − | − |
| LM (TK⁻) | − | − | − |
| F34 | | − | − |
| MP | + | + + + | + |

somes remained essentially the same, but one chromosome, the X, was never observed in late cultures and other chromosomes were missing or present in only one copy (fig. 2).

The chromosome constitution of PAZG, LM(TK⁻), and PAZG × LM(TK⁻) hybrids (fusion 34-(F)-Cl-4 and (J) is shown in table II. In both (F) and (J), about 7–15 chromosomes were lost, mostly the acrocentrics. Marker chromosomes derived from both parents are present in both (F) and (J) (fig. 3).

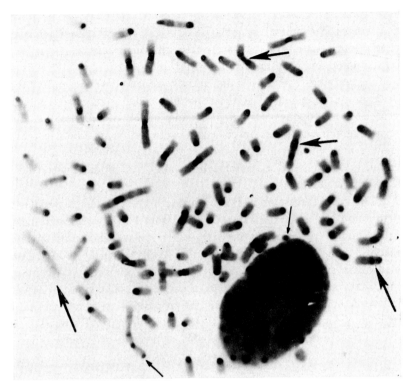

*Fig. 3.* Metaphase spread of PAZG × LM(TK⁻). C bands. Thin arrows indicate PAZG marker chromosomes; thick arrows, LM(TK⁻) markers.

When the chromosomes of cells in primary cultures made from tumors produced by injections of F34-(F) or (J) into F$_1$ hybrid mice were analyzed, (F) showed no chromosome reduction, but (J) had 5–10 chromosomes less than their respective cells before this one passage *in vivo*. Again, acrocentrics rather than biarmed chromosomes decreased in number (table III).

Melanogenesis

The melanogenic activities of different cell lines are summarized in table IV.

Both LM(TK⁻) and CH were nonmelanogenic; when they were fused with the melanogenic PAZG cells, the hybrids were all nonpigmented.

Tumorigenicity

Among the animal systems used by us to test tumorigenicity, the cheek pouch system of the cortisone-conditioned hamster gave the most reproducible and clear-cut results. After injections of $2.5 \times 10^6$ cells, small nodules varying from 1 to 4 mm usually appeared at the end of 7 days. With nontumorigenic cells, these nodules usually regressed and disappeared in 10–14 days. Histological examination of nodules that did not regress at the end of 2–3 weeks, but were less than 5 mm in diameter, showed mononuclear inflammatory cell infiltrate with either a few degenerated tumor cells or no tumor cells at all. These nodules were therefore scored as negative.

The cells were scored as tumorigenic if they produced nodules more than 5 mm in diameter, increased in size from 1 to 3 weeks, and histologically showed proliferative activity in the hosts. The tumors generally reached their maximum at the end of 3 weeks when the growth rate leveled off in spite of the continuation of immunosuppressive treatment. In fact, many animals died at the end of 6–8 weeks. The cause of death varied; some appeared to die of infectious processes – necropsy showed hemorrhagic colitis, proliferative ileitis, pyelonephritis, and abscesses in the liver, mesenteries, and jaws – probably as a result of complications from immunosuppressive measures. In those that survived, the tumors did not increase in size.

Neonate mice did not prove to be a satisfactory system because the mortality rate among them was high and the injected cell suspension tended to leak out of the injection site.

In the adult mouse system, tumor production was frequently delayed but not completely abolished. For example, the F34 hybrid cells did not produce tumors in the $F_1$ hybrid mice until 70–75 days after injections, whereas the PAZG cells always produced tumors at 30 days. Had we terminated the experiment at the end of 60 days, or at the same time as we examined the PAZG tumors (30 days), we would have concluded that the hybrid cells were nontumorigenic.

Even though the results in these two systems (hamster and mouse) were not identical, they were somewhat parallel; i.e. if one cell line was nontumorigenic in the hamsters, it was either nontumorigenic or only slightly tumorigenic in the mice. At no time was one cell line highly tumorigenic in one system and nontumorigenic in the other. But since the hamster system gave more clear-cut results, we used it exclusively for later experiments.

F57: PAZG × CH

When $1-2\times10^6$ (7) and (9) hybrid cells were injected into one-day-old newborn mice treated with either antithymocyte serum (ATS) or normal rabbit serum (NRS), no tumors had developed at the end of 89–90 days (0/12) or 104 days (0/4). In addition, no tumors were produced by $2.5\times10^6$ (7) cells at the end of 145 days in 14 adult male C57BL mice which had been treated with ATS or NRS. Among these, 9 mice had been reinoculated with $5\times10^6$ cells at 56, 70, or 83 days. Tumors were never observed in animals which had been treated with either NRS or PBS and then injected with F 57 cells (table I).

More than $5\times10^6$ (9) cells were inoculated into the cheek pouches of 5 unconditioned hamsters at about the same time as the neonate mouse injections, but no tumors were observed in 77 days (table I).

After another 4 or more months *in vitro*, these same cell lines were tested for tumorigenicity in cortisone-conditioned hamsters.

Table I summarizes the tumorigenicity and chromosome data for parental and F57 hybrid cells. Within 14–21 days, pigmented tumors were produced in conditioned hamsters by PAZG cells and nonpigmented tumors by hybrid cells, but none were formed by Chinese hamster cells. By contrast to the earlier results in the neonates and unconditioned hamsters, (9) produced nonpigmented tumors in 9/12 animals; these tumors increased in size up to 3 weeks when their growth rate leveled off. By this time, the tumors were usually noticeably necrotic and adhered to and eroded the pouch; the animals generally died at the end of 5–6 weeks. Necropsy showed no evidence of metastasis; death appeared to be due to infectious processes, which were probably the result of immunosuppressive measures. (7), on the other hand, produced small nodules in 4/7 hamsters; when examined histologically, these nodules showed essentially a granulomatous reaction. The tumor cells were mostly necrotic; only a few could be recognized. Apparently, the host had mounted an effective defense which ended in the partial destruction of the tumor cells. Therefore, (9) cells appeared to be tumorigenic, whereas (7) are not or at least are much less so.

F34: PAZG × LM(TK⁻)

Injections of $10^6$ PAZG cells into C57BL/6 mice and (C57BL/6 × C3H) $F_1$ hybrid male mice grew into tumors in about 25–30 days. The other parent, LM(TK⁻) cells, was not known to be tumorigenic, but when $2.5\times10^6$ cells were injected into conditioned Syrian hamster cheek pouches, hemorrhagic tumors were produced in 3/3 hamsters (table II). Although this incidence of tumors was comparable to that produced by PAZG cells, the degree of inflammatory reaction was different. When $2.5-5 \times 10^6$ LM(TK$^-$) cells were injected subcutaneously into 9 C3H mice, no tumors had been produced after 50 days, and when $5 \times 10^6$ LM(TK$^-$) cells were injected into 10 (C57BL/6 $\times$ C3H) F$_1$ hybrid mice, no tumors were produced after 40 days. Whether these cells will eventually produce tumors in these animals at a later date we cannot yet predict.

F34-(J) produced one nonpigmented tumor within 62 days in one of 3 injected mice, but no tumors were seen in the other two at the end of 183 days (table II).

When $2.5 \times 10^6$ to $5 \times 10^6$ F34-(F)-C1-4 cells were injected into 7 F$_1$ hybrid mice, no tumors were observed after 52 days, but 3 nonpigmented tumors formed after 75 days (table II). Similarly in conditioned hamster cheek pouches, small tumors formed only in 2 of the 7 hamsters injected. Therefore, it appeared that in the hamsters the hybrid cells were less tumorigenic than either of the parental cells.

### Discussion

Whether tumorigenicity can be defined as a dominant or recessive genetic trait in cell hybrids derived by fusing tumorigenic and nontumorigenic cells has been debatable. Earlier data [1, 10, 20] weighted the evidence in favor of dominance because of the apparent tumorigenicity of several tumorigenic × nontumorigenic cell hybrids. On the other hand, since these hybrids were characterized by chromosome loss, the data could just as easily be interpreted to reflect genetic loss rather than malignant parent dominance in the Mendelian sense. WIENER et al. [21–23], however, have suggested that tumorigenicity is really recessive because, whenever complete chromosome sets of both parents were retained, the hybrids were nontumorigenic and whatever tumors were produced contained cells with reduced chromosomes. Whenever tumorigenic × nontumorigenic hybrids are nontumorigenic, but become tumorigenic after chromosome reduction, we must hypothesize that on a cellular level, tumorigenicity is a recessively inherited trait. Of key importance is the reservation that in this case each parental chromosome must be unequivocally identified, and that there is some relationship between specific chromosome(s) loss from the nontumorigenic parent and the reexpression of

*Table V.* Melanogenesis and tumorgenesis in melanoma cells and their hybrids

| Fusion | Parent cells | | Hybrids | |
|---|---|---|---|---|
| | M | T | M | T |
| PAZG × LM (TK⁻) | + − | + + ? | − | decrease |
| PAZG × CH | + − | + − | − | increase |
| PAZG × Isogenic host cell | + − ? | + − | increase | negative |

M = Melanogenesis; T = tumorigenesis.

tumorigenicity. This relationship was verified in the extinction and the later reexpression of esterase-2 in RAG (mouse renal adenocarcinoma cells) × human cell hybrids [13].

Assuming that our initial test systems with ATS-treated newborn mice and unconditioned hamsters are comparable to our later contitioned hamster test system, our data from PAZG × CH hybrids support the view that tumorigenicity *is* a recessive trait. Although we, like others [2, 3], have not yet associated individual chromosome loss with tumorigenicity, future studies with the G-banding technique [19] may reveal such a correlation. *We have, however, clearly demonstrated that in spite of a drastic reduction in the number of PAZG chromosomes (from the expected 53–57 to 10–11) after prolonged* in vitro *cultivation of F57-(9), these hybrids were highly tumorigenic.*

Both LM(TK⁻) and PAZG were tumorigenic, but the tumorigenicity of their hybrids was greatly depressed. Despite the loss of approximately 15 chromosomes, except for the marker chromosomes, PAZG chromosomes could not be distinguished from those of LM(TK⁻). As a result, the question about which parental chromosomes were eventually deleted remains unanswerable.

Neither LM(TK⁻) nor CH cells are pigmented and neither is capable of forming melanin. Their hybrids, formed after the fusion with melanogenic PAZG cells, are also nonmelanogenic. These results support the general opinion that when differentiated cells are fused with cells that do not express that differentiated function, the hybrids resemble the undifferentiated parent [6]. But in both F34 and F57, there were apparent losses of genetic material which could be from PAZG, the melanogenic parent.

In another experiment which we reported elsewhere [11], however, hybrids (MP) formed by the *in vivo* fusion of PAZG and their isogenic host cells were melanogenic (table IV); indeed, they were more actively melanogenic than the parental PAZG cells. It appears, therefore, that crosses between differentiated and undifferentiated cells do not as a rule exclude the 'luxury' function (in this case, melanin pigmentation). One may argue that (1) MP cells may have formed from the fusion of PAZG cells with the pigment cells of the host, or (2) the gene(s) responsible for the regulation (suppression) of pigmentation is lost in this hybrid line. Both explanations, however, are unlikely because (1) the number of pigment cells in the tissue environment where the injected cells make contact is much less than that of the nonpigment-forming cells such as fibroblasts, macrophages, endothelial, and blood cells, and (2) there is little or no chromosome loss in these hybrid cells.

## Conclusion

Table V summarizes the expression of melanogenesis and tumorigenesis in PAZG and their hybrids.

Our results indicate that tumorigenicity and lack of pigmentation in the hybrids are related to chromosome loss from the parental cells. We are continuing to examine these hybrids as they proliferate in culture to determine whether any changes in these characteristics are related to specific chromosome losses.

## Summary

All hybrid cells derived from fusion of murine melanoma cells PAZG × Chinese hamster peritoneal cells (CH) and PAZG × LM(TK⁻) cells are nonpigmented; their tumorigenicity, however, varies.

It appears that tumorigenicity and lack of pigmentation in the hybrids are related to chromosome loss from the parental cells. Our data from PAZG × CH hybrids support the view that tumorigenicity is a recessive trait. We have, however, demonstrated that one hybrid line derived from PAZG × CH (F57-(9)) was highly tumorigenic in spite of a drastic reduction in the number of melanoma chromosomes.

## Acknowledgments

We are indebted to Dr. JAMES PALOTAY of the Department of Pathology, who performed the autopsy and searched for evidences of metastasis in the tumor-bearing hamsters; to DINAH TERAMURA, CORAL JEAN COTTERELL, and CATHY TAYLOR for expert technical assistance, and to MARGARET BARSS for careful editing of the manuscript.

Publication No. 861 of the Oregon Regional Primate Research Center supported in part by Grants CA 08499 of the National Cancer Institute, RR 00163 of the Animal Resources Branch, Division of Research Resources, and AM 08445 of the National Institute of Arthritis and Metabolic Diseases, National Institutes of Health.

## References

1   BARSKI, G.; BLANCHARD, M.-G.; YOUN, J. K., and LÉON, B.: Expression of malignancy in interspecies Chinese hamster × mouse cell hybrids. J. natn. Cancer Inst. *51:* 781–792 (1973).

2   BEREBBI, M. et MEYER, G.: Transformation cellulaire maligne et modification caryologiques: apport de l'hybridation somatique de lignées de hamster chinois. Int. J. Cancer *10:* 418–435 (1972).

3   BLANCHARD, M.; BARSKI, G.; LÉON, B. et HÉMON, D.: Expression du pouvoir tumorigène dans les clones cellulaires hybrides isologues de hamster chinois. Int. J. Cancer *11:* 178–185 (1973).

4   COON, H. G. and WEISS, M. C.: A quantitative comparison of formation of spontaneous and virus-produced viable hybrids. Proc. natn. Acad. Sci. USA *62:* 852–859 (1969).

5   DAVIDSON, R. L.: Regulation of melanin synthesis in mammalian cells, as studied by somatic hybridization. III. A method of increasing the frequency of cell fusion. Expl Cell Res. *55:* 424–426 (1969).

6   DAVIDSON, R. L.: Review. Control of expression of differentiated function in somatic cell hybrids; in DAVIDSON and DE LA CRUZ Somatic cell hybridization, pp. 131–146 (Raven Press, Hewlett 1974).

7   DAVIS, R. C.; COOPERBAND, S. R., and MANNICK, J. A.: Preparation and *in vitro* assay of effective and ineffective antilymphocyte sera. Surgery, St Louis *66:* 58–64 (1969).

8   DEAVEN, L. L. and PETERSON, D. F.: The chromosomes of CHO, an aneuploid hamster cell line: G-band, C-band and autoradiographic analyses. Chromosoma *41:* 129–144 (1973).

9   DEFENDI, V.; EPHRUSSI, B.; KOPROWSKI, H., and YOSHIDA, M. C.: Properties of hybrids between polyoma-transformed and normal mouse cells. Proc. natn. Acad. Sci. USA *57:* 299–305 (1967).

10  FOLEY, G. E.; HANDLER, A. H.; ADAM, R. A., and CRAIG, J. M.: Assessment of potential malignancy of cultured cells. Further observations on the differentia-

tion of 'normal' and 'neoplastic' cells maintained *in vitro* by heterotransplantation in Syrian hamsters. Natn. Cancer Inst. Monogr. *7:* 173–204 (1962).

11   Hu, F. and Pasztor, L. M.: *In vivo* hybridization of cultured melanoma cells and isogenic normal mouse cells. Differentiation *4:* 93–97 (1975).

12   Hu, F. and Lesney, P. F.: The isolation and cytology of two pigment cell strains from B16 mouse melanomas. Cancer Res. *24:* 1634–1643 (1964).

13   Klebe, R. J.; Chen, T. R., and Ruddle, F. H.: Mapping of a human genetic regulator element by somatic cell genetic analysis. Proc. natn. Acad. Sci. USA *66:* 1220–1227 (1970).

14   Laidlaw, G. F. and Blackberg, S. N.: Melanoma studies. II. A simple technique for the dopa reaction. Am. J. Path. *8:* 491–498 (1932).

15   Lowry, O. H.; Rosebrough, N. J.; Farr, A. L., and Randell, R. J.: Protein measurement with Folin phenol reagent. J. biol. Chem. *193:* 265–275 (1951).

16   Pasztor, L. M.; Hu, F.; Stankova, L., and Bigley, R.: 8-Azaguanine-resistant melanoma cells *in vitro* and *in vivo*. J. natn. Cancer Inst. *52:* 1143–1150 (1974).

17   Pasztor, L. M.; Hu, F., and White, R. L.: Distinctive C-bands as identification markers for B16 melanoma lines (this volume).

18   Pomerantz, S. H.: Tyrosine hydroxylation catalyzed by mammalian tyrosinase. An improved method of assay. Biochem. biophys. Res. Commun. *16:* 188–194 (1964).

19   Seabright, M.: A rapid banding technique for human chromosomes. Lancet *ii:* 971–972 (1971).

20   Silagi, S.: Hybridization of a malignant melanoma cell line with L cells *in vitro*. Cancer Res. *27:* 1953–1960 (1967).

21   Wiener, F.; Klein, G., and Harris, H.: The analysis of malignancy by cell fusion. III. Hybrids between diploid fibroblasts and other tumor cells. J. Cell Sci. *8:* 681–692 (1971).

22   Wiener, F.; Klein, G., and Harris, H.: The analysis of malignancy by cell fusion. IV. Hybrids between tumor cells and a malignant L cell derivative. J. Cell Sci. *12:* 253–261 (1973).

23   Wiener, F.; Klein, G., and Harris, H.: The analysis of malignancy by cell fusion. V. Further evidence of the ability of normal diploid cells to suppress malignancy. J. Cell Sci. *15:* 177–183 (1974).

F. Hu, MD, Oregon Regional Primate Research Center, 505 N.W. 185th Avenue, *Beaverton, OR 97005 (USA)*

Pigment Cell, vol. 2, pp. 47–58 (Karger, Basel 1976)

# Factors Responsible for
# Platyfish-Swordtail Hybrid Melanoma – Many or Few?

Michael J. Siciliano, Donald C. Morizot and David A. Wright[1]

The University of Texas System Cancer Center, M. D. Anderson Hospital and Tumor Institute, Houston, Tex.

*Introduction*

Since the original works of Gordon [10] and Kosswig [13], in 1927, hundreds of papers have appeared on various aspects of the melanoma produced as a result of the hybridization of platyfish *(Xiphophorus maculatus)*, which carry macromelanophore spotting genes, and swordtails *(X. helleri* or *X. clemenciae)* which do not have such genes. Many of these investigations, as summarized in the reviews of Gordon [11], Atz [5], and Anders [3], have demonstrated the genetic nature of this pigment cell neoplasm. The pertinent facts are these: (a) The macromelanophore *(Sd* for spotted dorsal will be used for an example here, although it is only one of a series of 6 co-dominant alleles, all of which react in the same basic way) spotting gene is sex-linked in the platyfish. (b) All $F_1$ hybrids (platy $\times$ swordtail) inheriting *Sd* develop atypical melanosis and/or melanoma. (c) Backcrossing a melanotic $F_1$ hybrid to swordtail produces broods 1/2 of which inherit *Sd* and have melanoma generally more severe than in the $F_1$ and 1/2 of which do not inherit *Sd* and are perfectly normal. (d) Backcrossing $F_1$ hybrids to platyfish produces *Sd* fish which have melanosis generally less severe than that seen in the $F_1$. (e) $F_2$ *Sd* fish (3/4 of those produced by crossing 2 $F_1$ hybrids) vary from least to most melanotic. (f) Abnormal hyperpigmentation is also seen in $F_1$ hybrids be-

1    The authors wish to acknowledge the financial support of the United States National Institutes of Health (grants GM-19513 and CA 16672) and the excellent technical support of Ms. Billie White and Mrs. Betty Young.

tween populations of *maculatus* from different river systems, although the melanosis is not as severe as seen in interspecific hybrids.

The classical interpretation of this information has been that the melanoma is caused by a 'genic imbalance' in the hybrids. The crosses and results summarized above suggest that lack of control of *Sd* is a function of the number of swordtail chromosomes located in the same genome. However, it has never been unequivocally established whether the atypically melanotic response is a function of *Sd* in conjunction with swordtail chromosomes in general, or due to certain specific factors on few swordtail chromosomes. If the latter is true, it suggests the presence of specific tumor genes or perhaps chromosomally located viral information modifying macromelanophore control. An answer to this question has great relevance to understanding human tumors of suspected genetic etiology since KNUDSON et al. [12] noted three characteristics in these – early age of onset, multiple primary lesions and tissue specificity – which are also features of the fish hybrid melanoma. The fish melanoma has also been shown to share certain characteristics with human hereditary melanoma in particular: histological appearance [7, 9], greater severity in males [1, 15], maternal effect in inheritance [4, 14], and tyrosinase activity [8].

There are two straightforward approaches to the question of how many factors are responsible for the melanoma – neither of which is open to experimental verification:

A. One could look at the *Sd* offspring of $F_1$ hybrids crossed back to the swordtail (HHM-BC). If only one pair of swordtail chromosomes carries factors responsible for melanoma induction, 1/2 of the *Sd* HHM-BC hybrids should have 1 platyfish and 1 swordtail chromosome of the pair endowing them with a level of melanosis comparable to that of the $F_1$ parent. The other half of the *Sd* fish should be homozygous for the swordtail chromosomes and therefore be very severely melanotic. The *Sd* HHM-BC hybrids should therefore fall into two discontinuous groups with respect to abnormal melanosis – more and less severe. If 2 swordtail loci are involved, 3 classes should be seen: more, intermediate, and less severe. However, there are obviously other epigenetic factors which modify *Sd* expression making such a determination very difficult. For one, there is clearly a sex effect on melanoma enhancement wherein males show an earlier age of onset and as adults have larger tumors, greater numbers of melanotic sites and more extensive invasion of neoplastic cells into normal tissue [15]. This has been studied in the $F_1$ hybrid. To compound the problem of evaluating *Sd* HHM-BC fish in light of the above is the fact that the hybridizations combine two different sex-inheriting mechanisms of the two parental species, resulting not only in terribly skewed sex ratios, but also, in fish of the same age being in all different stages of sexual maturity (many never undergo complete sexual differentiation). Various environmental factors, pH and salinity of the water, degree of crowding, etc., also appear to modify $Sd$ expression [3]. These points taken together indicate the difficulty of placing the $Sd$ HHM-BC fish into discontinuous groups with respect to extent of melanosis. This would be especially true if more than one, but still only a few, specific swordtail chromosomal loci were involved, since the number of genotypic classes would increase and one would not know what kind of interaction took place between the multiple factors.

B. The second method would be to put the $Sd$ HHM-BC fish into 2 groups (based on melanotic severity) even though there were some which were ambiguously classified. This would be possible if the percentage of fish falling into the ambiguous zone was small. ANDERS et al. [2] have reported that this can be done; our experience is also that it can be done, with no more than 20% of the fish in a 'difficult to classify' category. One would then examine the chromosomes of the fish in the two groups and look for homozygosity of specific swordtail chromosomes in more severely melanotic fish, as opposed to 1 platyfish and one swordtail chromosome of the pair in not-so-severely melanotic backcross hybrids. Unfortunately, platyfish and swordtail chromosomes are so small, so uniform and so alike [19] that such an analysis at present appears unfeasible.

Different approaches to the problem thus are required to answer the question. If clear genetic markers could be found to mark specific platyfish and swordtail chromosomes, studies could be conducted relating melanotic severity to the markers. We have been working over the last several years with vertical starch gel electrophoresis of *Xiphophorus* tissue homogenates followed by histochemical staining for a large number of enzyme loci products. Characterizations of 69 such loci have been recently reported [18]. Two aspects of this approach which relate to the question of the number of factors responsible for abnormal melanosis will be reported on here: (a) use of isozyme markers to relate specific swordtail chromosomes to melanotic severity in $Sd$ HHM-BC hybrids, and (b) use of variation at enzyme loci to determine the genetic distance between platyfish and different species and subspecies of swordtails used to produce $F_1$ hybrids with the platyfish and to relate that distance to severity of melanoma in the $Sd$ $F_1$ hybrids.

## Materials and Methods

A. Fish used and crosses made: All species, subspecies and strains of *Xiphophorus* (Poeciliid fish from the Atlantic coastal drainage of Central America and Mexico) used in this study were obtained from K. KALLMAN of the New York Zoological Society. These include:

*X. maculatus,* strain Jp 163A. This is a highly inbred strain, at least 50 brother-to-sister matings since capture in 1939, from the Rio Jamapa.

*X. helleri strigatus,* strain 501. Green swordtails maintained in closed colony since capture from the Rio Sarabia in 1963. Inbred brother to sister in our laboratory for 5 generations since 1971.

*X. helleri strigatus,* pedigree 2977. Green swordtails maintained in closed colony since capture from the Rio Sarabia in 1971.

*X. helleri guentheri,* pedigree 3062. Green swordtails maintained in closed colony since capture from Dolores, Guatemala in 1971.

*X. helleri helleri,* strain Cd 25. Green swordtails highly inbred (at least 25 brother-to-sister matings) since their capture from the Rio Jamapa.

*X. clemenciae,* pedigrees 3258 and 2985. Yellow swordtails maintained in closed colony since their capture from the Rio Sarabia in 1971.

Female 163A platyfish (homozygous for *Sd*) were artificially inseminated [6] with sperm from all the above groups of swordtails, and melanotic severity was measured as a function of rate of spot production in the $F_1$ [14]. Male $F_1$ hybrids from the crosses using 501 and 2977 swordtails were backcrossed to female 2977 swordtails producing HHM-BC broods numbered 44, 70 and 100. Female $F_1$ hybrids from the crosses using 3062 swordtails were backcrossed to male 3062 swordtails producing HHM-BC broods numbered 103 and 108. The *Sd* HHM-BC hybrids were classified into more severely or less severely melanotic groups, before they reached sexual maturity, by the extent of macromelanophore proliferation and production, and by the size and number of nodular lesions. Backcross to platyfish hybrids HMM-BC were also produced to add to the genetic analysis of the segregation of enzyme loci.

B. Biochemical genetics: Vertical starch gel electrophoresis was conducted on various tissue homogenates (liver, eye, brain, blood, and muscle) of parental strains and hybrids. After electrophoresis, gels were sliced and each slice stained histochemically for the enzymes and proteins listed in table I. Details of the electrophoretic and histochemical procedures have been meticulously described [17]. Characterization of the numbers of different genetic loci in the genus coding for each protein studied, the basis for those characterizations and the number of different loci with variant electrophoretic alleles have been described [18].

For the genetic distance determinations all loci coding for 6PGD, IDH, PGM, GPI, Fumarase, MP, ME, G6PDH, G3PDH, LDH, MDH, TO and AP were used. These represent the products of 26 loci. Genetic distance determinations did not include certain loci (*Est-1, Est-2, MPI, ADA, PIP,* and *Acon*) used in the linkage to melanotic potential experiments (all of which are listed in table II) since methods for the resolution of the products of these loci were not available at the time that the genetic distance study was in progress. Standard segregation and recombination

*Table I.* Enzymes, proteins and number of loci coding for each studied

| Enzyme or protein | Number of loci in *Xiphophorus* |
|---|---|
| 6-Phosphogluconate dehydrogenase (6PGD) | 1 |
| Isocitrate dehydrogenase (IDH) | 3 |
| Phosphoglucomutase (PGM) | 1 |
| Glucose phosphate isomerase (GPI) | 2 |
| Fumarase | 1 |
| Muscle protein (MP) | 5 |
| Malic enzyme (ME) | 1 |
| Glyceraldehyde-3-phosphate dehydrogenase (G₃PDH) | 2 |
| Glucose-6-phosphate dehydrogenase (G₆PDH) | 1 |
| Lactate dehydrogenase (LDH) | 3 |
| Malate dehydrogenase (MDH) | 3 |
| Tetrazolium oxidase (TO) | 2 |
| Acid phosphatase (AP) | 1 |
| Esterase (Est) | 2 |
| Mannose phosphate isomerase (MPI) | 1 |
| Adenosine deaminase (ADA) | 1 |
| Plasma protein (PlP) | 1 |
| Aconitase (ACON) | 1 |

*Table II.* Segregation of enzyme alleles into backcross hybrids

| Locus | Homozygotes | Heterozygotes | Total |
|---|---|---|---|
| EST-1 | 60 | 68 | 128 |
| EST-2 | 62 | 70 | 132 |
| G3PDH-1 | 121 | 119 | 240 |
| GPI-1 | 95 | 102 | 197 |
| MDH-2 | 19 | 12 | 31 |
| PGM | 91 | 97 | 188 |
| 6PGDH | 88 | 99 | 187 |
| G6PDH | 92 | 86 | 178 |
| MP-2 | 48 | 50 | 98 |
| MP-4 | 37 | 50 | 87 |
| MP-5 | 20 | 16 | 36 |
| IDH-1 | 74 | 83 | 157 |
| IDH-2 | 83 | 88 | 171 |
| MPI | 60 | 53 | 113 |
| ADA | 53 | 42 | 95 |
| PIP | 34 | 31 | 65 |
| LDH-3 | 19 | 28 | 47 |
| ACON | 29 | 36 | 65 |
| | 1,085 | 1,130 | 2,215 |

analyses were conducted on the enzyme loci variant between the platyfish and swordtails in HHM-BC and HMM-BC hybrids.

C. Genetic distance estimates: This procedure has been described in detail [16]. In brief, to calculate the distance between any 2 groups, in this case the 163A platyfish and any of the swordtail subspecies or species listed above, one first looks at any locus and determines the total of absolute differences in allele frequencies at that locus between the 2 forms. The overall distance between any two forms is then simply an average calculated from the distances observed over all the loci studied. Where 2 groups have the same alleles at the same frequency at every locus the distance equals 0.0. If completely different at every locus, the distance is 1.0.


## Results and Discussion

The three types of swordtails used for hybridization with platyfish to eventually produce both HHM-BC and HMM-BC hybrids differ from platyfish in the electrophoretic mobility of the products of a total of 18 enzyme loci tested in this study. These loci are listed in table II. As can be seen from the example zymogram (fig. 1), these markers clearly distinguish HHM-BC fish homozygous for swordtail alleles at the marked loci from those which are heterozygous (have 1 platyfish and 1 swordtail chromosome carrying the marked locus). Further evidence for this can be seen from the data on backcross to swordtail as well as backcross to platy broods (table II). Segregation of marker genes at each locus in either of these cases follows Mendelian expectations. In no case is there a significant difference from 1:1 homozygotes to heterozygotes in these backcrosses. The 1:1 ratio is also maintained for all loci combined. The fact of normal segregation, allowing these enzyme loci products to be used as markers for linkage to genes responsible for melanoma is not surprising, since we have seen the expected number of bivalents (24) in testis squashes obtained from $F_1$ hybrids (fig. 2).

As expected, 1/2 of the HHM-BC hybrids produced in all 5 crosses inherited the $Sd$ gene from the $F_1$ parent and were atypically melanotic. Consistent with the report of ANDERS et al. [2], these melanotic backcross hybrids could be placed into 2 fairly equal groups: more severely melanotic and less severely melanotic (table III). Using the marker loci in these, one can ask if the number of swordtail chromosomes carrying factors which enhance melanosis are few or many. If few, let us say one, for example, and if one of our enzyme markers is located on that same chromosome, and if the linkage of this marker with the factor is close enough,

GPI; HHM-BC hybrids

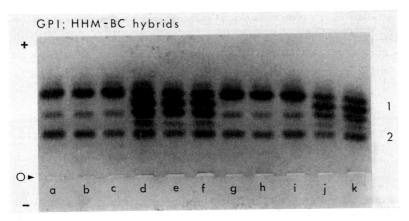

Fig. 1. Photograph of a starch gel specifically stained for GPI. Electrophoretic patterns from muscle extracts of individual backcross hybrids are visualized. There are two loci for GPI in *Xiphophorus*. Locus 2 is identical in the parental species, while electrophoretic differences are seen in locus 1. Fish a, b, c, g, and i are homozygous for the swordtail allele, while d, e, f, j, and k are heterozygous for this locus.

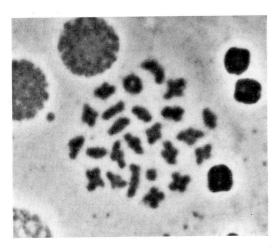

Fig. 2. Meiotic metaphase I squash of an $F_1$ hybrid testis after short-term culture. The expected number of bivalents (n = 24) predicts normal segregation of platyfish and swordtail chromosomes [19].

*Table III.* Numbers of more and less severely melanotic backcross swordtail hybrids

| Brood No. | More | Less | Total |
|---|---|---|---|
| 44 | 7 | 11 | 18 |
| 70 | 12 | 12 | 24 |
| 100 | 7 | 11 | 18 |
| 103 | 12 | 11 | 23 |
| 108 | 3 | 2 | 5 |
| | 41 | 47 | 88 |

one would expect the more severely melanotic fish to be homozygous for swordtail alleles at that enzyme locus and less severely melanotic fish to be heterozygous (1 platyfish and 1 swordtail allele). In a linkage analysis, such fish would be considered parental types. If the linkage is not absolute, crossovers between the locations of the factors responsible for abnormal melanosis and the alleles of the marker enzyme locus would be expected. This would generate severely melanotic fish heterozygous at that enzyme locus as well as less severely melanotic fish homozygous for swordtail alleles. These would be considered recombinant types. In order for the linkage to be detected, parental types must significantly outnumber recombinant types.

If the number of factors were many, scattered throughout the swordtail genome, with the number of fish tested here, we would not expect to find parental types for any single locus significantly greater than 50%, but might expect the number of parental types totaled from all loci to significantly outnumber recombinants.

Table IV presents the number of parental and recombinant types relative to extent of melanosis for each polymorphic enzyme locus for which we had a histochemical staining procedure at the time of the analysis. Backcross hybrids with greater melanosis while homozygous for swordtail alleles at the *Est-1* locus, plus those with lesser melanosis while heterozygous for *Est-1*, were produced in significantly ($p < 0.001$) greater numbers than recombinants, i.e. fish with greater melanosis while heterozygous for *Est-1*, plus those with lesser severity of melanosis while homozygous for swordtail alleles. This was the only case of significant difference between the number of parental versus recombinant types. It was also noted that the combined data for all broods and all loci show essentially the same number of recombinant versus parental types (these fig-

*Table IV.* Numbers of parental (par)[a] and recombinant (rec)[b] types of backcross swordtail hybrids, when enzyme locus genotypes are related to extent of melanosis.

| Brood No. | | Enzyme loci | | | | | | | | | | | | | | | | | | | Total for all loci |
|---|---|---|---|---|---|---|---|---|---|---|---|---|---|---|---|---|---|---|---|---|---|
| | | EST-1 | EST-2 | G3PD-1 | GPI-1 | PGM | 6PGD | G6PD | MP-2 | MP-4 | MP-5 | IDH-1 | IDH-2 | MPI | ADA | PLP | LDH-E | ACON | MDH-2 | |
| 44 | Par | 13 | —[c] | 10 | 6 | 3 | 7 | 6 | 8 | — | X[d] | 5 | 6 | — | — | — | X | — | 8 | 72 |
| | Rec | 5 | — | 8 | 4 | 3 | 3 | 3 | 2 | — | X | 5 | 4 | — | — | — | X | — | 10 | 47 |
| 70 | Par | 18 | 11 | 12 | 14 | 11 | 11 | 16 | 13 | 2 | X | 11 | 10 | 4 | 4 | 0 | X | 3 | X | 140 |
| | Rec | 6 | 9 | 12 | 10 | 13 | 12 | 7 | 11 | 3 | X | 3 | 11 | 1 | 1 | 4 | X | 2 | X | 110 |
| 100 | Par | 9 | 7 | 7 | X | 6 | 7 | 9 | 10 | 8 | X | 7 | 8 | 10 | 8 | 3 | X | 4 | X | 103 |
| | Rec | 3 | 10 | 11 | X | 12 | 11 | 9 | 8 | 10 | X | 10 | 9 | 8 | 10 | 5 | X | 4 | X | 120 |
| 103 | Par | X | 10 | 15 | 8 | 9 | 13 | 8 | X | 9 | 10 | 6 | 7 | 10 | 7 | 8 | 15 | 7 | X | 142 |
| | Rec | X | 8 | 8 | 15 | 14 | 10 | 15 | X | 9 | 8 | 12 | 11 | 13 | 11 | 10 | 8 | 11 | X | 163 |
| 108 | Par | X | 2 | 2 | 3 | 0 | 2 | 2 | X | 2 | 4 | 3 | 2 | X | 2 | 1 | 3 | 1 | X | 29 |
| | Rec | X | 3 | 3 | 2 | 5 | 3 | 3 | X | 3 | 1 | 1 | 3 | X | 3 | 4 | 1 | 3 | X | 38 |
| Total | Par | 40 | 30 | 46 | 31 | 29 | 40 | 41 | 31 | 21 | 14 | 32 | 33 | 24 | 21 | 12 | 18 | 15 | 8 | 486 |
| | Rec | 14 | 30 | 42 | 31 | 47 | 39 | 37 | 21 | 25 | 9 | 36 | 38 | 22 | 25 | 23 | 9 | 20 | 10 | 478 |

[a] Parentals represent the sum of: (1) more severely melanotic fish which are also homozygous for swordtail alleles, and (2) less severely melanotic fish which have 1 swordtail and 1 platyfish allele at the indicated locus.

[b] Recombinants represent the sum of: (1) more severely melanotic fish which have 1 swordtail and 1 platyfish allele at the indicated locus, and (2) less severely melanotic fish which are homozygous for swordtail alleles.

[c] No data since method for resolving product of locus was developed after brood was analyzed.

[d] X Non-informative cross at this locus since platyfish and swordtails used for hybridization producing this brood did not differ for this protein.

*Table V.* Rates of spot development in $F_1$ hybrids between female 163A platyfish and different taxa of swordtails

| Number of days after birth | Taxon of male swordtail parent | | | | | | | |
|---|---|---|---|---|---|---|---|---|
| | *Xiphophorus helleri guentheri* (3)[a] | | *Xiphophorus helleri strigatus* (24)[a] | | *Xiphophorus helleri helleri* (3)[a] | | *Xiphophorus clemenciae* (3)[a] | |
| | F[b] | % | F | % | F | % | F | % |
| 20 | 15/101 | 14.9 | 107/444 | 24.1 | 7/17 | 41.2 | 8/14 | 57.0 |
| 40 | 48/159 | 30.2 | 258/517 | 49.9 | 29/31 | 93.5 | 12/14 | 85.7 |
| 60 | 57/119 | 47.9 | 397/546 | 87.1 | 31/31 | 100.0 | 14/14 | 100.0 |
| 80 | 105/108 | 97.2 | 485/491 | 98.8 | 31/31 | 100.0 | 14/14 | 100.0 |

[a] Numbers in parentheses refer to the number of $F_1$ broods used in the analysis.
[b] F is the frequency of expression of macromelanophore spotting, i.e. the number of offspring expressing spot divided by the total number of offspring.

ures become practically identical if corrected for *Est-1*). The combined data suggest that abnormal melanosis in *Sd* backcross hybrids is not due simply to the combination of *Sd* with a greater number of swordtail chromosomes in general. If this were true, a greater number of melanotic fish would have more swordtail chromosomes and a greater number of not so severely melanotic fish would have less, and these two types together would appear in the 'parental types' in totals which should greatly outnumber the alternatives appearing in the recombinant class. The results, at least with respect to the chromosomes marked by the enzyme loci in this study, do not support that view. They suggest that a particular pair of chromosomes may carry factors responsible for modifying *Sd* expression. At this time, the *Est-1* locus appears to mark such a chromosome, the linked factor or factors accounting for much of the observed variation in melanotic severity. It may turn out that as more animals and more loci are studied, additional and/or different factors modifying macromelanophore expression may be exposed.

The data concerning the relationship of melanotic severity in $F_1$ hybrids to the genetic distance between the parental types used for the hybridization are also consistent with the above conclusions. As can be seen from table V, some swordtail stocks produce $F_1$ hybrids with the female 163A platyfish, in which development of atypical melanosis is much more rapid than in hybrids produced from swordtails of other stocks. The figures are very highly significantly different (p<0.001), particularly at 40

days after birth. The genetic distances, however, between the platyfish
and swordtail used in the crosses are in no way correlated with the severity of melanoma in the $F_1$ (*maculatus-guentheri*, genetic distance 0.41; *ma-
culatus-strigatus*, 0.35; *maculatus-helleri*, 0.33; *maculatus-clemenciae*,
0.39). Indeed, the swordtail with the greatest genetic distance from Jamapa platyfish *(guentheri)* produced $F_1$ hybrids with the slowest growing and
least severe melanoma. If the melanoma resulted from a general, non-specific loss of genetic control in hybrids produced by highly divergent fish,
one would expect the opposite result. The result obtained is consistent
with the view that the melanoma is due to factors at a small number of
loci.

## Summary

Earlier work largely by MYRON GORDON and KURT KOSSWIG has done much in
characterizing the inheritance of melanoma in fish of the genus *Xiphophorus*. However, the identification of the number and location of genes modifying macromelanophore expression was and has been inhibited by the lack of other specific genetic
markers. The understanding of the genetic distance between species used in crosses
to produce melanotic fish has also been retarded by the lack of such markers. Consequently, it has also not been feasible to relate the genetic distance between forms
and the severity of melanoma in their hybrids. Using starch gel electrophoresis of
homogenates of different tissues from *X. maculatus* (platyfish) and *X. helleri*
(swordtails) as well as their $F_1$, $F_2$ and backcross hybrids, followed by histochemical
staining for over 30 proteins, has enabled us to resolve the products of 64 genetic
loci in the genus. Analysis of the polymorphisms at these loci has thus far permitted
the recognition of 15 linkage groups within the system. The comparative frequency
of all allozymes at 26 loci in platyfish (strain 163A), compared to various subspecies
and species of swordtails to which 163A has been hybridized, reveals no relationship
between the genetic distance and severity of melanoma in the $F_1$. The significance
of these results with respect to the uncovering of specific genes responsible for melanoma is discussed.

## References

1   ALLEN, A. C.: The skin, pp. 987–991 (Grune & Stratton, New York 1967).
2   ANDERS, A.; ANDERS, F., and KLINKE, K.: Regulation of gene expression in the
    Gordon-Kosswig melanoma system. I. The distribution of controlling genes in
    the genome of the Xiphophorin fish, *Platypoecilus maculatus* and *Platypoecilus
    variatus*; in SCHRODER Genetics and mutagenesis of fish, pp. 33–52 (Springer,
    Berlin 1973).

3   Anders, F.: Tumour formation in platyfish-swordtail hybrids as a problem of gene regulation. Experientia 23: 1–10 (1967).

4   Anderson, D. E.: Inheritance of a genetic type of cutaneous melanoma in man; in Riley Pigmentation: its genesis and control, pp. 401–413 (Appleton Century Crofts, New York 1972).

5   Atz, J. W.: Effects of hybridization on pigmentation in fishes of the genus Xiphophorus. Zoologica 47: 153–181 (1962).

6   Clark, E.: A method for artificial insemination in viviparous fishes. Science 112: 722–723 (1950).

7   Erwin, R. and Gordon, M.: Regeneration of melanomas in fishes. Zoologica 40: 53–67 (1955).

8   Fitzpatrick, T. B.; Lerner, A. B.; Calkins, E., and Summerson, W. A.: Occurrence of tyrosinase in horse and fish melanomas. Proc. Soc. exp. Biol. Med. 75: 394–402 (1950).

9   Grand, C. G.; Gordon, M., and Cameron, G.: Neoplasm studies. VIII. Cell types in tissue culture of fish melanotic tumors compared with mammalian melanomas. Cancer Res. 1: 660–666 (1941).

10  Gordon, M.: The genetics of viviparous top-minnow Platypoecilus; the inheritance of two kinds of melanophores. Genetics 12: 253–283 (1927).

11  Gordon, M.: Genetic and correlated studies of normal and atypical pigment cell growth. 10th Growth Symp., 1951, pp. 153–219.

12  Knudson, A. G.; Strong, L. C., and Anderson, D. E.: Heredity and cancer in man. Prog. med. Genet., vol. 9, pp. 113–158 (Grune & Stratton, New York 1973).

13  Kosswig, C.: Über Bastarde der Teleostier. Platypoecilus und Xiphophorus. Z. indukt. Abstamm.-Vererb.-L. 44: 253 (1927).

14  Siciliano, M. J. and Perlmutter, A.: Maternal effect on development of melanoma in hybrid fish of the genus Xiphophorus. J. natn. Cancer Inst. 49: 415–421 (1972).

15  Siciliano, M. J.; Perlmutter, A., and Clark, E.: Effect of sex on the development of melanoma in hybrid fish of the genus Xiphophorus. Cancer Res. 31: 725–729 (1971).

16  Siciliano, M. J.; Wright, D. A.; George, S., and Shaw, C. R.: Inter- and intra-specific genetic distances among teleosts; in 17e Congr. Int. de Zoologie, 1973, thème No. 5, pp. 1–24.

17  Siciliano, M. J. and Shaw, C. R.: Separation and visualization of enzymes on gels; in Smith Chromatographic and electrophoretic techniques, vol. 2; 4th ed., pp. 185–209 (Heinemann, London 1976).

18  Siciliano, M. J. and Wright, D. A.: Biochemical genetics of platyfish-swordtail hybrid melanoma system. Prog. exp. Tumor Res., vol. 20, pp. 398–411 (Karger, Basel 1975).

19  Siciliano, M. J. and Hsu, T. C.: Unpublished data.

Michael J. Siciliano, PhD, The University of Texas System Cancer Center, Biology Department, Texas Medical Center, Houston, TX 77025 (USA)

Pigment Cell, vol. 2, pp. 59–68 (Karger, Basel 1976)

# Distinctive C-Bands as Identification Markers for B16 Melanoma Lines [1]

L. M. Pasztor, F. Hu and R. L. White [2]

Oregon Regional Primate Research Center, Beaverton, Oreg.

## Introduction

C-Banding patterns of mitotic chromosomes from *Mus musculus* have established that constitutive heterochromatin, which is rich in satellite DNA, is restricted to the centromeric region of each of the 40 acrocentric chromosomes except the Y [6]. On the one hand, several murine cell lines contained chromosomes with only centromeric C-bands [5]; on the other, two cell types possessed chromosomes with interstitial or terminal C-bands in addition to centromeric C-bands [4, 7].

Stephenson and Stephenson [9], who described the B16 karyotype before the C-banding technique was available, reported that whereas the stemline karyotype of the primary contained 41 chromosomes, including two metacentrics, one abnormally elongated acrocentric, one Y, and one minute, seventeenth passage cells appeared to incorporate an additional minute and become polyploid.

Having analyzed several primary cultures from B16 tumors, as well as long-term cell lines of this often-used melanoma, we determined that they are chromosomally heterogeneous with respect to constitutive heterochromatin patterns and modal chromosome number. Furthermore, in many cell lines, not only was constitutive heterochromatin distributed to

1 Publication No. 863 of the Oregon Regional Primate Research Center. Supported in part by Public Health Service, National Institutes of Health Grants RR00163 and RR05694 of the Animal Resources Branch, Division of Research Resources, and CA08499 of the National Cancer Institute.
2 We thank Cathy Taylor, Dinah Teramura, and Coral Jean Cotterell for expert technical assistance.

chromosomal regions where it is not normally found in the mouse, but also unique C-banded marker chromosomes evolved during culture *in vitro*. These distinctive C-banded chromosomes were also preserved after passage *in vivo*.

## Methods and Materials

*Cells.* A detailed history of the B16 murine melanoma tumors and cell lines studied is given in figure 1. The original B16 mouse melanoma arose spontaneously in the skin at the base of the ear of a C57BL mouse at the Jackson Laboratory in 1954 [2]. Two cell strains derived from the B16 melanoma were described by Hu and Lesney in 1964 [3] and since that time several pigmented as well as non-pigmented cell lines have been isolated. In addition, many laboratories maintain the B16 tumor *in vivo*. A brief description and abbreviations of the tumors and cell lines we examined are given in table I.

*Cell culture.* For primary cultures, tumors excised from mice were washed with Hanks' balanced salt solution and minced with curved scissors until a fine tumor mash was produced. This mash was then treated with 0.25% trypsin for 10 min at 37 °C, centrifuged with 0.5 ml fetal calf serum, and seeded into a 250 ml plastic culture flask (Falcon Plastics, Los Angeles, Calif.) or a Blake bottle containing Eagle's minimal essential medium (MEM) enriched with 30% fetal calf serum. These cultures were incubated at 37 °C and harvested for chromosome preparation after 48–72 h. B16 cell lines were grown in either Medium 199 or MEM supplemented with 10% fetal calf serum. Medium and serum were purchased from Grand Island Biological Co. (Grand Island, N. Y.).

*Karyology.* Chromosome preparation followed the standard air-drying technique [8]. Constitutive heterochromatin was demonstrated by the method of Arrighi and Hsu [1] with a few modifications. Instead of being incubated with 0.07 N NaOH for 2 min, the slides were treated for 45 sec with 0.035 N NaOH. As a final step, a 10% Gurr's Giemsa 'R66' (Biomedical Specialities, Los Angeles, Calif.) prepared with pH 6.8 buffer made with Gurr's buffer tablets) was applied for 8–9 min.

## Results

### Chromosome Analysis

*MF and M188.* These B16 tumors had been passaged *in vivo* at the Jackson Laboratory and sent to Dr. Morris Foster at different times (fig. 1). Both (fig. 2, 3) contained acrocentric and biarmed chromosomes with constitutive heterochromatin restricted to the centromeres, but differed significantly in their modal chromosome number. Only one each of

*Table I.* Tumor and cell line abbreviations

|  | Description |
|---|---|
| *Primary* | |
| MF | Nonpigmented; from M. FOSTER. Has never been *in vitro.* Obtained by M. FOSTER from the Jackson Laboratory. |
| M188 | Pigmented; given to V. RILEY by M. FOSTER, March 1972. Has had one passage *in vitro.* Obtained by M. FOSTER from the Jackson Laboratory. |
| V916A | Nonpigmented; passed *in vitro* since 1966 by K. ADACHI and V. RILEY. Derived from 21st passage of tumors that originated by inoculating cells that had been selected for non-pigmentation *in vitro* and *in vivo* for 22 months. |
| M34A | Pigmented; passaged *in vivo* since August 1969 by V. RILEY. Derived from 81st tumor passage. Tumor originated by inoculating cells that had been selected for pigmentation *in vitro* for 18 months. |
| *Cell line* | |
| NP/133/21 | Nonpigmented; derived from 133rd tumor passage. Tumor originated by inoculating cells that had been selected for non-pigmentation *in vitro* and *in vivo* for 22 months. *In vitro* since May 1972. |
| 440B/34/43/21/25 | Pigmented[1]; derived from B16 tumor in 2–63; frozen and thawed at intervals since May 1964. Subcultured a total of 123 times. |
| P/51/214 | Pigmented; derived from 51st tumor passage. Tumor originated by inoculating cells that had been selected for pigmentation and had been *in vitro* 18 months. *In vitro* since March 1968. |
| P/140/21 | Pigmented; derived from 140th tumor passage. Tumor originated by inoculating cells that had been selected for pigmentation and had been *in vitro* 18 months. *In vitro* since September 1972. |

1 Pigmentation ascertained by visual inspection of tumor *in situ* produced by inoculating cells into C57BL/6 mice.

the 2 pairs of biarmed chromosomes seen in MF (fig. 2) were present in M188 (fig. 3). This difference was also reflected in the modal number of biarmed chromosomes: 4 in the former but only 2 in the latter. The modal total chromosome number in MF was also approximately twice that of M188 (70–74 vs. 35–38). Less than 2% of the metaphases carried a chromosome which lacked a centromeric C-band and could be tentatively identified as a Y chromosome.

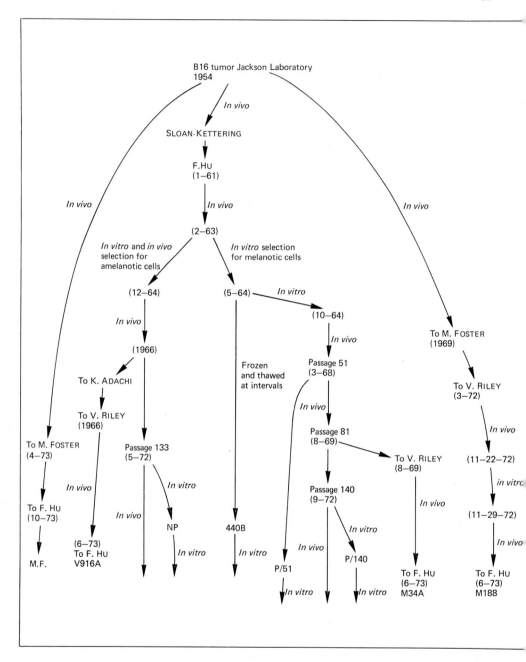

*Fig. 1.* History of B16 murine melanoma tumors and cell lines.

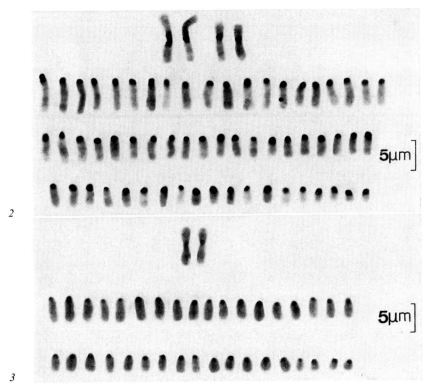

Fig. 2. MF chromosomes. C-Banded regions are restricted to centromeric regions.

Fig. 3. M188 chromosomes. C-Banded regions are restricted to centromeric regions.

*NP and V916A.* Chromosomes from cell line NP and a primary derived from tumor V916A were similar. Both shared the same type and number of biarmed chromosomes with centromeric C-bands (table II; fig. 4). This is not surprising since NP and V916A were derived from the same amelanotic B16 tumor line (fig. 1). NP and V916A had a modal chromosome number of 60–64 and could be differentiated easily from MF and M188 on the basis of chromosome number.

*440B and P/51.* Both of these were derived from the same B16 tumor (fig. 1). They had 4 types of marker chromosomes in common: (1) a medium-sized metacentric with terminal as well as centromeric C-bands, (2) an acrocentric with a large block of C-heterochromatin

Table II. Frequency of C-banded marker chromosomes

| Cell Line | | | | | | | | | Number of metaphases analyzed |
|---|---|---|---|---|---|---|---|---|---|
| 440B/34/43/21/25 | 0.80 | 0 | 0.66 | 0.86 | 1.0 | 0.66 | 0 | 0.16 | 50 |
| P/51/214 | 0.03 | 0.94 | 0.72 | 0 | 1.0 | 0.46 | 0 | 0.01 | 80 |
| P/140/21 | 0.77 | 0 | 0.82 | 0 | 0.96 | 0 | 0.88 | 0.91 | 65 |
| NP/133/21 | 0 | 0 | 0 | 0 | 1.0 | 0 | 0 | 0 | 114 |
| | | | | | | | | | |
| Primary | | | | | | | | | |
| M34A | 0.75 | 0 | 0.68 | 0 | 1.0 | 0 | 0 | 0.49 | 59 |
| V916A | 0 | 0 | 0 | 0 | 1.0 | 0 | 0 | 0 | 50 |
| M188 | 0 | 0 | 0 | 0 | 1.0 | 0 | 0 | 0 | 56 |
| MF | 0 | 0 | 0 | 0 | 1.0 | 0 | 0 | 0 | 50 |

slightly distal to the centromere, (3) a small metacentric with a centromeric C-band, and (4) an elongated acrocentric with a dark centromeric C-band and a lighter, distally located C-band (fig. 5). Marker chromosome frequencies were analogous except for type 1 (table II). In addition to these common chromosomes, each cell line has its own unique marker (table II; fig. 5, 6).

*P/140.* This cell line was closely related to P/51 (fig. 1) and shared with it and 440B types 1, 2, and 4 marker chromosomes, but lacked type 3 marker chromosome (table II). P/140 was also identified in by a special C-banded marker chromosome not found in any other cell line (table II; fig. 7).

*M34A.* Although this tumor had been passaged *in vivo* for almost 4 years in another laboratory (fig. 1), it contained types 1, 2, and 4 marker chromosomes (table II) that were also identified in 440B, P/51, and P/140 (table II).

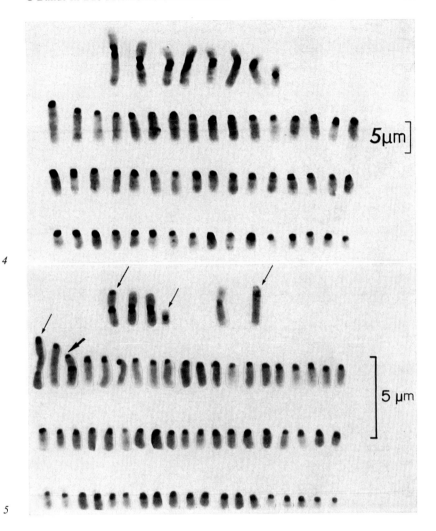

*Fig. 4.* NP chromosomes. C-Banded regions are restricted to centromeric regions.

*Fig. 5.* 440B chromosomes. Thin arrows indicate common marker chromosomes. Thick arrow indicates unique C-banded marker in this cell line.

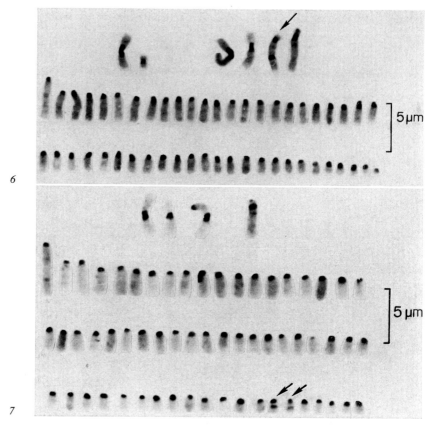

Fig. 6. P/51 chromosomes. Arrow indicates unique C-banded marker in this cell line.

Fig. 7. P/140 chromosomes. Arrows indicate two copies of the unique C-banded marker chromosome in this cell line.

## Discussion

We have established that several B16 tumors and cell lines are unique in their chromosome constitution or number and that these features can be used to identify each of them.

Two tumors, MF and M188, which had no history or only a limited history *in vitro* were similar in one respect to tumor V916A which had been derived from a long-term cell culture. All possessed biarmed chromosomes with centromeric C-bands, but their modal number of total chromosomes and biarmed chromosomes was very different and did not overlap. V916A tumor chromosomes, however, were identical to those of NP, the cell line from which it originated. M188 most closely adheres to the description STEPHENSON and STEPHENSON [9] reported for B16. Their analysis revealed a stemline of 41, including two biarmed chromosomes, a Y, and one minute. By contrast, M188 had a stemline of 38 chromosomes, less than 2% of the metaphases carried a Y, but all lacked a minute. In general morphology, the two metacentrics illustrated in that paper were similar to the two biarmed chromosomes we observed in M188.

Although NP, 440B, P/51, and P/140 cell lines originated from the same B16 tumor, NP has diverged markedly from the others. NP has no marker chromosomes with anomalous C-banded regions whereas the other three shared three chromosomes in which C-heterochromatin was not restricted to the centromere. That these markers were a stable feature of the karyotype was supported by the observations that they have been identified in (1) tumors after several years of passage *in vivo* and (2) in these 3 cell lines at different subcultures over a period of 2 years. More importantly, 440B, P/51, and P/140 were distinguished individually by unique C-banded marker chromosomes.

### Summary

When B16 murine melanoma chromosomes were studied with the C-banding technique, the constitutive heterochromatin distribution was found to be dissimilar in some primary cultures and long-term cell lines. Primaries prepared from B16 tumors which had no history or only a limited history of cultivation *in vitro* possessed two or four biarmed chromosomes in which constitutive heterochromatin was restricted to the centromeric region. By contrast, cell lines which had grown *in vitro* for several months or years, as well as tumors derived by inoculating C57BL mice with such cells, were often characterized by unique chromosomes with interstitial or terminal C-bands.

### References

1    ARRIGHI, F. and HSU, T. C.: Localization of heterochromatin in human chromosomes. Cytogenetics *10:* 81–86 (1971).
2    GREEN, E. L. (ed.): Handbook of genetically standardized Jax mice; 2nd ed. (Jackson Laboratory, Bar Harbor 1968).

3 HU, F. and LESNEY, P. F.: The isolation and cytology of two pigment cell strains from B16 mouse melanomas. Cancer Res. *24:* 1634–1643 (1964).

4 NATARAJAN, A. T.; AHNSTRÖM, G., and RAPOSA, T.: Distribution of constitutive heterochromatin in the chromosomes of MSWBS ascites tumor cells. J. natn. Cancer Inst. *50:* 1721–1726 (1973).

5 OLICINI, C. D.; EVANS, C. H., and DIPAOLO, J. A.: Chromosome patterns of nontransformed variants from chemically transformed Balb/3T3 cells. J. Cell Physiol. *83:* 401–408 (1974).

6 PARDUE, M. L. and GALL, J. G.: Chromosomal localization of mouse satellite DNAs. Science *170:* 1356–1358 (1970).

7 POPESCU, N. C. and DIPAOLO, J. A.: Heterochromatin, satellite DNA, and transformed neoplastic cells. J. natn. Cancer Inst. *49:* 603–606 (1972).

8 PRIEST, J. R.: Cytogenetics (Lea & Febiger, Philadelphia 1969).

9 STEPHENSON, E. M. and STEPHENSON, N. G.: Karyotype analysis of the B16 mouse melanoma with reassessment of the normal mouse idiogram. J. natn. Cancer Inst. *45:* 789–800 (1970).

Dr. L. M. PASZTOR, Oregon Regional Primate Research Center, 505 N. W. 185th Avenue, *Beaverton, OR 97005* (USA)

Pigment Cell, vol. 2, pp. 69–78 (Karger, Basel 1976)

# Biochemical, Immunological, and Morphological Changes Correlated with Loss of Tumorigenicity in 5-Bromodeoxyuridine-Grown Melanoma Cells

S. Silagi, E. W. Newcomb, J. R. Wrathall and J. K. Christman

Cell Genetics Laboratory, Department of Obstetrics and Gynecology, Cornell University Medical College, and Department of Pediatrics, Mount Sinai School of Medicine, New York, N. Y.

*Effects of Continuous Growth in Bromodeoxyuridine (1 $\mu g/ml$)*

Highly tumorigenic and pigmented clone $B_5 59$ of B16 mouse melanoma [3, 12, 14] forms few or no tumors after growth in cell culture in medium containing low concentrations of the thymidine analog, 5-bromodeoxyuridine (BrdU) [15]. From cells grown for 9 months in 1 $\mu g$ of BrdU/ml, we have selected a clone, $C_3 471$, which is completely nontumorigenic in adult mice and is highly immunogenic, protecting 70–100% of mice against an inevitably tumor-producing dose of untreated $B_5 59$ melanoma cells when those mice had previously received 3 weekly subcutaneous (s.c.) injections of $C_3 471$ cells [13]. Plating efficiencies and growth rate of both clonally derived lines are approximately equal. Differences between the 2 lines which may be related to the diametrically opposite tumorigenic potentials are the high immunogenicity of the $C_3 471$ cells as opposed to its apparent absence in the $B_5 59$ cells [13, 14]; the flat, 'contact-inhibited' fibroblastic morphology of $C_3 471$ cells versus the piled semicolonial melanocytic morphology of $B_5 59$ cells [12]; the high titer of C-type virus, gs-1 and gs-3 viral antigens, and Gross cell-surface antigen in $C_3 471$ vs their undetectability in $B_5 59$ cells [14]; increase in H-$2^b$ antigen titer; and the absence from $C_3 471$ cells of plasminogen activator, a proteolytic enzyme activity found in virtually all solid tumors tested [6, 7], as contrasted with abundant secretion by $B_5 59$ melanoma cells [2]. A change unrelated to oncogenicity is the complete loss of melanin, melanosomes, and tyrosinase [15, 20]. Preliminary data (table I) from our laboratory indicate that $C_3 471$ cells have 2- to 3-fold

*Table I.* Comparison of control, 72-hr BrdU-treated (3 $\mu$g/ml) and cells grown continuously in BrdU (1 $\mu$g/ml)

| | Control B$_5$59 cells[a] | 72-hour-treated: 3 $\mu$g/ml[b] | C$_3$471: 1 $\mu$g/ml continuous[c] |
|---|---|---|---|
| Tumorigenicity, % | 100 | 2.5 (1/40) | 0 |
| Morphology | piling, melanocytic | flattened | flattened, fibroblastic |
| % BU substituted for T[d] | 0 | 45.2 | 22.0 |
| C-type virus (pfu/ml)[e] | 0 | ND | $4.5 \times 10^3$ |
| Immunogenicity[f] | 0 | 50 | 70–100 |
| Gross cell-surface antigen[g] | 0 | ND | present |
| Sialic acid ($\mu$mol $\times 10^{-3}/10^6$ cells)[h] | $11 \pm 1.6$ | ND | $5 \pm 0.6$ |
| Plasminogen activator[i], % of control | 100 | 6 | 0 |
| Plating efficiency, % of control | 100 | 65 | 70–115 |
| Viability, mean % | 89 | 85 | 91 |

[a] Control cells grown in RM or RM + $10^{-5}$ M thymidine; mean of many experiments.
[b] Tumorigenicity data: mean of 4 experiments. Rest of data from single experiment, except for plasminogen activator (see footnote [i]).
[c] Passages 2–15: mean or range of many experiments.
[d] In DNA (X-ray fluorescence method of ZEITZ and LEE [22]).
[e] XC plaque assay method [9].
[f] Immunogenicity refers to % animals protected against challenge with $2 \times 10^5$ untreated B$_5$59 melanoma cells, inoculated s.c. 7 days after final inoculation of $10^6$ BrdU-grown cells or $10^4$ untreated B$_5$59 cells injected s.c. 3 times at 7-day intervals. All preinjections used nontumorigenic doses, whereas challenge dose was inevitably tumor-producing in unimmunized adult mice. Data for B$_5$59 and C$_3$471 cells in part from SILAGI *et al.* [14]; 72-hour-treated cells and additional C$_3$471 data from previously unpublished experiments.
[g] Data from SILAGI *et al.* [16].
[h] Sialic acid assay of trypsinized cells by method of WARREN [18].
[i] Data from CHRISTMAN *et al.* [2]. Assay by release of counts from $^{125}$I-fibrin-coated Petri dishes.
ND = Not done.

lower sialic acid content than do the tumorigenic $B_5$59 cells. Rios and Simmons [8] and Bekesi et al. [1] have shown that some tumor cells become more immunogenic and less oncogenic after release of sialic acid residues by treatment with *Vibrio cholorae* neuraminidase. Thus, the increased immunogenicity and decreased oncogenicity of the long-term BrdU-grown melanoma cells may, at least in part, be related to their lower sialic acid content. Related to this is the finding that $C_3$471 cells are able to grow in neonates and in adult mice immunologically compromised by repeated injections of antithymocyte serum [16]. Another difference between $C_3$471 cells and their parental melanoma cells is an alteration in amino acid pools and molar percentage of 5 amino acids in cellular proteins [11].

We have been measuring the fractional replacement of thymine (T) by 5-bromouracil (BU) in the DNA by X-ray fluorescence spectroscopy [19, 22], through the courtesy of Dr. Zeitz. The DNA is prepared by a modification of Marmur's [5] method. The DNA of nontumorigenic passages 7–15 contained 22% BU substitution for T (table I).

### Growth in BrdU (3 µg/ml) for 72 h

In order to look at early events in the changeover from the tumorigenic (and melanotic) state of these cells to the nontumorigenic, immunogenic (and amelanotic) state, we have been studying them after 24, 48, and 72 h of growth in BrdU. Preliminary experiments indicated that maximal effect with minimal toxicity was obtained with the concentration of 3 µg of BrdU per ml ($10^{-5}$ M). The results obtained after 72 h (approximately 3 cell divisions) are shown in table I. Animals inoculated subcutaneously (s.c.) with $2 \times 10^5$ control untreated viable cells (vc) all had palpable tumors by day 24 postinjection (pi), whereas no animals injected once with $2 \times 10^5$ vc (0/10) or 3 times (0/10) with $10^6$ treated vc developed palpable tumors. Animals that did not develop tumors were kept for 70 days, sacrificed and the site of injection dissected. One tiny mass was found in 1 of 20 animals after dissection. In later experiments, no tumors were found, even upon dissection on day 70, in 20 additional mice injected with $2 \times 10^5$ cells grown in BrdU (3 µg/ml) for 72 h. The animals injected 3 times at weekly intervals were challenged 7 days after the third injection with $2 \times 10^5$ untreated $B_5$59 melanoma vc on the opposite side of the animal. Five of the 10 developed $B_5$59 tumors, the

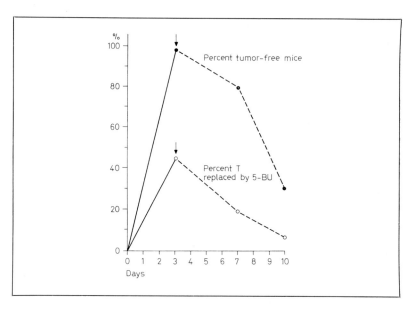

*Fig. 1.* Correlation of reduction in tumorigenicity (●) with changes in the percent of 5-bromouracil (5-BU) substituted for thymine (T) in the DNA of melanoma cells (O) grown for 72 h in medium containing BrdU (3 μg/ml) (——) and then allowed to grow in medium devoid of BrdU for 7 days (– – –); arrow indicates time when medium was changed. The data plotted were obtained from one experiment. Ten mice were inoculated s.c. ($2\times10^5$ viable cells/mouse) for each time point and the percent of mice remaining free of tumors for 70 days is shown.

first 2 on day 28 postchallenge, the third on day 38, the fourth on day 64, and the last, found on dissection, on day 70. Thus, even in the 50% that developed tumors, the latent period was considerably increased.

That the suppression of tumorigenic potential was reversible had been previously shown with animals injected with cells grown in BrdU for 7 days or more and then grown in normal medium [12]. We tested the kinetics of reversibility in 72-hour treated cells after growth in normal medium (RM) for 4 days and 7 days (fig. 1). Four-day reversed cells produced tumors in 2 of 10 animals, and 7-day reversed cells in 7 of 10. All tumors had an increased latent period compared with controls. Thus, as few as 3 days of growth in $10^{-5}$ M BrdU had a profound effect on both tumorigenicity and immunogenicity of the melanoma cells.

*Table II*. Reversible effects of one and two divisions in BrdU (3 μg/ml) on mouse melanoma cells

|  | Controls[a] | 24 h BRM | 24 h BRM + 6 days RM | 48 h 3 BRM | 48 h BRM + 5 days RM |
|---|---|---|---|---|---|
| Tumorigenicity, % | 100 | 55 | 95 | 15 | 93 |
| % BU substitution for T in DNA | 0 | 23 | 2 | 39 | 7 |
| Plasminogen activator[b], % of control | 100 | 38–79 | ND | 6–30 | 90–100 |
| Plating efficiency, % of control | 100 | 119 | 61 | 48 | 34 |
| Viability, mean % | 89 | 96 | 95 | 91 | 98 |

[a] Controls grown in RM or RM + $10^{-5}$ M TdR.
[b] Data from CHRISTMAN *et al.* [2].
BRM = RM + $10^{-5}$ M BrdU (3 μg/ml).

Reversal to high tumorigenicity, although not complete after 7 days' growth on RM, was considerable.

DNA substitution studies showed that 45% of T was replaced by BU after 72 h in BrdU. This was reduced after 4 days' growth in RM to 19% and by 7 days to 6%. As with $C_3471$ cells, there was a good correlation between effect on tumorigenicity and substitution in the DNA (fig. 1).

CHRISTMAN *et al.* [2] have recently shown that growth in BrdU greatly decreases the activity of plasminogen activator. Their data are given in tables I and II. We have found subsequently that the degree of reduction can vary from experiment to experiment, but is always in the same direction as published.

### Effects of 24 and 48 h of Growth in BrdU (3 μg/ml)

Table II summarizes the effects of 4 experiments in which $B_559$ cells were grown for 1 and 2 divisions (24 and 48 h) in BrdU-containing medium and then subcultured into RM. Figure 2a and b show respectively the effect of 24 and 48 h of BrdU treatment on tumor suppression and BU replacement. Comparison of figures 1 and 2 show that the de-

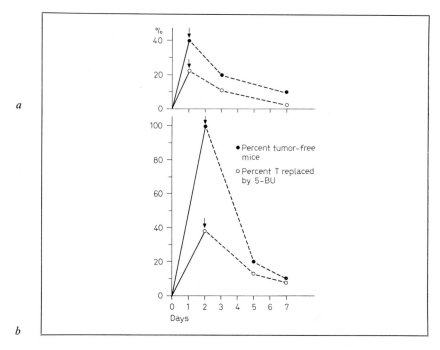

*Fig. 2.* Correlation of changes in tumorigenicity with changes in percent of 5-BU substituted for T in DNA of melanoma cells grown in medium containing BrdU (3 µg/ml) for: (a) 24 h, and (b) 48 h, and then in medium without BrdU as indicated. Data plotted were obtained from one representative experiment.

gree of BU incorporation and suppression of tumorigenicity increase with time of exposure to BrdU. This supports the hypothesis that BU incorporation into the DNA is a prerequisite for the suppression of tumorigenicity in melanoma cells grown in BrdU. Earlier experiments [12, 13] had shown that cell division and incorporation of the thymidine analog were necessary to produce the morphological effects occurring with growth in the presence of BrdU, and that these could be prevented by inhibition of DNA synthesis with cytosine arabinoside or by adding equimolar thymidine to medium containing BrdU. DNA synthesis is also essential for BrdU to suppress formation of plasminogen activator of $B_5$59 cells [4]. The data reported here and by Wrathall *et al.* [19] show that the degree of suppression of tumorigenicity is roughly proportional to the amount of BU in the DNA. A key question that remains unresolved is whether this is merely an effect of the quantity of BU in

DNA, or whether specific loci must contain substituted DNA, with the probability of those loci being 'hit' increased as the quantity of substitution in the cell population increases.

The regaining of tumorigenic potential upon growth of BrdU-treated cells in non-BrdU-containing medium is also roughly proportional to the decreased amount of BU left in the DNA as the cells divide in RM. Here, too, the question of specific substituted loci is unresolved. Cells treated for 72 h and allowed to grow in RM for 7 days still had 6% of their T replaced by BU and formed tumors in 70% of inoculated mice (fig. 1), whereas those treated for 48 h and grown in RM for 5 days had 7% of T replaced by BU but formed tumors in 93% of inoculated mice (table II). This would seem to indicate that some factor(s) in addition to the quantity of substitution may be the reason for tumor suppression and reversal.

WRATHALL et al. [17, 19, 21] have indicated that a single cell division (24 h) in BrdU is sufficient to produce a striking reduction in tyrosinase activity. The same is true for tumorigenicity and plasminogen activator (fig. 2b, table II) [2, 19]. Thus, substitution in only a single strand of the DNA is sufficient to produce significant suppression. A more extended discussion of the phenomenon of 'unifilar dominance' can be found in the work of RUTTER et al. [10] and WRATHALL et al. [19].

## Conclusions

This and previous work with these melanoma cells grown in medium containing 1–3 $\mu$g/ml of BrdU shows that they are able to continue growth in analog-containing medium with little toxic effect. At the same time, profound changes take place in morphology, melanogenesis, cell membranes, including sialic acid content and Gross cell-surface antigen, plasminogen activator, C-type virus, and in the immunogenic and tumorigenic potential of the cells. Kinetic studies during the first 3 cell divisions in BrdU (3 $\mu$g/ml) indicate that substitution of BU for T in the DNA occurs, going from 0 in untreated cells to 23, 39, and 45% with each day. This is correlated with decrease in tumorigenicity from 100% in untreated cells to 55, 15, and 2.5% with each day's growth in BrdU. Decrease in the proteolytic enzyme, plasminogen activator [2], follows a similar time course.

By 3 days, the cells have become immunogenic and capable of protecting 50% of the mice against a tumorigenic dose of untreated cells. Other phenomena seen in cells grown for months in 1 $\mu$g/ml of BrdU and not in untreated B$_5$59 melanoma cells are C-type virus production, with concomitant production of Gross cell-surface antigen as well as gs-1 and gs-3 viral antigens [14], decrease in sialic acid content and increase in H-2$^b$ antigen titer [16]. Study of these phenomena is now proceeding in the short-term treated cells.

All of these findings indicate that this model system is proving useful in elucidating and defining parameters related to changes in tumorigenic potential.

## Summary

Suppression of malignant potential is a consistent effect of growth of clone B$_5$59 of B16 mouse melanoma in culture medium containing 1–3 $\mu$g/ml of 5-bromodeoxyuridine (BrdU). Nontumorigenic clone C$_3$471 was selected from B$_5$59 cells which had grown for 9 months in 1 $\mu$g/ml of BrdU. Differences between the 2 cell lines which may be related to the diametrically opposite tumorigenic potentials are the high immunogenicity of C$_3$471 cells as opposed to its apparent absence in B$_5$59 cells; the absence from C$_3$471 cells of plasminogen activator, a proteolytic enzyme activity found in virtually all solid tumors tested, as contrasted with abundant secretion by B$_5$59 melanoma cells; decreased sialic acid content and increased H-2$^b$ antigen titer of C$_3$471 cells over the tumorigenic cells, and finally the presence of C-type virus, gs-1, gs-3 and Gross cell-surface antigens in C$_3$471 contrasted with their undetectability in B$_5$59 cells. C$_3$471 cells are 'contact inhibited' fibroblast-like, whereas B$_5$59 cells grow as piled melanocytes. C$_3$471 cells during the first 15 passages are nontumorigenic and have 22% of thymine (T) residues in the DNA replaced by 5-bromouracil (BU). In order to study early events in the changeover, we have grown B$_5$59 cells in medium containing BrdU (3 $\mu$g/ml) for 24, 48, and 72 h, corresponding to approximately 1, 2, and 3 cell divisions, and then allowed them to revert in normal medium for up to 7 days. After a 24-hour treatment, tumors grew in 55% of mice injected with 2×10$^5$ cells, correlated with 23% substitution of BU for T; at 48 h, tumors grew in 15%, and at 72 h, in 2.5% of the injected mice and BU substitution was 39 and 45%, respectively. All mice inoculated with 2×10$^5$ untreated B$_5$59 cells developed tumors (TD$_{50}$ = 5×10$^4$ viable cells). When cells were grown in medium without BrdU, they gradually reversed to high tumor production and their DNA gradually diluted out the BU. They also gradually regained the parental morphology after having flattened out upon growth for 48–72 h in BrdU. Plasminogen activator also decreases with growth in BrdU and increases when the cells reverse in normal medium. Growth of these melanoma cells in BrdU is thus proving useful as a model system in probing factors related to the malignant change.

## Acknowledgments

This work was supported in part by USPHS-NCI Grants CA 10095, CA 16890 and Damon Runyon-Walter Winchell Memorial Foundation Grant 1095. S. SILAGI is a recipient of Faculty Award PRA-77 from the American Cancer Society. We wish to thank R. BALINT for preparing the DNA and performing the X-ray fluorescence spectrometry, L. ZEITZ for his cooperation and assistance, and N. CORTEZ for her expert technical assistance.

## References

1  BEKESI, J. G.; ST.-ARNEAULT, G.; WALTER, L., and HOLLAND, J. F.: Immunogenicity of leukemia L1210 cells after neuraminidase treatment. J. natn. Cancer Inst. *49:* 107–118 (1972).

2  CHRISTMAN, J. K.; SILAGI, S.; NEWCOMB, E. W.; SILVERSTEIN, S. C., and ACS, G.: Correlation of 5-bromodeoxyuridine suppression of tumorigenicity and plasminogen activator in mouse melanoma cells. Proc. natn. Acad. Sci. USA *72:* 41–50 (1975).

3  HU, F. and LESNEY, P. F.: The isolation and cytology of two pigmented cell strains from $B_{16}$ mouse melanoma. Cancer Res. *24:* 1634–1643 (1964).

4  KYNER, D. S.; CHRISTMAN, J. K.; NEWCOMB, E. W.; SILAGI, S., and SILVERSTEIN, S. C.: Effect of cell division, cell fusion and cocultivation on the release of plasminogen activator by mouse melanoma. Fed. Proc. Fed. Am. Socs exp. Biol. *34:* 532 (1975).

5  MARMUR, J.: A procedure for the isolation of deoxyribonucleic acid from micro-organisms. J. molec. Biol. *3:* 208–218 (1961).

6  OSSOWSKI, L.; UNKELESS, J.; TOBIAS, A.; QUIGLEY, J. P.; RIFKIN, D. B., and REICH, E.: An enzymatic function associated with transformation of fibroblasts by oncogenic viruses (II). J. exp. Med. *137:* 112–126 (1973).

7  RIFKIN, D. B.; LOEB, J. N.; MOORE, G., and REICH, E.: Properties of plasminogen activators formed by neoplastic human cell cultures. J. exp. Med. *139:* 1317–1328 (1974).

8  RIOS, A. and SIMMONS, R. L.: Immunospecific regression of various syngeneic mouse tumors in response to neuraminidase-treated tumor cells. J. natn. Cancer Inst. *51:* 637–644 (1973).

9  ROWE, W. P.; PUGH, W. E., and HARTLEY, J. W.: Plaque assay technique for murine leukemia viruses. Virology *42:* 1136–1139 (1970).

10  RUTTER, W. J.; PICTET, R. L., and MORRIS, P. W.: Toward molecular mechanisms of developmental processes. A. Rev. Biochem. *42:* 601–646 (1973).

11  SCHULMAN, J. D.; WRATHALL, J. R.; SILAGI, S., and DOORES, L.: Altered amino acid concentrations accompanying suppression of malignancy of mouse melanoma cells by 5-bromodeoxyuridine. J. natn. Cancer Inst. *52:* 275–277 (1974).

12  SILAGI, S.: Control of pigment production in mouse melanoma cells *in vitro.* J. Cell Biol. *43:* 263–274 (1969).

13 SILAGI, S.: Modification of malignancy by 5-bromodeoxyuridine. Studies of reversibility and immunological effects. In Vitro 7: 105–114 (1971).

14 SILAGI, S.; BEJU, D.; WRATHALL, J., and DEHARVEN, E.: Tumorigenicity, immunogenicity and virus production in mouse melanoma cells treated with 5-bromodeoxyuridine. Proc. natn. Acad. Sci. USA 69: 3443–3447 (1972).

15 SILAGI, S. and BRUCE, S. A.: Suppression of malignancy and differentiation in melanotic melanoma cells. Proc. natn. Acad. Sci. USA 66: 72–78 (1970).

16 SILAGI, S.; NEWCOMB, E. W., and WEKSLER, M. E.: Relationship of antigenicity of melanoma cells grown in 5-bromodeoxyuridine to reduced tumorigenicity. Cancer Res. 34: 100–104 (1974).

17 SILAGI, S. and WRATHALL, J. R.: Reversible suppression of differentiation and malignancy in bromodeoxyuridine-treated melanoma cells. 4th Int. Symp. Princess Takamatsu Research Fund, pp. 369–395 (University of Tokyo Press, Tokyo 1974).

18 WARREN, L.: The thiobarbituric acid assay of sialic acid. J. biol. Chem. 234: 1971–1975 (1959).

19 WRATHALL, J. R.; NEWCOMB, E. W.; BALINT, R.; ZEITZ, L., and SILAGI, S.: Suppression of melanoma cell tyrosinase activity and tumorigenicity after incorporation of bromouracil for one or two cell divisions. J. Cell Physiol. 86: 581–592 (1975).

20 WRATHALL, J. R.; OLIVER, C.; SILAGI, S., and ESSNER, E.: Suppression of pigmentation in mouse melanoma cells by 5-bromodeoxyuridine. Effects on tyrosinase activity and melanosome formation. J. Cell Biol. 57: 406–432 (1973).

21 WRATHALL, J. R. and SILAGI, S.: Suppression of melanoma cell tyrosinase activity after incorporation of 5-bromodeoxyuridine during one round of DNA Synthesis (this volume).

22 ZEITZ, L. and LEE, R.: Element analysis in labeled DNA by X-ray fluorescence. Analyt. Biochem. 23: 442–458 (1968).

Dr. S. SILAGI, Cell Genetics Laboratory, Department of Obstetrics and Gynecology, Cornell University Medical College, New York, NY 10021 (USA)

Pigment Cell, vol. 2, pp. 79–93 (Karger, Basel 1976)

# Morphological, Cytogenetic and Ultrastructural Observations on Three Lines of Human Melanoma Cells Kept in Long-Term Culture

ANNE KREMENTZ ZIMMERING, PETER W. A. MANSELL,
ROBIN S. DIETRICH and CAROL O'NEIL

Department of Surgery, Tulane University School of Medicine, New Orleans, La.

Recent interest has been focused on the use of cultured human malignant cells as target cells in the immunological evaluation of the host response to malignant disease and also for use in immunotherapy [3, 8, 13, 21]. Attention has been drawn by several workers to the fact that cells that have been in culture for long periods of time may not only differ markedly from the tissue of origin, insofar as cell surface antigens are concerned, but may also vary from passage to passage [7, 14].

Three lines of malignant melanoma cells have been kept in continuous culture at this centre for three years and have been used not only as target cells, but also as immunogens for the raising of antibodies of xenogeneic hosts [10, 11] as agents in immunotherapeutic procedures when sufficient numbers of the autologous cells were not available for autoimmunization.

This study was undertaken in order to investigate the morphological, cytogenetic, and ultrastructural features of these cell lines, in order to find out in what ways, if any, they differ from primary malignant melanoma cells.

## Methods and Materials

Fresh biopsy specimens of tumor were minced and set up, in 4- or 20-oz. glass prescription bottles in either Medium 199, Earle's salt base, or RPMI 1640, both of which were supplemented with 15% fetal bovine serum (FCS) 1 ml antibiotic/antimycotic mixture per 100 ml medium and 1.8 ml L-glutamine per 500 ml medium. The medium was changed twice weekly under strictly sterile conditions. Cultures were incubated in a Napco 1000 series incubator, model 332, at 37 °C in an atmosphere of 95% air with 5% $CO_2$ in a humid atmosphere.

Confluent monolayers of cells were passaged either by means of mechanical disaggregation or using 0.125% trypsin in culture medium without FCS. Trypsin was left in contact with the monolayer at 37 °C for a maximum of 5 min and then the cells were gently agitated and washed off with fresh medium. Cells were stored for future use in medium with 20% FCS and 10% dimethylsulphoxide, sealed in glass ampules and stored in gas phase liquid nitrogen after being frozen in a Linde BF-5 Biological Freezer for 2 h.

For cytogenetic investigation, the cells were harvested 48 h after passage using the technique of TIJO and LEVAN [22]. The cells were arrested in metaphase with colcemid. Harvesting was accomplished by trypsinization. Hypotonic treatment with distilled water was followed by fixation in methanol-acetic acid. Slides were prepared by air drying and the chromosomes were stained with buffered Giemsa stain. Preparations of the three cell lines were scanned for metaphase plates; the range of chromosome number and the modal number of chromosomes per cell in each line were determined. Karyotypes were prepared and assessed for numerical and/or structural aberrations of the chromosomes.

For electron microscopy, confluent monolayers of cells were gently scraped off the culture bottle and washed three times with cacodylate buffer [17] or SORENSEN's [20] buffer. The cells were centrifuged and the pellet was fixed for 2 h with buffered glutaraldehyde at 5 °C (1.5% glutaraldehyde in cacodylate or 3% glutaraldehyde in Sorensen's buffer). The cells were washed twice and postfixed with 1% osmium tetroxide in buffer. The cell pellets were then dehydrated with an ethanol series followed by propylene oxide, infiltrated with a 1:1 solution of propylene oxide: maraglas followed by pure maraglas infiltration at 5 °C for 48 h. Ultrathin sections were cut with a diamond knife on a Porter-Blum MT-2 ultramicrotome (Sorvall), and doubly stained with saturated aqueous uranyl acetate and lead citrate [9, 18]. The sections, mounted on copper grids, were examined in a Siemens 1 and Phillips EM-300 electron microscope.

## Results

*Morphology.* Two of the cell lines, TC and TM, are virtually indistinguishable to ordinary microscopic examination. They both show a predominantly epithelioid appearance, the cells are small and grow to confluence after passage in 5–6 days in both cases. Occasionally, both cell lines could be subcultured twice a week. On close examination, however, there were several differences between the 2 lines. The line TM was isolated from a metastatic lesion on a 48-year-old white male in June, 1970. The cells were originally grown in RPMI 1640 and in late 1972 were changed, without trouble, into TC 199 medium. When stained with Giemsa *in situ* (fig. 1A) the cells show a fairly abundant cytoplasm with an ill-defined

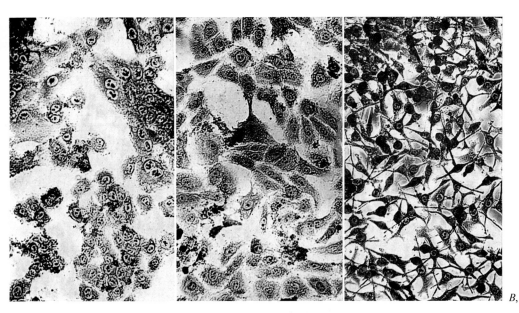

B, C

*Fig. 1. A* Light micrograph of cell line TM stained *in situ*. Giemsa. × 155. *B* Light micrograph of cell line TC stained *in situ*. Giemsa. × 155. *C* Light micrograph of cell line TB *in situ*. Giemsa. × 155.

cell membrane; the cytoplasm contains occasional vacuoles and has a finely reticular pattern; there is no evidence of pigmentation. The nucleus is large and oval with up to 3 very prominent nucleoli. This line of cells grew as a flat monolayer with no piling up of the cells. Occasional spindle-shaped cells were seen.

The line TC was isolated from the nonpigmented lung metastasis in a white female aged 24 on July 14, 1970. This patient was subsequently treated with immunotherapy and remains alive with no evidence of disease at the present day [15]. The cells of this line are very similar to those of TM except that they have a more granular cytoplasm with no evidence of pigment (fig. 1B). These cells, however, grow in small clumps and show loss of contact inhibition when confluent. There is a wide variation in the size of both the whole cells and the nuclei. In recent months, this line has shown an increasing number of bipolar spindle cells in the population. Both this line and TM are very resistant to trypsinization, usually needing to be mechanically removed from the glass surface.

Cell line TB was isolated in RPMI 1640 from the deeply pigmented metastasis of a white male aged 38 on Nov. 5, 1970. This patient has since died from his disease. An attempt was made to change this line to TC 199 medium, but the cells would not tolerate it and it had to be returned to RPMI 1640 as a result of which a remarkable change occurred in the cell morphology. Whereas the TB cells had resembled those of the other 2 lines, TM and TC, the cells that survived the change in medium and are now regarded as line TB have a quite different distinctive appearance (fig. 1C). The cells are small and stellate in form with scanty cytoplasm which has a reticular pattern, there are vacuoles seen in many of the cells and the cells are obviously pigmented although the pigmentation is not uniform, some cells being more deeply pigmented than others while others are nonpigmented. The nuclei are small and round with large deeply staining nucleoli. Occasional cells are seen with less dense cytoplasm and larger, or multiple, nuclei. There is very obvious piling up of the cells and this line is very easily removed from the glass with a minimum exposure to trypsin. These cells grow more slowly than the other two lines and only require subculture once a week.

### Cytogenetics

*Line TB.* 25 metaphases were counted and 23 cells had a near tetraploid chromosome number. One cell was decaploid with 222 chromosomes and one was near heptaploid with 177 chromosomes; no diploid cells were seen in the metaphase preparations. In the near tetraploid cells, the range of chromosome number per cell was 85–96 and the modal number 90. Karyotypes of these near tetraploid cells showed a consistent lack of one or more of the G chromosomes (fig. 2). Occasional trisomies of the B, C, and D groups yield pseudo-tetraploid or hypertetraploid chromosomal complements. The lack of the 'y' chromosome in the karyotype of TB (fig. 2) was the only sex chromosome abnormality seen in any of the 3 cell lines. Many TB cells showed a large submetacentric marker chromosome with a distinct and elongated secondary constriction near the centromere; this marker was, in most cases, paired with an identical marker. The first pair of chromosomes in group A also had distinct secondary constrictions (fig. 2, arrow). Occasional chromatid gaps and frequent small, unpaired chromosome fragments were noted in the metaphase plates of this line.

*Line TC.* Metaphase counts show a high degree of chromosomal aneuploidy in this line. In 36 metaphase plates there was a range of

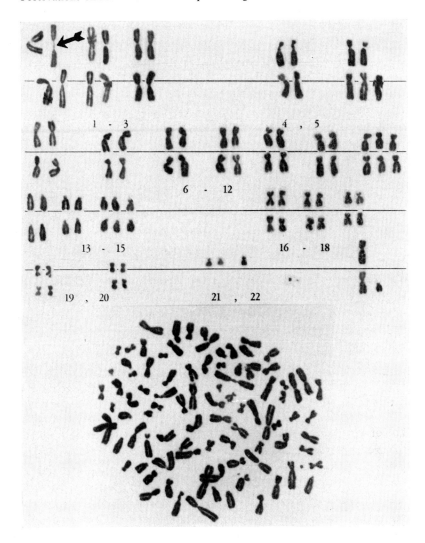

*Fig. 2.* Karyotype with metaphase plate from cell line TB. Arrow points to secondary constriction typical of this cell line.

36–93 chromosomes per cell. Three cells had a normal diploid number of 46, 12 cells (33%) had a hyperdiploid range of 49–52, and 13 cells (36%) had a near tetraploid number varying from 88 to 93 per cell.

Chromosomal irregularities are abundant in this cell line. Deletions, chromatid gaps, and chromatid breaks were frequently seen, but did not occur in a regular pattern. With the exception of 1 cell, all metaphase plates had 1 or more isochromatid fragments; these fragments occasionally had an appearance similar to very small acrocentric or metacentric chromosomes. One cell was noted in which extensive chromosomal breakage had resulted in a recombination of the fragments to form quadriradial configurations. Figure 3 (arrow) demonstrates the large unpaired submetacentric marker chromosome which was observed in 2 of 9 karyotypes from this line. Satellites of the D and G group chromosomes were prominent and satellite association among these chromosomes occurred often.

Numerical abnormalities were also frequent in the TC line. A highly irregular pattern of monosomies and trisomies was seen. A peculiar phenomenon was observed in two cells in which the group C chromosomes and the sex chromosomes were diploid whereas almost all other chromosomes in the cell were tetraploid (fig. 3).

*Line TM.* Metaphase plates of 50 cells were counted for this line and a modal number of 50 was measured. The range of chromosome number varied from 44 to 54, but 70% of the cells had 49–51 chromosomes per cell. Although most of the cells had a hyperdiploid modal number the karyotypes were not always identical. Five karyotypes showed a wide range of structural and numerical abnormalities. Figure 4 (arrow) shows a pair of large acrocentric marker chromosomes; these markers did not occur in all the TM cells. Trisomies were noted in groups A, B, C, and D and nullosomy of a pair of F chromosomes was noted. Chromosome pulverization was apparent in several metaphase plates. Terminal deletions, isochromatid fragments and satellite association were also frequent.

Ultrastructure

Of the 3 cell lines, only line TB demonstrated readily identifiable melanosomes. The TC line cells have what may be a highly aberrant type of pigment producing melanosome and the TM cells are undifferentiated and do not appear to contain any type of pigment producing cytoplasmic organelle.

*Line TB.* The cytoplasm of this line shows many membrane-bounded

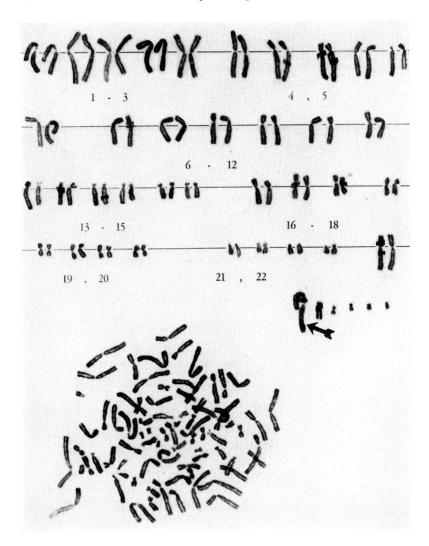

*Fig. 3.* Karyotype with metaphase plate from cell line TC. Arrow indicates unpaired submetacentric marker chromosome.

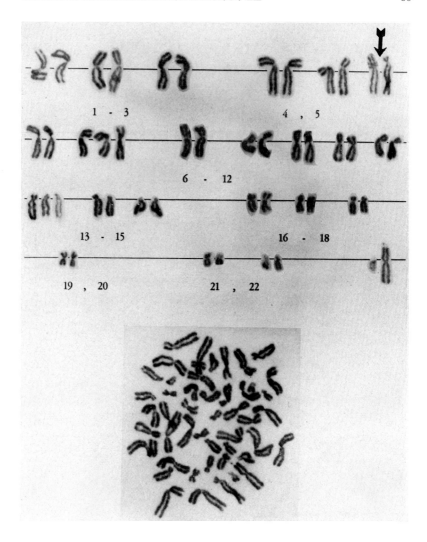

*Fig. 4.* Karyotype with metaphase plate from cell line TM. Arrow indicates pair of acrocentric marker chromosomes.

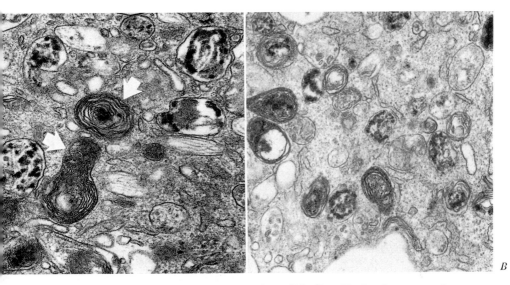

*Fig. 5. A* Electron micrograph of part of a cell in line TB showing scattered melanosomes. Arrows point to myelin bodies. × 39,600. *B* Electron micrograph of part of a cell in line TB, showing melanosomes. × 30,900.

lipid droplets and prominent mitochondria. Abnormally large amounts of Golgi apparatus are seen and are associated with numbers of small cytoplasmic vesicles. Well-developed annulate lammellae are seen associated with the Golgi apparatus, and the evolution of the Golgi could be seen from an annulate lammellus. The cytoplasm contains abundant microfilaments, and only small amounts of endoplasmic reticulum are seen. Multilamellelar myelin bodies were occasionally noted in the cytoplasm (fig. 5A, arrows). The cell membrane is extended into long tortuous microvilli. The nuclei of these cells contain granular chromatin with little heterochromatin except for a few condensations along the nuclear membrane. The nucleolus may be multiple and is usually large and lobulated.

An abnormal form of melanosome was seen in this line. The melanosomes were not uniform in shape or size, but were usually cigar shaped or circular in section, most often being irregularly circular. These membrane-bound melanosomes (fig. 5A, B) contain an array of periodically cross striated filaments, arranged either in concentric rings or in a disorganized array. Melanosomes are seen in all stages of pigment synthesis and deposition, some having no pigment and some with well-marked pigment granules deposited on the filaments. In some organelles, the filaments are

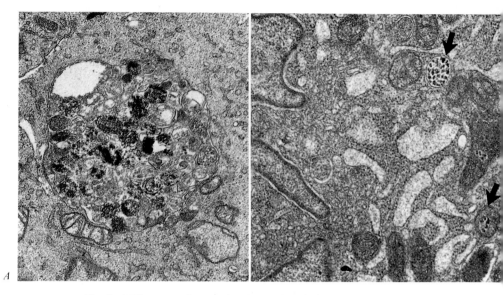

*Fig. 6. A* Electron micrograph of cytoplasmic inclusion seen in line TB. The inclusion contains intact melanosomes and melanosomal debris. × 15,680. *B* Electron micrograph of representative part of a cell in line TC. Arrows point to compound granular type organelles which may contain pigment. × 25,900.

completely occluded by large quantities of deposited pigment. This cell line also exhibited large cytoplasmic inclusions (fig. 6A) bounded by an intact membrane and containing numbers of melanosomes and melanosomal debris. This type of inclusion may be an autophagosome or it may have a lysosomal origin. Large amounts of fine microtubules were also seen in this cell line. These cells appear to correspond to type II cells of CLARK [6].

*Line TC.* The cells of this line resemble those of line TB very closely except that no well-defined cytoplasmic melanosomes were seen. The cytoplasm of these cells contained exuberant Golgi bodies, lamellar organelles and granular organelles. The latter (fig. 6B, arrows) are considered to be aberrant forms of melanosomes; therefore, we would classify these cells as type III cells [6]. Mitochondria, rough-surfaced endoplasmic reticulum and membrane-bounded lipid droplets were all seen in the cytoplasm of these cells. TC cells have irregular nuclei with finely granular chromatin and single or occasionally double nucleoli.

*Line TM.* The cells of this line are less differentiated than the other cells. The cytoplasm contains no melanosomal organelles of any type. In common with the other cell lines, the TM line shows elaborate Golgi apparatus and the presence of the membrane-bound lamellar organelle, thought to be of lysosomal origin. Mitochondria and rough-surfaced endoplasmic reticulum are also seen.

The irregularly shaped nuclei of the TM line are of 2 types; one has heterochromatin lining the nuclear membrane and also small clumps of heterochromatin scattered throughout the nucleus. The other type of nucleus has finely granular chromatin and no heterochromatin. The nucleolus may be single or double and on occasion may be so large as to occupy almost the whole of the nucleus. These cells would be classified as the undifferentiated type IV cell [6].

### Discussion

The results of these studies show that although there is a morphological resemblance of the TC and the TM lines there are great differences to be seen both cytogenetically and ultrastructurally. The TB line differs in almost every respect from the other two lines.

The line TB, which is so very different from TM and TC, underwent a change in morphology as a result of a change in tissue culture conditions. It appears that this brought about the outgrowth of a clone which differed from that which had been dominant earlier in the history of the culture. It is very probable that this process of cloning is occurring regularly throughout the life of a culture and that it is this that accounts for the reported changes in the cell surface antigens as well as the changes in the naked eye appearance of cultures. The ultrastructural observation of 2 types of nucleus in the line TM may well be the result of 2 different clones of cells growing alongside one another so that there is a heterogenous population of cells in this line. It also appears possible that the TC line has more than one cell type since recently an increasing proportion of bipolar cells has been noted in this culture.

The difference between these 3 cultures is well emphasized by the results of the electron microscopy. The TB cells are type II cells with obvious melanosomes and a regular homogenous pattern to the cells. Line TC is composed of type III cells with some aberrant melanosomes of the compound granular organelle type; although it differs relatively little in its ultrastructure from the type II TB cell, it is easily distinguishable by light microscopy. The third line, TM, is a nondifferentiated cell line of type IV cells resembling TC when viewed by light microscopy, but clearly very different and also composed of two clones.

Electron microscopy indicates that we have long-term human malignant melanoma tissue culture cells that have not dedifferentiated and continue to produce pigment and that the cells which do not produce pigment still have a large amount of Golgi apparatus and many vesicles in their cytoplasm. The presence of excess Golgi material and cytoplasmic vesicles may reflect the potential to produce melanosomes.

A summary of the cytogenetic survey of these melanoma cells is as follows. None of the three cell lines had a diploid chromosomal complement; however, each line demonstrated one or two modal ranges of chromosome number per cell. There were frequent structural and numerical chromosomal abnormalities in each line and marker chromosomes were noted in all three lines. Although we have observed a number of chromosomal variations that have not been reported for melanoma cells, the cytogenetics of these three lines of malignant melanoma cells are similar to those described for other melanoma cells both *in vivo* and in long- and short-term cultures [1, 4, 5, 12, 19, 23].

None of the cells examined in the electron microscope in this study, nor a large number examined by one of us (PWAM) in an earlier unpublished study showed any evidence of the presence of viruses. The observation in no way rules out the presence of virus-like particles, such as have been recently described by PARSONS et al. [16] or viral nucleic acid, described by BIRKMAYER et al. [2].

The results of HL-A typing of the TC cell line compared with those for normal fibroblasts from the same patient and normal lymphocytes from the patient are of considerable interest. The lymphocytes showed the pattern (2, 3, 7, 17), the normal cultured fibroblasts (2, 3 7) and the line of melanoma cells, TC (2, 3, 7, 12). Thus, there appears to have been a deletion of a locus in the fibroblast with an addition of a locus not found either on the lymphocyte or the fibroblast on the melanoma cell. It is hard to assign any particular significance to this finding, except to say that if the surface antigens of cells can be shown to differ in this way, it is not hard to imagine that they may also differ with respect to other antigens and that different clones may differ within the same line of cells.

In general, the conclusions to be drawn from this study are that even though cell lines may appear, grossly, to resemble one another, they can be shown to differ from each other in many ways. These differences can probably be induced relatively easily by such crude events as changes in the conditions of tissue culture and there are probably several different clones of cells resident in any line at the same time. It may be that these changes are increasing in number and magnitude with the length of time the cells have been in culture. Yet despite the changes that may occur in tumor cells from passage to passage, we have observed long-term cultured melanoma cells that have remained differentiated in respect to melanogenesis. Also, we observed in these long-term culture cells chromosomal changes that are similar to what has been observed in primary malignant melanoma. While we have noted gross morphological changes in these cells over a long period of cell culture, we believe that these long-term human malignant melanoma cells have retained a few, if not more, similarities to primary malignant melanoma cells.

## Summary

Three lines of human melanoma cells have been kept in culture for 3 years. Morphologically 2 of them resemble epithelial cells, neither of them show gross pigmentation. The third line is composed of small stellate cells and shows clumps of pigmented cells. Cytogenetic studies have shown that none of the 3 lines are now diploid and that each of them displays regular abnormalities unique to the line but not shared by the others. No common genetic abnormality has been found. Electron microscopy has shown melanin formation in the pigmented line and rudimentary premelanosomes in one of the other lines; the third shows no evidence of melanin formation. All the lines show active Golgi apparatus and many microvilli. There is no evidence of virus in any of the lines.

## Acknowledgments

This work has been supported by US Public Health Service Grant No. CA05837-12 from NIH, and by the Ladies Auxiliary of the Veterans of Foreign Wars. The HL-A typings were kindly performed by Dr. MITSUO TAKASAGI, Department of Surgery, School of Medicine, The Centre for Health Sciences, Los Angeles. Dr. JAMES C. HARKIN, Department of Pathology, Tulane University School of Medicine, New Orleans, assisted with the electron microscopy. Dr. MARIA VARELA, Department of Anatomy, Tulane University School of Medicine, New Orleans, assisted with the cytogenetics. Mr. EDWARD BENES, Research Assistant of the Department of Surgery and presently in Department of Radiotherapy at the Charity Hospital of New Orleans, established the 3 lines of cells used in this study.

## References

1 BERGER, R.; LEJEUNE, J. et LACOURE, J.: Evolution chromosomique d'un melanome malin. Revue eur. Etud. clin. biol. *16:* 476–481 (1971).

2 BIRKMAYER, G. D.; BALADA, B. R., and MILLER, F.: Oncorna-viral information in human melanoma. Eur. J. Cancer *10:* 419–424 (1974).

3 BRUNNER, K. T.; MAUEL, J.; CEROTTINI, J. C., and CHAPUIS, B.: Quantitative assay of the lytic action of immune lymphoid cells on ⁵¹Cr-labelled allogeneic target cells *in vitro*; inhibition by isoantibody and by drugs. Immunology *14:* 181–196 (1968).

4 CHEN, T. R. and SHAW, M.: Stable chromosome changes in a human malignant melanoma. Cancer Res. *33:* 2042–2047 (1973).

5 CHERVONNAIA, L. V. and GLADUNOVA, Z. D.: Ploidy characteristics of malignant melanomas and nevi. Vop. Oncol. *18:* 9–11 (1972).

6 CLARK, W. H.: Four types of cellular fine structure associated with human amelanotic melanoma. Yale J. Biol. Med. *46:* 428 (1973).

7 DEVRIES, J.: Personal commun. (1974).

8 DEVRIES, J.; RÜMKE, P., and BERNHEIM, J. L.: Cytotoxic lymphocytes in melanoma patients. Int. J. Cancer *9:* 567–576 (1972).

9 GIBBONS, I. R. and GRIMSTONE, A. V.: On flagella structure in certain flagellates. J. biophys. biochem. Cytol. *7:* 697–710 (1960).

10 GOODWIN, D. P.; HORNUNG, M. O.; LEONG, S. P. L., and KREMENTZ, E. T.: Immune responses induced by human malignant melanoma in the rabbit. Surgery, St Louis *72:* 737–743 (1972).

11 HORNUNG, M. O. and KREMENTZ, E. T.: Specific tissue and tumor responses of chimpanzees following immunization against human melanoma. Surgery, St Louis *75:* 477–486 (1974).

12 KATAYAMA, K. P.; WOODRUFF, J. D.; JONES, H. W., and PRESTON, E.: Chromosomes of condyloma accuminatum, Paget's disease, *in situ* carcinoma, invasive squamous cell carcinoma and malignant melanoma of the human vulva. Obstet. Gynaecol. *39:* 348–350 (1972).

13 LEVY, N. L.; MAHALEY, M. S., and DAY, E. D.: *In vitro* demonstration of cell-mediated immunity to human brain tumors. Cancer Res. *32:* 477–482 (1972).

14 LEWIS, M. G.: Immunology and melanomas; in current topics in microbiology and immunology, vol. 63, pp. 49–84 (Springer, Berlin 1974).

15 MANSELL, P. W. A.; KREMENTZ, E. T., and DILUZIO, N. R.: Clinical experiences with immunotherapy of melanoma; in Behring Institute Research Communications – Immunological reactions to melanoma antigens (in press 1975).

16 PARSONS, P. G.; GOSS, P., and POPE, J. H.: Detection in human melanoma cell lines of particles with some properties in common with RNA tumour viruses. Int. J. Cancer *13:* 606–618 (1974).

17 PLUMEL, M.: Tampon au cacodylate de sodium. Bull. Soc. Chim. Biol. *30:* 129–130 (1948).

18 REYNOLDS, E. W.: The use of the lead citrate at high pH as an electron opaque stain in electron microscopy. J. Cell Biol. *17:* 208–212 (1963).

19  SANDBURG, A. A.; TAKAGI, N., and KATO, H.: Cytogenetic studies of normal and neoplastic cells *in vitro;* in The proliferation and spread of neoplastic cells, pp. 99–136 (Williams & Wilkins, Baltimore 1968).

20  SORENSEN, S. P. L.: in COLOWICK and KAPLAN Methods of enzymology, vol. 1, p. 143 (Academic Press, New York 1955).

21  TAKASUGI, M. and KLEIN, E.: A micro-assay for cell-mediated immunity. Transplantation *9:* 219–227 (1970).

22  TIJO, J. H. and LEVAN, A.: The chromosome number of man. Hereditas *42:* 1–6 (1956).

23  WHANG-PENG, J.; CHRETIEN, P., and KNUTSEN, T.: Polyploidy in malignant melanoma. Cancer *25:* 1216–1223 (1970).

ANNE KREMENTZ ZIMMERING, Tulane University School of Medicine, 1430 Tulane Avenue, *New Orleans, LA 70112* (USA)

Pigment Cell, vol. 2, pp. 94–107 (Karger, Basel 1976)

# Relation between Surface Structures and Cell Shape during the Cell Cycle of Mouse Melanoma Cells in a Monolayer Culture

J. Matsumoto and A. Oikawa

Department of Biology, Keio University, Yokohama-Hiyoshi, and Biochemistry Division, National Cancer Center Research Institute, Tokyo

*Introduction*

Vertebrate melanocytes are characterized with an asymmetric, extremely dendritic, broadly spreading shape. Cumulative knowledge of the development of these cells indicates that they originate in and migrate from the neural crest, and thereafter settle in a given area of the integument where differentiation of cell shape is completed [25].

Thus far, little is known regarding the problem of how pigment cells manipulate their shape during the course of the development. In the present study, an attempt has been made, using mouse melanoma cells in a monolayer culture, to determine the fundamental events relating to cell shape formation during the cell's cycle. We used these specimens primarily because of the ease in repeating a unit process, and also because of the assumption that the basic procedure utilized by these transformed cells could be extrapolated to normal melanocytes.

Recent progress in scanning electron microscopy has made it possible to survey the cell surface of cultured cells, yielding much important information on its role in cell shape formation [5, 7–9, 14, 18–21, 26]. Therefore, emphasis of this study has been on elucidation of the behavior of the surface structures occurring in association with changes in cell shape during the cell's cycle. In conjunction with these analyses, the possible participation of intracytoplasmic skeletons, such as microtubules and microfilaments, to these cell's shaping is also examined by transmission electron microscopy. The influence of cytochalasin B and colchicine, both of which are regarded as being specific disintegrating agents for cytoskeleton [2, 24], is also examined.

## Experimental Procedures

The cells from a clonal melanotic cell line ($C_2M$) of mouse melanoma B16 were cultured according to a monolayer technique, in Eagle's minimum essential medium supplemented with 10% calf serum and 50 $\mu$g/ml of Kanamycine [16, 17]. The cell suspension for experimental cultures was prepared by treating cells with 0.25% trypsin, washing them with the culture medium, and then adjusting the cell count (approx. $1 \times 10^5$ cell/ml). When 2 drops of the suspension were seeded at the center of a 35 mm Falcon plastic dish containing 2 ml of the culture medium, and then allowed to stand for 24 h at 30 °C in humidified air supplemented with 5% $CO_2$, a monolayer exhibiting a radial gradient of population density was obtained. For scanning electron microscopy, cells were grown on glass cover slips placed in Falcon dishes. The effect of cytochalasin B was examined at a concentration of 10 $\mu$g/ml, whereas that of colchicine was at a concentration of 1 mM or 1 $\mu$M.

Cells were fixed in 2.5% glutaraldehyde in 0.1 M sodium cacodylate buffer at pH 7.2 for 2 h at room temperature and then rinsed in the same buffer for several hours. Postfixation was carried out in 1% $OsO_4$ in 0.1 M sodium cacodylate buffer for 2 h in the cold. Subsequent dehydration was processed in a graded series of ethanol.

For scanning electron microscopy, specimens thus treated were rinsed twice in absolute amylacetate and then in liquid $CO_2$. They were dried in a critical point drying device by gradually raising the temperature of a chamber up to 45 °C [3, 19, 20]. Dried specimens were lightly coated with carbon and then gold. Observations were carried out using a JEOL-S 1 scanning electron microscope operated at 10 kV.

For transmission electron microscopy, specimens subjected to dehydration were embedded without passing propylene oxide into Epon 812 in Falcon dishes. Thin sections were made on a LKB ultramicrotome, stained doubly with uranyl acetate and lead citrate and then examined in a Hitachi HS-7 electron microscope operated at 50 kV.

The surface area of the cells were estimated on scanning electron micrographs using an Amsler's planimeter.

## Observations and Discussion

### Assembly of Surface Structures and Cytoskeletons in Cell Shape Formation in Interphase Cells

Interphase cells, numerically predominant in the nonsynchronous cultures, are specified with an irregularly polygonal, broadly spreading and flat shape (fig. 1).[1] Scanning electron microscopy indicated that most cells at this stage exhibit a smooth appearance and lack any surface activities

1     Figures 1–23 are scanning and transmission electron micrographs of cultured mouse melanoma cells. The procedure applied is given by the abbreviations S (scanning) or T (transmission) in parentheses following magnification.

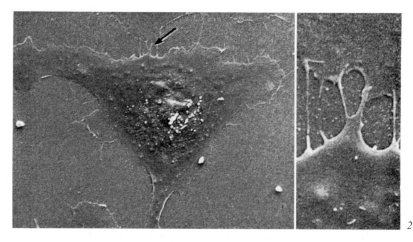

Fig. 1. An interphase cell. Note a smooth appearance of the cell surface and the presence of slender finger-like projections along its margins. × 1,350 (S).

Fig. 2. Magnified view of figure 1 (arrow). × 4,950 (S).

over their thin cell margins. The occurrence of bulbous excrescences or microvilli in these cells is limited to the perinuclear surface (fig. 1). Along their margins, large numbers of finger-like extensions were observed (fig. 2). Occasionally, a few cells in this stage show active ruffling along their peripheries which is an indication of locomotive activities [13].

Transmission electron microscopy indicates that a number of contact specializations are found along the cell's surface closely apposing neighboring cells or a substrate (fig. 3–6). In a section cut transversely through a substrate, these specializations occur more frequently in the marginal portions and possibly correspond to finger-like extensions or pointed corners, whereas they appear less frequently in the basal portions of the main cell body. Thus, it is likely that the slender finger-like extensions in the cell's periphery function as an apparatus for attachment. These attachment devices are specified with a localized accumulation of cytoplasmic filaments inside and along the plasma membrane, and accompany a plaque outside on the substrate apposing to them (fig. 3–6). These specializations, when formed between the surrounding cells, assume an image of junctional complex of zonula adherence type (fig. 4, 6). The presence of contact specialization of this kind has been found in cultured chicken retinal pigment epithelia [6, 15] and fibroblasts from varying sources [5, 8, 12, 18].

In close approximation to these contact specializations, several numbers of microtubules occur in a bundle form (fig. 4, 6). Even though numerous microtubules appear separately in random orientation within the cytoplasm, these microtubules are presumed to be arrayed specifically for cell adhesion. When interphase cells are detached by trypsin treatments, they assume an irregularly polygonal shape for a certain length of time and then gradually, not immediately as in other cells [7], round up.

In the thin cell margins of mouse melanoma cells, innumerable microfilaments, measuring 6–7 nm in thickness, are observed (fig. 7). Apparently, most of them are components of cytoplasmic cortex and some are involved in the formation or maintenance of knobby and microvilli-like surface configurations which have been observed in various types of cultured cells [1, 2, 14, 23, 25].

The interphase cells, when exposed to cytochalasin B for 3–8 h, exhibit a multidendritic satellite shape with a convoluted central cell body (fig. 8). This phenomenon usually has been observed in mesenchymal cells [14, 22, 26] and often is designated as arborization [22]. In these drug-exposed cells, the presence of internal skeletons stretching radially from the central portions is fairly clearly visualized (fig. 9). If the numbers of drug-induced arms are counted along their outermost periphery, they $(172 \pm 30)^2$ agree with the numbers of the finger-like extensions present along the cell margins of the normal interphase cells $(164 \pm 21)$. This indicates that the adhesivity of attachment devices remains unchanged under the treatment, notching cell margins firmly to the substrate. Within these artificially induced arms, microfilaments and microtubules run along the axis (fig. 11). Therefore, it appears that the connection of microtubules and attachment devices is superimposed upon the so-called arborization. An organization of this kind is reminiscent of the fundamental architectural assembly of normal pigment cells in general [4].

When the surface area of a normal interphase cell is expressed in terms of the spreading in a flat plane (approximately $36 \times 10^2 \ \mu m^2$) and when that of cytochalasin-treated cells is regarded as being composed of flat cell margins plus a hemisphere (approximately $20 \times 10^2 \mu m^2$), it is shown that the total cell surface is reduced by about half upon drug treatment. Although the idea that an elevation of cell body under cytochalasin treatment is brought about by the surfacial contraction has been set forth by MIRANDA et al. [14], this is clearly proven with the mouse melanoma cells.

2    Mean $\pm$ standard deviation. The number of cells examined was 9 for the control and 7 for experimental treatment both in the interphase and divisional phase.

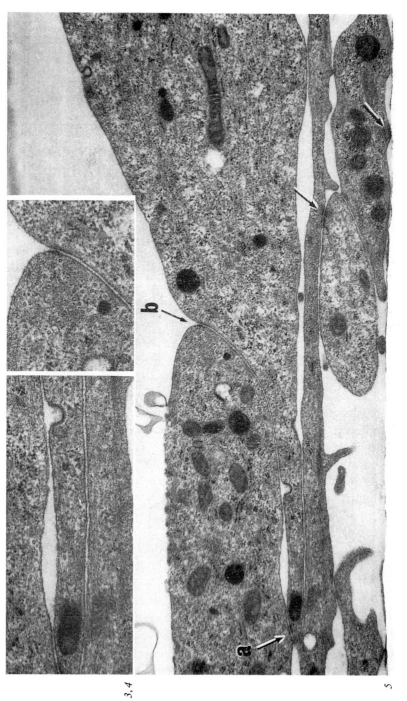

*Fig. 3.* A highly magnified transverse-sectional view of peripheral projections (fig. 5a). Note close approximation of microtubules to the tip of a finger-like extensions. × 30,000 (T).

*Fig. 4.* A highly magnified transverse-sectional view of contact specialization (fig. 5b). Note appearance of a cross-sectional profile of microtubules. × 30,000 (T).

*Fig. 5.* A transverse section of thin cell margins of the melanoma cells in a confluent phase. Note the occurrence of contact specialization (arrow) and their associated microtubules along the cell surface. The bottom of the picture is a Falcon plastic substrate (detached). × 6,500 (T).

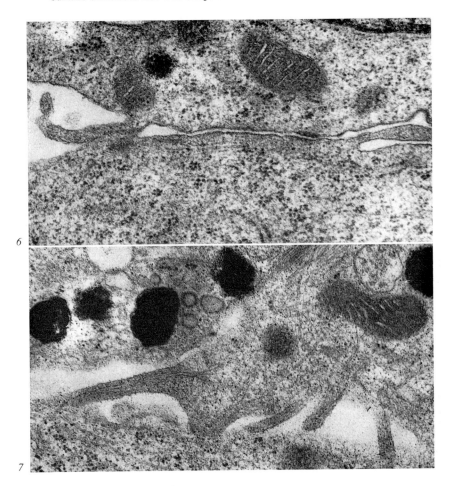

Fig. 6. An image of horizontally sectioned contact specialization (junctional complex) which is formed between the neighboring cells. Note a close approximation of microtubules in a form of bundle to it. × 30,000 (T).

Fig. 7. Horizontally sectioned cell periphery. The presence of microfilaments in cytoplasmic cortex is apparent. They appear to participate in the shaping or maintenance of surface structures. × 30,000 (T).

Colchicine treatment causes few changes in the morphology of the surface structures and cell shape, except for a certain degree of loss in surface tenacity. Since microtubules in these treated cells occur in a form of short fragments, it appears that the function of microtubules in the maintenance of cell shape is additional and possibly covered by the lining of cortical microfilaments.

From these observations, an assumption is drawn for the possible sequence of events regarding cell shaping in interphase cells: When a cell settles on the substrate, contact specializations are organized along the tips of the spreading thin cell margins. With slight retraction of plasma membrane, finger-like projections appear from the contact specializations involving their associated microtubules. An alignment of contact specializations and microtubules provides fulcra and supporting skeletons for the formation of an irregularly polygonal shape. In the meanwhile, cortical microfilaments serving with a moderate degree of tension to cell surface would keep the cell surface smooth.

### Changes in Surface Structures in a Course of Rounding of Mitotic Cells

The cells in stages of mitosis are characterized by a spherical shape at late prophase to metaphase, or varying transposal forms to and from it. With the onset of rounding, the cells begin to retract their thin cell margins (fig. 12–15). Simultaneously, innumerable filopodia appear from the positions where the cell margins are located, and a large number of microvilli and blebs come to occupy the free surface (fig. 12). When the cell establishes a spherical shape, a radially stretching framework of filopodia (approximately 100 nm in the tip and 250 nm near the cell body in width) firmly anchors its cell body to the substrate (fig. 16, 17). The occurrence of filopodial attachment in spherically shaped mitotic fibroblasts and others has been reported by several investigators [5, 7–10], but little is avail-

---

*Fig. 8.* An interphase cell exposed to cytochalasin B for 8 h. Typical arborization is observed. × 1,350 (S).

*Fig. 9.* Magnified view of figure 8. × 4,050 (S).

*Fig. 10.* The cell at stages of mitosis in a cytochalasin B-containing medium. The surface structures abundant in the normally mitotic cell almost completely disappear. Note an irregularly deformed cell shape. × 4,050 (S).

*Fig. 11.* A transverse section of arms of a cytochalasin B-exposed cell. Note the presence of microtubules and fragmentary microfilaments within them. × 30,000 (T).

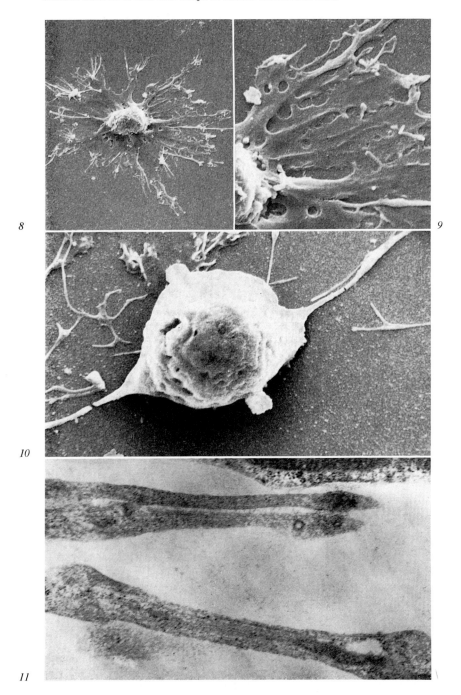

able so far regarding its formative processes as resolved under scanning microscopy.

The dimension of spreading of these filopodia ($16.4 \pm 3.8 \times 10^2$ $\mu m^2$) is found to coincide with that of the normal interphase cell ($18.0 \pm 2.4 \times 10^2$ $\mu m^2$). The number of filopodia in the furthermost tip ($145 \pm 35$) also agrees with that of marginal finger-like projections installed in the interphase cells ($164 \pm 21$). This indicates that the attachment devices present at the onset of mitosis are left in their original positions providing a starting site for filopodia formation.

During late prophase to metaphase, the exposed surface of the spherical cell body is completely covered with innumerable blebs of varying size (fig. 17). At these stages, microvilli are relatively less in number. When the surface area of a spherical cell body is determined on the basis of its average diameter (approximately $3.3 \times 10^2$ $\mu m^2$), it is apparent that total area reduction during rounding ranges from 1/8 to 1/10, as compared to the interphase cell. It is probable that most of these area reductions are adsorbed in the formation of microvilli and blebs, not in the formation of pleats or foldings, although an accurate calculation remains to be done. A recent study has indicated that membrane contents double during interphase [11]. If the estimates of surface area given herein represent an average value in the middle of interphase, the surface reduction must be larger than the above-mentioned one.

It is also noted that morphological changes occurring in cell margins during a course of rounding are similar, as seen in the scanning microscope, to those of cytochalasine-exposed cells (fig. 9, 12). This implies that the regression of cell margins is effected by surface contraction.

Observations on sections of mitotic cells indicate that microtubules, irrespective of their predominant occurrence near chromosomes, are scarcely observable inside the filopodia. The finding that filopodia are al-

---

Fig. 12. A cell at an earlier stage of rounding. Note appearance of numerous filopodia in the periphery and of microvilli and blebs over its exposed surface. $\times$ 1,350 (S).

Fig. 13. Magnified view of figure 12 (arrow). $\times$ 4,950 (S).

Fig. 14. A cell at an advanced stage of rounding. $\times$ 1,350 (S).

Fig. 15. Magnified view of figure 14. Filopodia are stepwise bound to thicker bundles with retraction of cell margins. $\times$ 3,480 (S).

Fig. 16. The cell that establishes a spherical shape (possibly in prophase to metaphase). $\times$ 1,350 (S).

Fig. 17. Magnified view of figure 16. Note the presence of innumerable blebs over the cell body and of a radially stretching system of filopodia. $\times$ 4,500 (S).

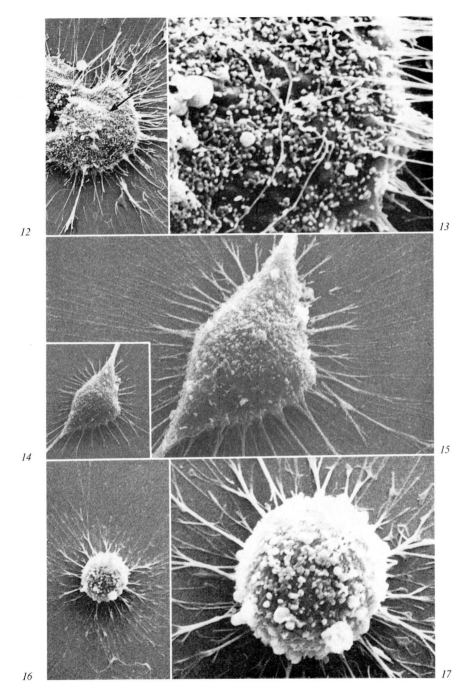

most completely destroyed upon exposure to cytochalasin B, whereas they remain unchanged under colchicine treatment, may also substantiate an absence of microtubule involvement.

The cells undergoing mitosis in the presence of cytochalasin B are devoid of any surface structures, exhibiting an irregularly distorted globular shape (fig. 10). If cytochalasin B modifies the integrity of cortical microfilaments, as proposed by several investigators [2, 14, 22, 23, 26], it appears reasonable to consider that microfilaments play an important role in the formation of surface structures as well as the maintenance of a regular spherical shape of the cell body. It appears that the increased contractility of cytoplasmic cortex is essential for regular spherical shaping.

Following cytokinesis (fig. 18, 19), daughter cells start to spread (fig. 20–23). While the cell body flattens, the surface structures gradually disappear. The relationship between surface structures and cell shape observed herein is essentially the same in surface behaviors, but opposite in sequence, to that occurring in a course of rounding. During a phase following cytokinesis, the cell seems to take a widely spreading shape, the surface of which is still covered with a certain number of microvilli.

## Summary

The changes in surface structures, cytoplasmic skeleton assembly and cell shape during cell cycle in a monolayer culture of the B16 mouse melanoma were examined by means of combined scanning and transmission electron microscopy. The interphase cell displays a smooth-surface, irregularly polygonal, widely spreading, flat shape which is attributed by peripheral attachment devices, their associated microtubules, and cortical microfilaments in a relaxed state.

With the onset of mitosis, the cell begins to round up, pulling in its thin margins and forming innumerable excrescences such as microvilli and blebs in the exposed surface. Since these changes accompany remarkable area diminution in total cell surface, and since microfilaments engage in the formation or maintenance of surface configurations, it is probable that the development of microvilli and blebs in a course of rounding not only provides a storage site for the plasma membrane, but

---

*Fig. 18.* A cell undergoing cytokinesis. × 1,350 (S).

*Fig. 19.* Magnified view of figure 18. × 3,510 (S).

*Fig. 20.* Two sister cells at the end of cytokinesis. × 1,350 (S).

*Fig. 21.* Magnified view of figure 20. They represent a surfacial image similar to figure 13. × 4,950 (S).

*Fig. 22.* The cells spreading over a substrate after cytokinesis. × 1,350 (S).

*Fig. 23.* Magnified view of figure 22. × 3,000 (S).

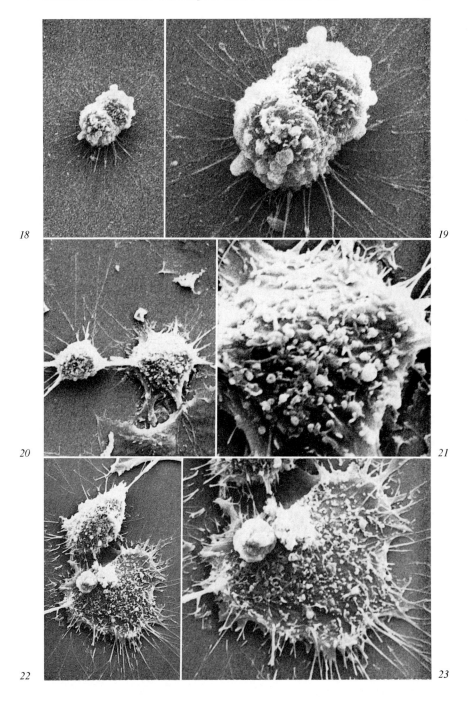

also reflects an increased activity of cortical microfilaments. The spreading of sister cells after cytokinesis follows processes which are opposite in sequence, but essentially the same in the relationship between surface structures and cell shape. The possible role of surface structures in cell shaping of mouse melanoma cells is discussed.

## Acknowledgments

The authors are very grateful to Mrs. YOSHIKO HORIKAWA and MICHIE NAKAYASU for their collaboration in the present study. They would also like to thank Mr. TATSUJI FUJIWARA for his technical advice in scanning electron microscopy. This work was supported by grants from Keio University and from the Ministry of Education (901006, 901026).

## References

1   ABERCROMBIE, M.; HEAYSMAN, J. E. M., and PEGRUM, S. M.: The locomotion of fibroblasts in culture. IV. Electron microscopy of the leading lamella. Expl Cell Res. *67:* 359–367 (1971).

2   ALLISON, A. C.: The role of microfilaments and microtubules in cell movement, endocytosis and exocytosis. Locomotion of tissue cells. Ciba Found. Symp., vol. 14, pp. 109–143 (Elsevier, Amsterdam 1973).

3   ANDERSON, T. F.: Technique for the preservation of three-dimensional structure in preparing specimens for the electron microscope. Trans. N.Y. Acad. Sci. Ser. II *13:* 130 (1951).

4   BIKLE, D.; TILNEY, L. G., and PORTER, K. R.: Microtubules and pigment migration in the melanophores of *Fundulus heteroclitus.* Protoplasma *61:* 322–345 (1966).

5   BOYDE, A.; WEISS, R. A., and VESELY, P.: Scanning electron microscopy of cells in culture. Expl Cell Res. *71:* 313–324 (1972).

6   CRAWFORD, B.; CLONEY, R. A., and CAHN, R. D.: Cloned pigmented retinal cells. The effects of cytochalasin B on ultrastructure and behaviour. Z. Zellforsch. mikrosk. Anat. *130:* 135–151 (1972).

7   DALEN, H. and TODD, P.: Surface morphology of trypsinized human cells *in vitro.* Expl Cell Res. *66:* 353–361 (1971).

8   DALEN, H. and SCHEIE, P.: Two types of long microextensions from cultivated liver cells. Expl Cell Res. *53:* 670–674 (1969).

9   EVERHART, L. P., jr. and RUBIN, R. W.: Cyclic changes in the cell surface. II. The effect of cytochalasin B on the surface morphology of synchronized Chinese hamster ovary cells. J. Cell Biol. *60:* 442–447 (1974).

10  GEY, G. O.: Some aspects of the constitution and behavior of normal and malignant cells maintained in continuous culture. The Harvey lecture (Academic Press, New York 1956).

11  GRAHAM, J. M.; SUMNER, M. C. B.; CURTIS, D. H., and PASTERNAK, C. A.: Sequence of events in plasma membrane assembly during the cell cycle. Nature, Lond. *246:* 291–295 (1973).

12 HARRIS, A.: Location of cellular adhesions to solid substrata. Devl Biol. *35:* 97–114 (1973).

13 HARRIS, A. K.: Cell surface movements related to cell locomotion. Locomotion of tissue cells. Ciba Found. Symp., vol. 14, pp. 3–20 (Elsevier, Amsterdam 1973).

14 MIRANDA, A. F.; GODMAN, G. C.; DEITCH, A. D., and TANENBAUM, S. W.: Action of cytochalasin D on cells of established lines. J. Cell Biol. *61:* 481–500 (1974).

15 NEWSOME, D. A.; FLETCHER, R. T.; ROBISON, W. G., jr.; KENYON, K. R., and CHADER, G. J.: Effects of cyclic AMP and Sephadex fractions of chick embryo extract on cloned retinal pigmented epithelium in tissue culture. J. Cell Biol. *61:* 369–382 (1974).

16 OIKAWA, A.; NAKAYASU, M.; CLAUNCH, C., and TCHEN, T. T.: Two types of melanogenesis in monolayer cultures of melanoma cells. Cell Different. *1:* 149–155 (1972).

17 OIKAWA, A.; NAKAYASU, M., and NOHARA, M.: Tyrosinase activities of cell-free extracts and living cells of cultured melanoma cells. Devl Biol. *30:* 198–205 (1973).

18 PORTER, K. R.; FONTE, V., and WEISS, G.: A scanning microscope study of the topography of HeLa cells. Cancer Res. *34:* 1385–1394 (1974).

19 PORTER, K. R.; KELLEY, D., and ANDREWS, P. M.: The preparation of cultured cells and soft tissues for scanning electron microscopy. Scanning electron microscopy (IIT Research Institute, Chicago 1972).

20 PORTER, K. R.; PRESCOTT, D., and FRYE, J.: Changes in surface morphology of Chinese hamster overy cells during the cell cycle. J. Cell Biol. *57:* 815–836 (1973).

21 RUBIN, R. W. and EVERHART, L. P.: The effect of cell-to-cell contact on the surface morphology of Chinese hamster ovary cells. J. Cell Biol. *57:* 837–844 (1973).

22 SANGER, J. W. and HOLTZER, H.: Cytochalasin B. Effects on cell morphology, cell adhesion, and mucopolysaccharide synthesis. Proc. natn. Acad. Sci. USA *69:* 253–257 (1972).

23 WESSELLS, N. K.; SPOONER, B. S., and LUDUENA, M. A.: Surface movements, microfilaments and cell locomotion. Locomotion of tissue cells. Ciba Found. Symp., vol. 14, pp. 53–82 (Elsevier, Amsterdam 1973).

24 WESSELLS, N. K.; SPOONER, B. S.; ASH, J. F.; BRADLEY, M. O.; LUDUENA, M. A.; TAYLOR, E. L.; WRENN, J. T., and YAMADA, K. M.: Microfilaments in cellular and developmental processes. Science, N. Y. *171:* 135–143 (1971).

25 WESTON, J. A.: The migration and differentiation of neural crest cells. Adv. Morphogenesis, vol. 8, pp. 41–114 (Academic Press, New York 1970).

26 UKENA, T. E.; BORYSENKO, J. Z.; KARNOVSKY, M. J., and BERLIN, R. D.: Effects of colchicine, cytochalasin B, and 2-deoxyglucose on the topographical organization of surface-bound concanavalin A in normal and transformed fibroblasts. J. Cell Biol. *61:* 70–82 (1974).

Dr. J. MATSUMOTO, Department of Biology, Keio University, Hiyoshi, Kohoku-ku, *Yokohama 223* (Japan)

Pigment Cell, vol. 2, pp. 108–115 (Karger, Basel 1976)

# Selective Lethal Effect of Substituted Phenols on Cell Cultures of Malignant Melanocytes[1]

STANLEY S. BLEEHEN

Hallamshire Hospital and University of Sheffield, Sheffield

Previous studies have shown that a number of substituted phenols have a selective lethal effect on mammalian melanocytes both *in vivo* [1, 3–5] and *in vitro* [6]. Of the compounds tested, 4-isopropylcatechol (4-IPC) and 4-hydroxyanisole (4-OHA) were found to be very potent in their melanocytotoxic effect. Both these compounds also have a toxic effect on melanomas. 4-IPC, when injected intraperitoneally into mice bearing the Harding-Passey melanoma, significantly prolonged mean survival time of the animals when compared with similar saline-injected controls [2]. WHITEHEAD and LITTLE [7] found that *p*-methoxyphenol was toxic when tested against two cell lines of human malignant melanoma.

The purpose of this paper is to report that both 4-IPC and 4-OHA have a lethal effect on Harding-Passey, B16, and human melanoma cells grown in tissue culture. Melanoma cells that are pigmented appear to be more susceptible to damage even after short exposures to very low concentrations of these compounds.

## Materials and Methods

The Harding-Passey and B16 melanomas have, over several years, been serially transplanted into C57 BL mice. Both of these melanomas were very black. Cell suspensions were prepared by the mechanical disaggregation of portions of the tumors which, after washing with Hanks BSS, were then seeded into Falcon flasks and also into Petri dishes. The cells were cultured in 199 medium supplemented with 10–20% fetal bovine serum, to which was also added penicillin 100 IU/ml and streptomycin 100 $\mu$g/ml. Primary cell cultures of these melanomas, between 5 and 21 days, were

1 This investigation was supported by grants from the Medical Research Council and the Endowment Fund of the United Sheffield Hospitals.

used for all experiments. Cell lines derived from two primary human malignant melanomas (1 nodular melanoma and 1 superficial spreading melanoma) were also
used. Both these primary cell lines were pigmented.

The effects of 4-IPC and 4-OHA on these monolayer cell cultures were studied
using phase microscopy and the changes observed directly and by means of time-
lapse photography. The cultures were exposed for varying lengths of time to varying concentrations of either 4-IPC or 4-OHA and the changes compared with control cultures. Mouse and human fibroblast cultures were also exposed to these compounds. After treatment with these compounds, a number of cultures were fixed using 3% gluteraldehyde. The monolayers of melanoma cells were embedded in epon
*in situ,* and ultrathin sections of selected colonies of cells were cut and stained and
these were viewed using transmission electron microscopy. Cells were also grown on
glass cover slips in Petri dishes and, after treatment with either 4-IPC or 4-OHA,
were fixed with gluteraldehyde and then coated for scanning electron microscopy.

### *Results*

### Light Microscopy

4-IPC and 4-OHA were found to be extremely toxic to primary cultures of Harding-Passey melanoma cells (table I). Both compounds were
toxic to B16 melanoma cells (table II) and to two pigmented cell lines derived from primary cutaneous human malignant melanomas (table III).

Marked damage to Harding-Passey, B16, and human melanoma cells
was observed within 30 min of exposure to these compounds when used
in a final concentration of $10^{-3}$ M. However, these compounds had no effect in this concentration on mouse and human fibroblast cultures. Even
at a concentration of $10^{-5}$ M, both 4-IPC and 4-OHA had a marked lethal
effect on Harding-Passey and B16 melanoma cells, especially on those
cells that were pigmented.

The sequence of events as observed by phase microscopy, directly
and by means of time-lapse photographs was as follows. Shortly after
these melanocytotoxic compounds were added to the nutrient medium,
bulges appeared on the cytoplasmic surface of the melanoma cells (fig. 1).
When 4-IPC or 4-OHA were used in a concentration of $10^{-3}$ M, these
changes occurred within 5 min. Later beading and breaks of the dendrites
occurred which frequently lost their attachments to the wall of the culture
vessel (fig. 2). Vacuoles appeared in the cytoplasm of the cell and the melanin granules tended to form clumps around a nucleus that later became
pyknotic. Some cells developed breaks of their outer limiting membrane
and extruded cytoplasmic contents into the nutrient medium.

*Table I.* Effect of 4-IPC and 4-OHA on Harding-Passey melanoma cells

| Compound | Concentration, M | Time of exposure | Damage to cells |
|---|---|---|---|
| 4-IPC | $1 \times 10^{-3}$ | 30 min | + + + |
| 4-OHA | $1 \times 10^{-3}$ | 30 min | + + + |
| 4-OHA | $1 \times 10^{-4}$ | 30 min | + + |
| 4-IPC | $1 \times 10^{-5}$ | 30 min | + |
| 4-IPC | $1 \times 10^{-5}$ | 60 min | + + |
| 4-OHA | $1 \times 10^{-5}$ | 60 min | + + |
| 4-OHA | $1 \times 10^{-6}$ | 60 min | + |
| 4-IPC | $1 \times 10^{-7}$ | 4 h | + |
| 4-IPC | $1 \times 10^{-7}$ | 12 h | + |
| 4-IPC | $1 \times 10^{-8}$ | 24 h | + |

*Table II.* Effect of 4-IPC and 4-OHA on B16 melanoma cells

| Compound | Concentration, M | Time of exposure, min | Damage to cells |
|---|---|---|---|
| 4-IPC | $1 \times 10^{-3}$ | 30 | + + |
| 4-OHA | $1 \times 10^{-3}$ | 30 | + + |
| 4-IPC | $1 \times 10^{-4}$ | 30 | + |
| 4-IPC | $1 \times 10^{-5}$ | 60 | + |
| 4-OHA | $1 \times 10^{-5}$ | 60 | + |

*Table III.* Effect of 4-IPC and 4-OHA on primary human melanoma cells

| Type of melanoma | Compound | Concentration, M | Time of exposure, min | Damage to cells |
|---|---|---|---|---|
| Superficial spreading melanoma | 4-IPC | $1 \times 10^{-3}$ | 30 | + + |
|  | 4-OHA | $1 \times 10^{-3}$ | 30 | + + |
| Nodular melanoma | 4-IPC | $1 \times 10^{-3}$ | 30 | + + |
|  | 4-IPC | $1 \times 10^{-4}$ | 30 | + |
|  | 4-IPC | $1 \times 10^{-5}$ | 60 | + |

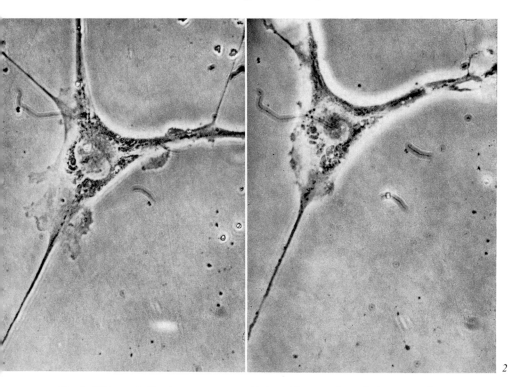

*Fig. 1.* Effect of 10-min exposure to $10^{-4}$ M 4-isopropylcatechol on Harding-Passey melanoma cell. Phase contrast. $\times$ 530.

*Fig. 2.* Same cell after 60-min exposure showing disruption of cytoplasm and nucleus and the loss of dendrites and their attachments. Phase contrast. $\times$ 530.

## Transmission Electron Microscopy

With concentrations of 4-IPC or 4-OHA in the range $10^{-3}$ to $10^{-5}$ M, many melanoma cells showed, after an exposure of 30 min or less, a considerable disruption of their subcellular architecture. The changes were most marked at the periphery of the cell near the outer limiting membrane, which showed frequent breaks in its continuity. Many vacuoles were to be found within the cytoplasm, most of them bounded by an ill-defined unit membrane. The outer limiting membrane of melanosomes and melanosomal complexes were often disrupted, as were those of other cytoplasmic organelles (fig. 3). Abnormal melanosomes were frequently found in the 4-IPC- and 4-OHA-treated melanoma cells, these being membrane-bounded electron-dense, rounded or elongated bodies with a finely granular internal matrix. Lamellated bodies with coiled filiaments were also present (fig. 4).

Longer exposures to 4-IPC or 4-OHA produced more disruption of the cytoplasm and nucleus of the melanoma cells. Cells with few melanosomal structures were only slightly damaged, and cultures of fibroblasts were unaffected by these compounds.

### Scanning Electron Microscopy

Striking cell surface changes were observed in cultures of melanoma cells exposed to these compounds. The cells showed a loss of dendrites and microvilli, and the surface had a jagged and tattered appearance (fig. 5, 6) and cellular debris was scattered around the cells.

### Comment

A dose-dependant cytotoxic effect by two substituted phenols, 4-IPC and 4-OHA, has been observed on pigmented melanoma cell lines. Both of these compounds produce considerable disruption and lytic changes of the membranes and organelles of functional malignant melanocytes. Previous studies [1, 5, 6] have indicated that the probable mode of action of these melanocytotoxic compounds is that they act as substrates for tyrosinase and are oxidized to form toxic free radicals which initiate lipid peroxidation, and that this chain reaction results in destroying the membraneous organelles of the cell. Cytolytic changes similar to that observed in this study have been reported by RILEY [6] on guinea pig melanocytes treated *in vitro* with 4-OHA and other substituted phenols. More recently, ultrastructural studies to determine the mechanism of depigmentation by hydroquinone [4] have shown that this compound produces a preferential disorganization of functional guinea pig melanocytes when applied topically or injected subcutaneously. Melanocyte necrosis appeared to be initiated by the disruption and degradation of membraneous organelles.

Though melanoma cells that were only lightly pigmented were relatively unaffected by either 4-IPC or 4-OHA, these compounds could be

---

*Fig. 3.* Electron micrograph of portion of Harding-Passey cell exposed for 15 min to $10^{-4}$ M 4-OHA showing damage to outer membranes of melanosomes. $\times$ 19,000.

*Fig. 4.* Electron micrograph of portions of B16 melanoma cells exposed for 45 min to $10^{-4}$ M 4-IPC, showing considerable disruption of their subcellular architecture. $\times$ 29,000.

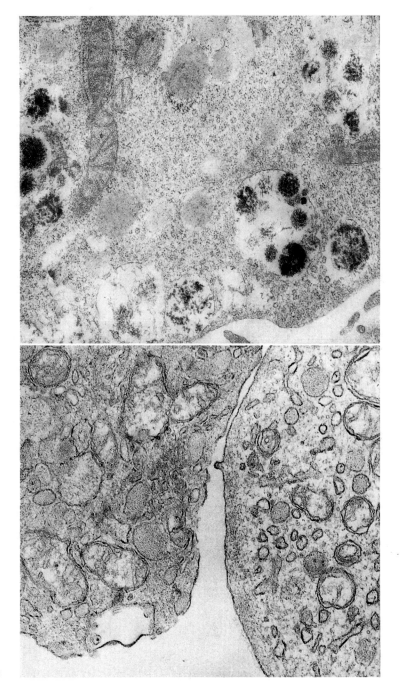

3

4

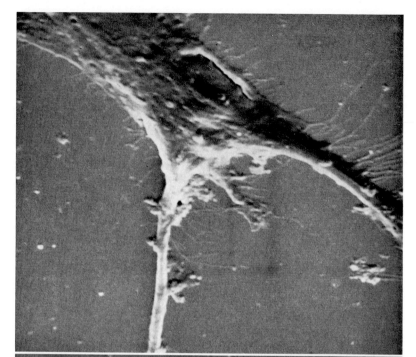

5

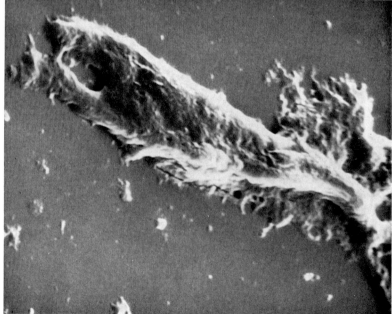

6

*Fig. 5.* Scanning electron micrograph of Harding-Passey melanoma cell showing normal appearance. $\times$ 1,600.

*Fig. 6.* Scanning electron micrograph of Harding-Passey melanoma cell after exposure to $10^{-3}$ M 4-IPC for 60 min. $\times$ 1,600.

of use in the therapy of human malignant melanomas that have tyroxinase activity and are pigmented. Further studies are required to determine whether these substituted phenols could be administered for the specific chemotherapy of melanoma in man.

## Summary

In this study, the effects of 4-isopropylcatechol (4-IPC) and 4-hydroxyanisole (4-OHA) have been observed on primary cultures of Harding-Passey and B16 mouse melanomas and cultures of two primary human cutaneous melanomas. Both 4-IPC and 4-OHA in concentrations of $10^{-3}$ M were very toxic to melanoma cells, especially those that were more pigmented. These substituted phenols were found to have a selective lethal effect on functional melanocytes producing considerable disruption of their subcellular architecture, even after short exposures to low concentrations of the compounds.

## References

1   BLEEHEN, S. S.; PATHAK, M. A.; HORI, Y., and FITZPATRICK, T. B.: Depigmentation of the skin with 4-isopropylcatechol, mercaptoamines and other compounds. J. invest. Derm. *50:* 103–117 (1968).

2   BLEEHEN, S. S.: The effect of 4-isopropylcatechol on the Harding-Passey melanoma. Pigment Cell, vol. 1, pp. 202–207 (Karger, Basel 1973).

3   FRENK, E. and OTT, F.: Evaluation of the toxicity of the mono-ethyl ether of hydroquinone for mammalian melanocytes and melanoma cells. J. invest. Derm. *56:* 287–293 (1971).

4   JIMBOW, K.; OBATA, H.; PATHAK, M. A., and FITZPATRICK, T. B.: Mechanism of depigmentation by hydroquinone. J. invest. Derm. *62:* 436–449 (1974).

5   RILEY, P. A.: Hydroxyanisole depigmentation. *In vivo* studies. J. Path. *97:* 185–191 (1969).

6   RILEY, P. A.: Mechanism of pigment-cell toxicity produced by hydroxyanisole. J. Path. *101:* 163–169 (1970).

7   WHITEHEAD, R. H. and LITTLE, J. H.: Tissue culture studies on human malignant melanoma. Pigment Cell, vol. 1, pp. 382–389 (Karger, Basel 1973).

Dr. S. S. BLEEHEN, Rupert Hallam Department of Dermatology, Hallamshire Hospital, *Sheffield S10 2JF* (England)

Pigment Cell, vol. 2, pp. 116–123 (Karger, Basel 1976)

# Suppression of Melanoma Cell Tyrosinase Activity after Incorporation of 5-Bromodeoxyuridine during One Round of DNA Synthesis

J. R. Wrathall and S. Silagi

Cell Genetics Laboratory, Department of Obstetrics and Gynecology, Cornell University Medical College, New York, N. Y.

*Introduction*

Culture of a variety of cell types with low concentrations of 5-bromo-deoxyuridine (BrdU) results in the suppression of cell-specific functions without significant disturbance of maintenance functions required for continued cell division (for review, see RUTTER *et al.* [5]. Such preferential suppression of differentiated functions by BrdU are generally reversible upon culture of BrdU-grown cells in medium devoid of the drug. Incorporation of BrdU into DNA as an analog of thymine is generally requisite for such suppression, but the exact molecular basis of these effects is still unknown. Nevertheless, BrdU provides a tool with which the expression of many cell-specific functions may be experimentally manipulated and therefore studied more closely.

The production of melanin by either embryonic melanocytes [2, 6, 11] or melanoma cells [6] is suppressed by growth in the presence of BrdU. We have reported [8] that culture of highly pigmented melanoma cells (clone $B_559$, derived from the B16 mouse melanoma) with BrdU (3 $\mu$g/ml, $10^{-5}$ M) for 7 days results in virtually amelanotic cells in which no evidence of premelanosome formation is seen and in which tyrosinase activity is usually undetectable. The suppression of pigmentation in these cells may be prevented by inclusion of equimolar or greater concentrations of thymidine in the medium along with the BrdU, or by preventing DNA synthesis during exposure to BrdU [6]. The suppression is reversible and pigmented cells reappear after growth of BrdU-treated cells in medium without the drug.

Recently, KRIEDER *et al.* [3] reported that a significant suppression of melanin production resulted from exposure of synchronized B16 melanoma cells to BrdU ($10^{-5}$ M) for a single DNA synthetic period. In the clone of B16 cells studied by these workers, melanogenesis is initiated after cultures have reached confluency. In our clone ($B_5 59$), melanin is produced continuously throughout the culture cycle. It was therefore of interest to determine whether melanogenesis would be significantly suppressed by exposure of $B_5 59$ cells to BrdU during a period consistent with incorporation of the drug during one synthetic cycle and to compare the degree of suppression after one or two such periods to that seen after 7 days of continuous culture with BrdU.

*Results*

Control $B_5 59$ cells (fig. 1C) grow in a piled reticulated manner. Virtually every cell is pigmented and melanin is dispersed through the cells and their cytoplasmic processes. After 3 days culture with BrdU (fig. 1A), some disassociation of cell piles and indications of cell flattening were seen. In addition, a striking alteration in the distribution of melanin was observed. Granules were concentrated in a juxtanuclear position and cytoplasmic processes were largely free of pigment. By 7 days (fig. 1B), most cells were unpigmented though some retained an indication of melanin near the nucleus. The cells were flattened, and the piled growth pattern of control cells was no longer evident. In cells exposed to BrdU for only 30 h, then grown in BrdU-free medium (fig. 1D and E), the morphological effects were similar in timing and extent to those resulting from 7 days of continuous growth with BrdU. Seven days after the BrdU 'pulse', the cells were largely amelanotic, but subsequently reversal began and pigmented cells reappeared (fig. 1F).

The suppression of melanogenesis can be quantitated by assaying cell homogenates for tyrosinase activity as previously described [8]. In figure 2, the time course of decrease in tyrosinase activity resulting from continuous growth with BrdU is compared to that resulting from exposure to BrdU for 24, 30, or 48 h then grown in medium without the drug. The kinetics of decrease were very similar, and tyrosinase activity approached levels undetectable by our assay after about one week, whether the cells had grown in BrdU for the entire period or for as little as 24 h. The experiment in which cells were 'pulsed' for 30 h (photographs of these cells are shown in fig. 1D, E, and F) was extended to document the return of tyrosinase activity in cultures during reversal of the BrdU effects. These cultures had no detectable tyrosinase activity 7 days after BrdU treatment, but by day 10 some activity was discernable, and by day 17 cultures had more than 50% of the activity of control cultures that had never been exposed to BrdU.

In all these experiments, cell cultures were set up 1–2 days prior to the addition of BrdU, so that cultures would be in logarithmic phase during exposure to BrdU. Under these conditions, cell counts showed the population doubled in number during the first 24 h with BrdU and doubled again between 24 and 48 h. When tritiated BrdU (BrdU-6-$^3$H, New England Nuclear, final activity 0.3 $\mu$Ci/ml) was included in the medium, autoradiography indicated that over 85% of the cells incorporated BrdU into their nuclei during the period 0–24 h or 24–48 h. Thus, for the population as a whole, growth with BrdU for 24 or 48 h appeared to represent incorporation during one or two rounds of DNA synthesis, respectively. This has been confirmed by preliminary results from Dr. MARY HAMILTON who has performed buoyant density analysis on purified DNA from cells grown with BrdU. More than 80% of the DNA from cells exposed to BrdU for 24 h had a density shift consistent with bromouracil substitution in one strand of the DNA. No 'heavy-heavy' peak of DNA was detected. In this experiment, tyrosinase activity reached undetectable levels after cultures exposed to BrdU for 24 h were grown in medium without the drug for 6 additional days (fig. 2).

The extent of bromouracil (BU) substitution for thymine (T) in these BrdU-treated cells was determined by the X-ray fluorescence method of ZEITZ and LEE [10] in which the ratio of bromine to phosphorus atoms is measured. DNA for analysis was purified by a modification of the MARMUR [4] procedure designed to minimize RNA contamination. Calculation of mole percent BU substitution for T was made on the basis of a T con-

---

*Fig. 1.* Photographs of living B$_5$59 melanoma cells. *A, B* Cells grown continuously with BrdU (3 $\mu$g/ml). *A* At 3 days melanin granules are concentrated near the nuclei. $\times$ 207. *B* At 7 days cells are flattened and little pigment remains. $\times$ 207. *C* Control cells growing in medium without BrdU grow in a piled manner and pigment is dispersed throughout the cytoplasm. $\times$ 127. *D–F* Cells 'pulsed' for 30 h with BrdU (3 $\mu$g/ml) then grown in medium without the drug. *D, E* 2 and 7 days after the 'pulse', the cells resemble those grown continuously with BrdU for 3 or 7 days, respectively. $\times$ 207. *F* 17 days after the BrdU 'pulse' many of the cells are again pigmented. $\times$ 127.

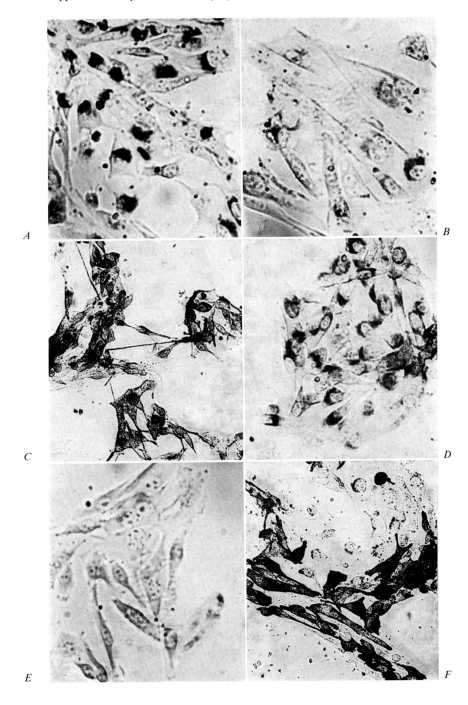

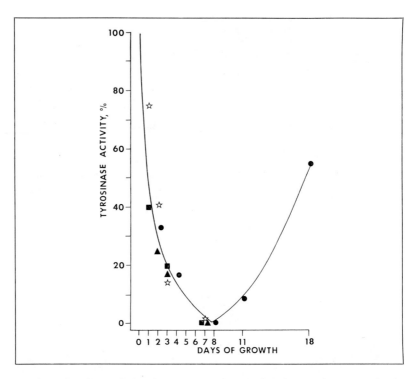

*Fig. 2.* Comparison of the time course of reduction in tyrosinase activity in cultures grown continuously with BrdU (3 μg/ml) for 7 days (☆), to that when cultures were exposed to BrdU for 24 h (■), 30 h (●), or 48 h (▲), then changed to medium without the drug. Tyrosinase activity is expressed as a percent of the specific activity of replicate control cultures in each experiment. The values for 7 days continuous culture with BrdU (☆) represent the average from 10 experiments as reported previously [8].

tent of 28.4 mol% in DNA from untreated $B_5$59 cells, as estimated by buoyant density analysis in neutral CsCl. Overall BU substitution was found to be about 23% after 24 h and almost 40% after 48 h exposure to BrdU. In cells grown for 24 h with BrdU this corresponds to at least 46% substitution in newly synthesized strands. During subsequent growth of BrdU-treated cultures in BrdU-free medium, the overall BU substitution decreased at a rate consistent with conservation of BU-substituted strands, but the dilution of this DNA by strands synthesized in the absence of BrdU.

## Discussion

These results demonstrate that the control of tyrosinase activity and pigmentation in these melanoma cells is highly sensitive to BrdU. Complete suppression of detectable tyrosinase activity can result from a 24-hour period of exposure to BrdU which allows incorporation during a single DNA synthetic period, and thus only single strand substitution. In additional experiments to be reported elsewhere [9], variability in the degree of suppression of tyrosinase activity has been seen, including one experiment in which cells treated with BrdU for 24 h retained 57% tyrosinase activity on day 7 of the experiment. Except for this puzzling instance, all our experiments have shown that tyrosinase activity is decreased by significantly more than 50% after incorporation of BrdU for 24 h, i.e. during one DNA synthetic period. Thus, BU substitution in one, and either, strand of the DNA duplex appears to be sufficient for suppression of tyrosinase activity. Such 'unifilar dominance' [5] has also been found in the suppression by BrdU of myoblast fusion [1] and the synthesis of tyrosine aminotransferase in hepatoma cells [7]. This unifilar dominance must be considered in developing models for the molecular basis of the preferential suppression of differentiated functions by BrdU.

In all experiments, tyrosinase activity of melanoma cells exposed to BrdU for 24–48 h continued to decline after the cultures were changed to BrdU-free medium and reached minimal values about one week after the initial addition of BrdU. An explanation for the relatively lengthy period required for the full manifestation of this effect of BrdU will require studies on the rate of tyrosinase synthesis and degradation in both control and BrdU-treated cells.

These results will facilitate the use of this system to probe normal regulation of melanogenesis. Brief exposure to BrdU minimizes possible secondary effects such as the increased cell doubling time seen by 7 days of continuous culture with BrdU. More importantly, we have now delimited a narrower band of time in which the primary regulatory events leading to suppression of melanogenesis probably occur.

## Summary

Culture of melanotic mouse melanoma cells (clone B$_5$59) with 5-bromodeoxyuridine (BrdU, 3 $\mu$g/ml) for 24 h (one DNA synthetic period) and subsequent growth for 6 days in medium without BrdU resulted in unpigmented cells without detectable tyrosinase activity. The kinetics of reduction of tyrosinase activity was indistinguishable from that when cells were grown for 48 h (2 rounds of DNA synthesis) or continuously for 7 days with BrdU. Thus, control of tyrosinase activity is highly sensitive to BrdU and incorporation of bromouracil into either strand of the DNA duplex is probably sufficient for suppression of tyrosinase activity.

## Acknowledgments

This work was supported in part by NCI grants CA-10095 and CA-08748. Dr. SELMA SILAGI is a recipient of Faculty Award PRA-77 from the American Cancer Society.

We wish to thank ROBERT BALINT for excellent technical assistance and Dr. LOUIS ZEITZ for instruction in, and the use of, his equipment for X-ray fluorescence analysis. Buoyant density analysis of DNA was performed through the kindness of Dr. MARY HAMILTON.

## References

1 BISCHOFF, R. and HOLTZER, H.: Inhibition of myoblast fusion after one round of DNA synthesis in 5-bromodeoxyuridine. J. Cell Biol. 44: 134–150 (1970).
2 COLEMAN, A. W.; COLEMAN, J. R.; KANKEL, D., and WERNER, I.: The reversible control of animal cell differentiation by the thymidine analog, 5-bromodeoxyuridine. Expl Cell Res. 59: 319–328 (1970).
3 KREIDER, J. W.; MATHESON, D. W.; BELTZ, B., and ROSENTHAL, M.: Inhibition of melanogenesis with 5-bromodeoxyuridine treatment in a single period of DNA synthesis. J. natn. Cancer Inst. 52: 1537–1540 (1974).
4 MARMUR, J.: A procedure for the isolation of deoxyribonucleic acid from micro-organisms. J. molec. Biol. 3: 208–218 (1961).
5 RUTTER, W. J.; PICTET, R. L., and MORRIS, P. W.: Toward molecular mechanisms of developmental processes. A. Rev. Biochem. 42: 601–646 (1973).
6 SILAGI, S. and BRUCE, S. A.: Suppression of malignancy and differentiation in melanotic melanoma cells. Proc. natn. Acad. Sci. USA 66: 72–78 (1970).
7 STELLWAGEN, R. H. and TOMKINS, G. M.: Preferential inhibition by 5-bromodeoxyuridine of the synthesis of tyrosine aminotransferase in hepatoma cell cultures. J. molec. Biol. 56: 167–182 (1971).
8 WRATHALL, J. R.; OLIVER, C.; SILAGI, S., and ESSNER, E.: Suppression of pigmentation in mouse melanoma cells by 5-bromodeoxyuridine. Effects on tyrosinase activity and melanosome formation. J. Cell Biol. 57: 406–423 (1973).
9 WRATHALL, J. R.; NEWCOMB, E. W.; BALINT, R.; ZEITZ, L., and SILAGI, S.: Suppression of melanoma cell tyrosinase activity and tumorigenicity after incorporation of bromouracil for one or two cell divisions. J. Cell Physiol. 86: 581–592 (1975).

10  ZEITZ, L. and LEE, R.: Element analysis in labeled DNA by X-ray fluorescence. Analyt. Biochem. *23:* 442–458 (1968).
11  ZIMMERMAN, J.; BBRUMBRAUGH, J.; BIEHL, J., and HOLTZER, H.: The effect of 5-bromodeoxyuridine on the differentiation of chick embryo pigment cells. Exp. Cell Res. *83:* 159–165 (1974).

J. R. WRATHALL, Department of Anatomy, Georgetown University Schools of Medicine and Dentistry, 3900 Reservoir Road, N.W., *Washington, DC 20007* (USA)

Pigment Cell, vol. 2, pp. 124–133 (Karger, Basel 1976)

# Cytotoxic Lymphocytes

*III. Cross-Reactions between Melanoma and Sarcoma Cells as Expressed by Lymphocytes and Serum Factors of Patients with Melanoma and Sarcoma and of Normal Healthy Donors*

H. THOTA, J. G. SINKOVICS, S. K. CARRIER, J. J. ROMERO and H. D. KAY

Section of Clinical Tumor Virology and Immunology, Department of Medicine, The University of Texas System Cancer Center M. D. Anderson Hospital and Tumor Institute, Houston, Tex.

*Introduction*

Two main principles seem to have dominated conceptually human tumor immunology as based on extensive *in vitro* studies [4–6, 8–12]: (1) the lymphocytes of patients reacted better than the lymphocytes of normal healthy donors to cultured tumor cells corresponding histologically to the patients' tumor type, and (2) cross-reactivity between histologically related and absence of cross-reactivity between histologically unrelated tumors occurred. Several disturbing early observations contrary to this picture remained unexplained [17, 30–32]. These were the occasional strong reactivity of healthy individuals to cultured tumor cells; the possibility of nonspecific activation of lymphocytes in culture by bovine proteins and/or antibiotics [15], and the poor growth of primary cultures of tumors often yielding colonies of fibroblasts instead of tumor cells and the uneven expression of tumor antigens by passaged tumor cells [22]. Recent data showed that normal healthy donors circulated lymphocytes and serum factors that were cytotoxic to cultured tumor cells [12, 16, 34, 35] and cross-reactivity occurred between histologically unrelated tumors [35].

Immunofluorescent and immunoelectron microscopy studies, using sera of patients with melanoma, revealed the presence of cytoplasmic,

membrane [8, 18, 19, 23–25, 28, 36] and nucleolar antigens [21] associated with melanoma cells. In over 60% of sera from patients with melanoma, there were antibodies reacting in immunofluorescence tests with
a melanoma cell line; only 10% of sera from patients with pathological
conditions other than melanoma contained this antibody [26]. When antibodies reacting with melanoma cells were detected in normal sera, the titer was always significantly lower than that in sera of patients with melanoma [36], however, the reactivity of normal sera has been repeatedly observed [23, 28]. Cytotoxicity to or inhibition of the growth of autologous
or allogeneic melanoma cells by the lymphocytes of patients with melanoma was higher than the reactivity of lymphocytes of melanoma patients
to nonmelanoma cells or to normal fibroblasts; the lymphocytes of normal healthy donors expressed low degree of reactivity to melanoma cells
[2–4, 6, 8–11, 13, 25, 37].

A Lab-Tek chamber/slide assay was designed in our laboratory to
monitor the immune reactions of patients to tumors [29]. We found that
the leukocytes, and serum in combination with leukocytes, of a patient
with melanoma expressed cross-reactivity between melanoma and sarcoma cells. In order to determine the extent of cross-reactions, these studies were extended by testing the lymphocytes and sera of patients with
melanoma, sarcoma, and of normal healthy donors against established
melanoma, sarcoma, and carcinoma cell lines.

## Materials and Methods

### The Lymphocyte-Mediated Cytotoxicity Assay

Established human cell lines derived from 3 sarcomas, 3 melanomas, and 1
squamous carcinoma (table I) were used in this study. Tumor cells were grown in
disposable plastic T-flasks (Falcon Plastics, Oxnard, Calif.) containing 100 ml of
Ham's F10 medium supplemented with 10–20% heat-inactivated fetal calf serum, 15
mM of L-glutamine, 0.5 mg each of D-Ca pantothenate, choline chloride, folic acid,
nicotinamide, pyridoxal HCL, and thiamine HCL, 1 mg of inositol, 500 $\mu$g of ribof-
lavin, 10 mg of neomycin, 14 mg of streptomycin, and $10^5$ units of penicillin G per
liter of medium. Cells from 2- to 3-day-old culture were collected by trypsinization,
washed twice with medium, and suspended in the tissue culture medium.

Buffy coat leukocytes were collected by dextran sedimentation of defibrinated
blood. Lymphocytes were purified by Ficoll-Hypaque technique [1].

The assays were performed using Lab-Tek chamber/slides with 8 flat square
wells. Suspensions of $2 \times 10^3$ target cells per well were dispensed into the wells in
triplicates. The control consisted of target cells in the presence of tissue culture me-

*Table I.* Established cell lines used as target cells

| Protocol No. | Description | Reference |
|---|---|---|
| *Sarcomas* | | |
| 2089 | rhabdomyosarcoma | [20] |
| 2291 | malignant fibrous histiocytoma (formerly believed to be rhabdomyosarcoma) | [32] |
| 2322 | chondrosarcoma | [32] |
| *Carcinomas* | | |
| 2043 | squamous cell carcinoma of the uterine cervix | [33] |
| *Melanomas* | | |
| 2124 | malignant melanoma | SCTVI |
| 2278 | malignant melanoma | SCTVI |
| 5145 | malignant melanoma | Bionetics Laboratories |

SCTVI = Cell line developed at the Section of Clinical Tumor Virology and Immunology, M.D. Anderson Hospital [unpublished].

dium. The slides were set in an incubator maintained with 5% $CO_2$ and humidity, for 30 min to 1 h. Heated (56 °C 30 min) sera were dispensed in appropriate wells; then attacker cells (leukocytes or lymphocytes) were added at a ratio of 300 attacker cells to 1 target cell, and the cultures were incubated in the humidified incubator. Slides were removed at the end of days 2, 3, and 4, and the supernatant fluid was discarded; the wells were rinsed with Dulbecco's phosphate buffered saline and fixed with methanol for 5–10 min. The slides were then stained using Wright's procedure.

### Cross-Reactivity Index (CRI)

Cross-reactivity between histologically unrelated tumors was expressed as CRI. CRI was calculated by dividing the percent reduction of target cells of histologically unrelated tumors by the percent reduction of target cells corresponding histologically to the patients' tumor type and multiplying by 100. CRI of 80–120 was considered to represent significant cross-reactivity. The percent reduction of target cells exposed to lymphocytes or serum was calculated by using the formula: % R = [(C-T)/C] × 100, where R represented the reduction, C the number of cells in the control, and T the number of cells in the treated wells.

## Results

The leukocytes (L) alone and in combination with sera (SeL) of Mr. C. K. (No. 90640), a patient with malignant melanoma, were tested

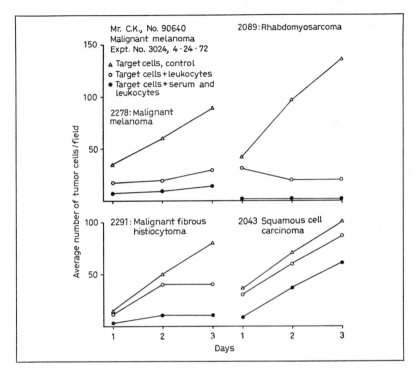

*Fig. 1.* Effect of leukocytes with and without serum of a patient with malignant melanoma on the growth of target tumor cells.

against established melanoma, sarcoma, and squamous carcinoma cell lines. The results are shown in figure 1. The L and SeL of Mr. C. K. were cytotoxic to melanoma, sarcoma, and malignant fibrous histiocytoma cells to the same extent but not to carcinoma cells. The extent of cross-reactivity is shown in table II. The data show that the L and SeL of Mr. C. K. expressed significant cross-reactivity between melanoma and sarcoma cells and were nonreactive to carcinoma cells.

The lymphocytes (Ly) alone and in combination with sera (SeLy) of 6 other patients with melanoma were tested in the same fashion and the data are shown in table III. While the Ly and SeLy expressed significant cross-reactivity between melanoma and sarcoma cells in 63 and 85% of the tests, respectively, the same Ly and SeLy preparations expressed cross-reactivity between melanoma and carcinoma cells in 23 and 31% of

*Table II.* Cross-reactions of cell-mediated cytotoxicity elicited by leukocytes and serum factors of a patient with malignant melanoma

| Cross-reaction with | Mean CRI mediated by: | |
| --- | --- | --- |
| | leukocytes | serum and leukocytes |
| Sarcoma | 80 | 105 |
| Carcinoma | 18 | 51 |

*Table III.* Extent and incidence of cross-reactivity between melanoma and sarcoma cells as expressed by lymphocytes and serum factors of patients with malignant melanoma

| Cross-reacting with | Lymphocytes | | Serum and lymphocytes | |
| --- | --- | --- | --- | --- |
| | CRI | incidence[a] (%) | CRI | incidence[a] (%) |
| Sarcoma | 84 | 7/11 (63) | 88 | 11/13 (85) |
| Carcinoma | 61 | 3/13 (23) | 57 | 4/13 (31) |

[a] Number of tests expressing significant CRI/number of times tested.

*Table IV.* Lymphocytes and serum factors of patients with sarcoma and of normal healthy donors express significant cross-reactivity between melanoma and sarcoma cells

| Cross-reacting with | Mean CRI mediated by: | | | |
| --- | --- | --- | --- | --- |
| | lymphocytes of | | serum and lymphocytes of | |
| | normal | sarcoma patient | normal | sarcoma patient |
| Melanoma | 105 (5/5) | 99 | 106 | 116 |
| Carcinoma | 42 (0/3) | 7 | 71 (1/3) | 27 |

Results in parentheses represent the number of tests expressing significant cross-reactivity/number of times tested.

the tests, respectively. The data were analyzed by computer using Student's *t* test [27]. The differences between CRI of sarcoma and carcinoma were found to be significant ($p < 0.002$).

The extensive cross-reactions observed between melanoma and sarcoma cells as expressed by lymphocytes and serum of patients with melanomas prompted us to test the reactivity of lymphocytes and serum of patients with sarcoma and normal healthy donors. The data of table IV clearly demonstrated that the lymphocytes and sera of patients with sarcomas and normal healthy donors also expressed cross-reactivity between melanoma and sarcoma cells and were nonreactive to carcinoma cells.

## *Discussion*

The results obtained by using Lab-Tek chamber/slide assay show that the lymphocytes and serum factors of patients with malignant melanoma, sarcoma, and of normal healthy donors expressed significant cross-reactivity between established melanoma and sarcoma cells and were not reactive to carcinoma cells. This might mean that (1) the patients and normal healthy donors develop immunity specifically to cross-reacting antigens associated with melanoma and sarcoma cells and express this immunity *in vitro*, or (2) melanoma and sarcoma cells are more susceptible to cytotoxic lymphocytes than carcinoma cells because of biological and metabolic but not immunological factors. However, the squamous carcinoma cells used in this study were susceptible to cytotoxic lymphocytes of patients with squamous cell carcinoma of the uterine cervix [7]. The first interpretation appears to be more likely, because immunological tests other than those that measure cytotoxicity, such as immunofluorescence and immunoelectron microscopy, demonstrated the presence of specific antigens on sarcoma and melanoma cells [21–23, 26, 28, 32, 36]. Other investigators, by using immunofluorescence, obtained results similar to ours. Cytoplasmic antigens associated with melanoma cells were detected by using the sera of patients with melanoma and normal healthy persons [23, 28]. More interestingly, antibodies to melanoma cells were detected in the sera of patients with melanoma, or with other malignancies, and of normal healthy persons [26, 36].

The fact that our cell lines were free from mycoplasma contamination excludes the possibility that the cross-reactivity was directed to mycoplasma antigens on the cell surface.

Cell line No. 2043 (table I) released large amounts of carcinoembryonic antigen in the tissue culture fluid but the sarcoma cell lines did not; however, cytotoxicity was not evident to cell line No. 2043 in the present study. Therefore, cross-reactivity on account of carcinoembryonic antigen expression is unlikely, because carcinoembryonic antigen-directed cytotoxicity should have been expressed toward cell line No. 2043. However, a different class of carcinoembryonic antigen may be expressed by both melanoma and sarcoma cells but not by carcinoma cells. Sarcoma-associated fetal antigens have been described [14].

Clearly recognizable morphologic differences between cell lines Nos. 2089, 2124, and 2043 as well as the other cultures used in this study (table I), makes the possibility of accidental mix-up of cell lines remote and most unlikely.

In order to identify the cross-reacting antigen in melanoma and sarcoma cells, the cell lines and the attacker lymphocytes will be analyzed for histocompatibility antigens. If cross-reactivity between sarcoma and melanoma cells will be established by immunofluorescence, the sera will be cross-absorbed with tumor cells, fetal cells, and guinea pig kidney cells.

## Summary

A Lab-Tek chamber/slide assay was used to determine the extent of cross-reactivity between melanoma (MM) and sarcoma (Sc) cells expressed as cross-reactivity index (CRI). Leukocytes (L) and lymphocytes (Ly) either alone or in combination with sera (Se) of patients (Pts) with malignant melanoma (MM), Ly, and SeLy of Pts with Sc and of normal healthy donors (NHD) were more cytotoxic to MM and Sc cells than to carcinoma (Cc) cells. These Ly and Se preparations expressed statistically significant cross-reactivity between MM and Sc cells and no cross-reactivity between Sc and Cc, and between MM and Cc cells. The cross-reactivity between MM and Sc cells might be due to a combination of tumor-specific, histocompatibility, and nonspecific cross-reacting antigens.

## Acknowledgments

The authors are grateful to Dr. Dennis A. Johnston, Biomathematician, Department of Biomathematics, for statistical analysis of data. The authors are obliged to Dr. Clifton D. Howe for support.

This work was supported by Contract No. 1-CP-33292 within the Virus Cancer program of the National Cancer Institute.

## References

1 BOYUM, A.: Separation of leukocytes from blood and bone marrow. Scand. J. clin. Lab. Invest. 21: suppl. 97 (1968).

2 BYRNE, M.; HEPPNER, G.; STOLBACH, L.; CUMMINGS, F.; McDONOUGH, E., and CALABRESI, P.: Tumor immunity in melanoma patients as assessed by colony inhibition and microcytotoxicity tests. A preliminary report. Natn. Cancer Inst. Monogr. 37: 3–8 (1973).

3 CLARK, D. A. and NATHANSON, L.: Cellular immunity in malignant melanoma; in RILEY Pigment Cell, vol. 1, pp. 350–359 (Karger, Basel 1973).

4 CURRIE, G. A. and BASHAM, C.: Serum mediated inhibition of the immunological reactions of the patient to his own tumor. A possible role for circulating antigen. Br. J. Cancer 26: 427–438 (1972).

5 DE VRIES, J. E.; RÜMKE, P., and BERNHEIM, J. L.: Cytotoxic lymphocytes in melanoma patients. Int. J. Cancer 9: 567–576 (1972).

6 DE VRIES, J. E.; CORNAIN, S., and RÜMKE, P.: Cytotoxicity of non-T versus T-lymphocytes from melanoma patients and healthy donors on short- and long-term cultured melanoma cells. Int. J. Cancer 14: 427–434 (1974).

7 DI SAIA, P. J.; SINKOVICS, J. G.; RUTLEDGE, F. N., and SMITH, J. P.: Cell-mediated immunity to human malignant cells. Am. J. Obstet. Gynec. 114: 979–989 (1972).

8 FOSSATI, G.; COLNAGHI, M. I.; DELLA PORTA, G.; CASCINELLI, N., and VERONESI, U.: Cellular and humoral immunity against human malignant melanoma. Int. J. Cancer 8: 344–350 (1971).

9 HELLSTRÖM, I.; HELLSTRÖM, K. E.; SJÖGREN, H. O., and WARNER, G. A.: Demonstration of cell-mediated immunity to human neoplasia of various histological types. Int. J. Cancer 7: 1–16 (1971).

10 HELLSTRÖM, I. and HELLSTRÖM, K. E.: Some recent studies on cellular immunity to melanomas. Fed. Proc. Fed. Am. Socs exp. Biol. 32: 156–159 (1973).

11 HELLSTRÖM, I.; WARNER, G. A.; HELLSTRÖM, K. E., and SJÖGREN, H. O.: Sequential studies on cell-mediated tumor immunity and blocking serum activity in ten patients with malignant melanoma. Int. J. Cancer 11: 280–292 (1973).

12 HELLSTRÖM, I.; HELLSTRÖM, K. E.; SJÖGREN, H. O., and WARNER, G. A.: Destruction of cultivated melanoma cells by lymphocytes from healthy black (North American Negro) donors. Int. J. Cancer 11: 116–122 (1973).

13 HEPPNER, G. H.; STOLBACH, L.; BYRNE, M.; CUMMINGS, F. J.; McDONOUGH, E., and CALABREST, P.: Cell-mediated and serum blocking reactivity to tumor antigens in patients with malignant melanoma. Int. J. Cancer 11: 245–260 (1973).

14 HIRSHAUT, Y.; PEI, D. T.; MARCOVE, R. C.; MUKHERJE, B.; SPIELVOGEL, A. R., and ESSNER, E.: Seroepidemiology of human sarcoma antigens (S1). New Engl. J. Med. 291: 1103–1107 (1974).

15 JOHNSON, G. J. and RUSSELL, P. S.: Reaction of human lymphocytes in culture to components of the medium. Nature, Lond. 208: 343–345 (1965).

16 KAY, H. D. and SINKOVICS, J. G.: Cytotoxic lymphocytes from normal donors. Lancet ii: 296–297 (1974).

17 LEVY, N. L.: Use of in vitro microcytotoxicity test to assess human tumor-spe-

cific cell-mediated immunity and its serum-mediated abrogation. Natn. Cancer Inst. Monogr. *37:* 85–92 (1973).

18  LEWIS, M. G.; IKONOPISOV, R. L.; NAIRN, R. C.; PHILLIPS, T. M.; FAIRLEY, G. H.; BODENHAM, D. C., and ALEXANDER, P.: Tumor-specific antibodies in human malignant melanoma and their relationship to the extent of the disease. Br. med. J. *iii:* 547–552 (1969).

19  LEWIS, M. G. and PHILLIPS, T. M.: The specificity of surface membrane immunofluorescence in human malignant melanoma. Int. J. Cancer *10:* 105–111 (1972).

20  MCALLISTER, R. M.; MELNYK, J.; FINKLESTEIN, J. Z.; ADAMS, E., and GARDNER, M. B.: Cultivation *in vitro* of cells derived from a human rhabdomyosarcoma. Cancer *24:* 520–526 (1969).

21  MCBRIDE, C. M.; BOWEN, J. M., and DMOCHOWSKI, L.: Antinucleolar antibodies in the sera of patients with malignant melanoma. Surg. Forum *23:* 92–93 (1972).

22  MOORE, M.; WITHEROW, P. J.; PRICE, C. H. G., and CLOUGH, S. A.: Detection by immunofluorescence of intracytoplasmic antigens in cell lines derived from human sarcomas. Int. J. Cancer *12:* 428–437 (1973).

23  MORTON, D. L.; MALMGREN, R. A.; HOLMES, E. C., and KETCHAM, A. S.: Demonstration of antibodies against human malignant melanoma by immunofluorescence. Surgery, St Louis *64:* 233–240 (1968).

24  MUNA, N. M.; MARCUS, S., and SMART, C.: Detection by immunofluorescence of antibodies specific for human malignant melanoma cells. Cancer *23:* 88–93 (1969).

25  NAIRN, R. C.; NIND, A. P. P.; GULI, E. P. G.; DAVIES, D. J.; LITTLE, J. H.; DAVIS, N. C., and WHITEHEAD, R. H.: Antitumor immunoreactivity in patients with malignant melanoma. Med. J. Aust. *i:* 397–403 (1972).

26  OETTGEN, H. F.; AOKI, T.; OLD, L. J.; BOYSE, E. A.; DeHARVEN, E., and MILLS, G. M.: Suspension culture of a pigment-producing cell line derived from a human malignant melanoma. J. natn. Cancer Inst. *41:* 827–843 (1968).

27  REMINGTON, R. D. and SCHORK, M. A.: Statistics with applications to the biological and health sciences, pp. 210–214 (Prentice Hall, Englewood Cliffs 1970).

28  ROMSDAHL, M. M. and COX, I. S.: Human malignant melanoma antibodies demonstrated by immunofluorescence. Archs Surg., Chicago *100:* 491–497 (1970).

29  SINKOVICS, J. G.; AHMED, N.; HRGOVCIC, M. J.; CABINESS, J. R., and WILBUR, J. R.: Cytotoxic lymphocytes. II. Antagonism and synergism between serum factors and lymphocytes of patients with sarcomas as tested against cultured tumor cells. Tex. Rep. Biol. Med. *30:* 347–360 (1972).

30  SINKOVICS, J. G.; CABINESS, J. R., and SHULLENBERGER, C. C.: Monitoring *in vitro* immune reactions to solid tumors; in VAETH Front. Radiat. Ther. Onc., vol. 7, pp. 99–119 (Karger, Basel 1972).

31  SINKOVICS, J. G.; TEBBI, K., and CABINESS, J. R.: Cytotoxicity of lymphocytes to established cultures of human tumors. Evidence for specificity. Natn. Cancer Inst. Monogr. *37:* 9–18 (1973).

32 SINKOVICS, J. G.; CAMPOS, L. T.; KAY, H. D.; CABINESS, J. R.; GONZALEZ, F.; LOH, K. K.; ERVIN, F., and GYÖRKEY, F.: Immunological studies with sarcomas. Effects of immunization and chemotherapy on cell- and antibody-mediated immune reactions. 26th Ann. Symp. Fundamental Cancer Research (Williams & Wilkins, Baltimore 1974).

33 SYKES, J. A.; WHITESCARVER, J. W.; JERNSTROM, P.; NOLAN, J. F., and BYATT, P.: Some properties of a new cell line of human origin. J. natn. Cancer Inst. 45: 107–115 (1970).

34 TAKASUGI, M.; MICKEY, M. R., and TERASAKI, P. I.: Reactivity of lymphocytes from normal persons on cultured tumor cells. Cancer Res. 33: 2898–2902 (1973).

35 TAKASUGI, M.; MICKEY, M. R., and TERASAKI, P. I.: Studies on specificity of cell-mediated immunity to human tumors. J. natn. Cancer Inst. (1974).

36 WOOD, G. W. and BARTH, R. F.: Immunofluorescent studies of the serologic reactivity of patients with malignant melanoma against tumor-associated cytoplasmic antigens. J. natn. Cancer Inst. 53: 309–316 (1974).

37 WYBRAN, J.; HELLSTRÖM, I.; HELLSTRÖM, K. E., and FUDENBERG, H. H.: Cytotoxicity of human rosette-forming blood lymphocytes on cultivated human tumor cells. Int. J. Cancer 13: 515–521 (1974).

Dr. H. THOTA, The University of Texas System Cancer Center, M. D. Anderson Hospital and Tumor Institute, *Houston, TX 77025* (USA)

Pigment Cell, vol. 2, pp. 134–139 (Karger, Basel 1976)

# A Rapid Microassay for Melanoma Tumor Immunity[1]

B. J. WILSON, F. HU, A. MALLEY, D. BURGER and L. M. PASZTOR

Oregon Regional Primate Research Center, Beaverton, and VA Hospital, Portland, Oreg.

The problems of (1) nonspecificity, (2) difficulty of procedure, and (3) lack of significance in data from currently available assays for tumor immunity in melanoma led us to design the assay reported here.

In developing this microassay, we have used the methodology and techniques reported elsewhere [2–4]. As designed the assay requires no prelabeling of target cells and is very rapid in both the preparative and harvesting phases. We have not only defined the conditions for killing of B16 mouse melanoma cells during growth, but demonstrated a blocking factor in the sera of tumor-bearing mice.

## Materials and Methods

Target cells for this assay were cultured B16 mouse melanoma cells carried in culture by Dr. Hu since 1968 [1]. Control target cells were mouse mammary tumor cells (MMT-CCL-51) obtained from the type culture collection. The cells were grown to confluency in Eagle's minimal essential medium, trypsinized and poured off, pelleted (500 g), resuspended and counted. They were then washed once with RPMI with 40 mM Hepes and resuspended in complete media (RPMI-1640 + 40 mM Hepes + Pen-Strep + 20% FCS) at $10^6$ cells/ml [3].

Killer spleen cells were raised in C57BL$_6$ mice by injecting subcutaneously 0.1 ml of a melanoma tumor mince. Spleens were removed at various times after tumor injection, and the cells were rinsed from the spleen into media (RPMI-1640

1    Publication No. 864 of the Oregon Regional Primate Research Center supported in part by Grants CA 08499 of the National Cancer Institute; RR 00163 of the Animal Resources Branch, Division of Research Resources; AM 08512 and AM 08445 of the National Institute of Arthritis, Metabolism and Digestive Diseases, National Institutes of Health.

media with 40 mM Hepes) with a 1-ml syringe fitted with a 22-gauge needle [4]. The cells were then washed 3 times, suspended in complete media, counted, and diluted to the proper concentration in complete media. Blood was drawn from the retro-orbital sinus of tumor-bearing mice at approximately 1-week intervals. Sera were pooled and inactivated at 56 °C for 30 min. When used in blocking sera assay, 0.5 ml of a 1:2 dilution was added to each well.

Microcytoxicity assay: 100 ml of tumor cell suspension ($10^6$/ml was dispensed into triplicate culture wells (Linbro, Vineland, N. J.). For direct toxicity assays, spleen cells at various concentrations were added in 100 $\mu$l.

For blocking assays, spleen cells were first dispensed into the wells in 50 $\mu$l, and then 50 $\mu$l of a 1:2 dilution of blocking or control sera were added. After the cells had incubated 1 h, 100 $\mu$l of tumor cells were added. For either assay, plates were covered loosely and incubated for 23 h in 95% air, 5% $CO_2$ at 37 °C and high humidity. Plates were then removed and 1 $\mu$Ci $^3$H-thymidine per well was dispensed. They were incubated one additional hour and then harvested with a multiple automated sample harvester (Otto Hiller, Madison, Wisc.) which aspirates culture contents onto a glass fiber strip. The glass fiber strips were then removed and dried at 125 °C for 15 min, and the areas where the culture contents were imposed were punched into 1-dram vials. 3 ml of Permafluor (Packard) was added and the vials placed in lidless scintillation vials for assay by a Packard liquid scintillation counter fitted with a punch tape. Data were usually available for analysis 48 h after the assay was begun.

## Results

Table I compares the incorporation of $^3$H-thymidine by melanoma cells and by spleen cells. During a 1-hour pulse, $10^5$ melanoma cells incorporated 35,051 counts whereas $10^5$ normal spleen cells incorporated only 175 counts. During tumor growth, the level of incorporation by the spleen cells changed only slightly. Even when as many as 10 times more spleen cells were added, they incorporated only 1,000 cpm.

The ability of spleen cells to inhibit melanoma cell growth during tumor growth is also shown in table I. This datum shows the percent of inhibition when equal numbers of spleen cells and tumor cells are cultured together. Normal C57BL$_6$ spleen cells inhibited thymidine incorporation by 48%. By day 7, the inhibiting ability of spleen cells from tumor-bearing mice had dropped to 21%. By day 14, it rose to a high of 64% and then dropped to 44% on day 21.

Figure 1 shows the percent of inhibition of thymidine incorporation during tumor growth at different spleen cell concentrations. At more than $5 \times 10^5$ spleen cells, the various spleen cell populations inhibited almost

*Table I.* Inhibition of $^3$H-thymidine incorporation of melanoma cells by spleen cells from tumor-bearing animals

|  | cpm | Percent inhibition |
|---|---|---|
| Melanoma cells | 35,051 | – |
| Normal spleen cells | 175 | |
| Melanoma cells + normal spleen cells | 18,511 | 48 |
| Spleen cells from tumor-bearing mice | | |
| Day 7 spleen cells | 343 | |
| Melanoma cells + day 7 spleen cells | 27,628 | 21 |
| Day 14 spleen cells | 60 | |
| Melanoma cells + day 14 spleen cells | 12,749 | 64 |
| Day 21 spleen cells | 121 | |
| Melanoma cells + day 21 spleen cells | 19,618 | 48 |

Total culture volume is 200 $\mu$l. Equal numbers ($10^5$) of spleen cells or melanoma cells were added to triplicate culture wells as indicated.

*Table II.* Blocking of spleen cell killing by sera from tumor-bearing mice

|  | cpm | Percent inhibition[a] | Percent blocking[b] |
|---|---|---|---|
| Melanoma cells | 35,501 | | |
| Melanoma cells + SCT-21[c] | 19,618 | 44 | |
| Melanoma cells + SCT-21 + BLS-6 | 19,316 | | – |
| Melanoma cells + SCT-21 + BLS-13 | 23,675 | | 21 |
| Melanoma cells + SCT-21 + BLS-22 | 29,980 | | 53 |

[a] Percent inhibition $= \dfrac{\text{Melanoma cells cpm} - \text{inhibited cpm}}{\text{melanoma cells alone} - \text{cpm}}$.

[b] Percent blocking $= \dfrac{\text{Protected cpm} - \text{inhibited cpm}}{\text{inhibited cpm}}$.

[c] SCT-21 = Spleen cells from mice injected with tumor mince 21 days before assay. BLS-6 = sera drawn from mice injected with tumor mince 6 days before assay. Blocking sera was added to $10^5$ spleen cells and incubated 1 h prior to addition of $10^5$ tumor cells.

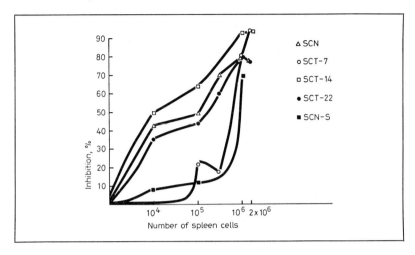

*Fig. 1.* Percent inhibition of incorporation of $^3$H-thymidine by melanoma cells co-cultured with varying numbers of different spleen cell populations. SCN = Spleen cells, normal (C57BL$_6$); SCT-7 = spleen cells drawn 7 days after tumor injection; SCN-S = normal spleen cells from Swiss Webster mice.

equally. The most significant finding in the inhibition experiments was that the inhibiting ability of spleen cells was much lower for day 7 spleen cells (SCT-7). Normal Swiss Webster mouse spleen cells were used as a specificity control. From 10$^4$ through 10$^6$ per well, low multiplicities, they inhibited only slightly, but at greater than 10$^6$ cells per well they inhibited as well as any of the other cell populations. Subsequent experiments were conducted with equal numbers of tumor and spleen cells.

Because of the high inhibiting level of normal spleen cells, the inhibition of a control cell line (MMT-CCL-51) was tested. Preliminary data indicate that the incorporation of $^3$H-thymidine by these cells was inhibited only slightly (20% or less) by either normal spleen cells or by spleen cells from day 14 tumor-bearing mice.

Table II shows how sera drawn during tumor growth blocked the inhibiting ability of spleen cells from day 21 tumor-bearing mice. This ability was not blocked in sera from mice injected with tumor cells 6 days before (BLS-6), but in sera from mice injected 13 days before (BLS-13) and from mice injected 22 days before (BLS-22), it was blocked by 21 and 53%, respectively.

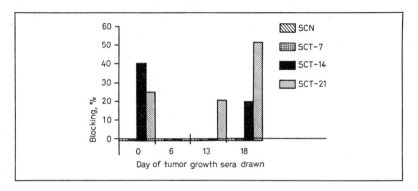

*Fig. 2.* Serum blocking of spleen cell inhibition of incorporation of ³H-thymidine by cultured melanoma cells. SCN = Spleen cells normal; SCT-7 = spleen cells from mice injected 7 days before with tumor mince. Blocking serum was taken from normal (day 0), and day 6, 13 or 18 tumor-carrying mice.

The percent of blocking measured in all populations of spleen cells and blocking sera is summarized in figure 2. Normal C57BL₆ mouse sera blocked killing by spleen cells taken from animals late in the course of tumor growth (day 14 or 21) but not by normal cells or those taken on day 7. Sera drawn on day 6 could not block any of the populations of cells tested, and sera drawn on day 13 could block day 21 spleen cells only at equivalence. The inhibiting ability of day 14 spleen cells was blocked at high multiplicities of spleen cells; day 18 sera could block inhibition by only day 14 or 21 spleen cells.

## Conclusions

From these experiments, we conclude that during tumor growth the ability of spleen cells from tumor-bearing animals to inhibit tumor growth varies little from that of normal spleen cells, although it appears to be specific for melanoma. Since Swiss Webster spleen cells have little effect in the lower range of spleen cell concentration, the effect would appear to be immunological. When equal numbers of spleen cells and tumor cells were used, the difference between normal spleen cells and spleen cells from tumor-bearing animals was most apparent. At higher multiplicities of spleen cells, the inhibition was nonspecific. The ability of spleen cells from a day 7 tumor-bearing mouse to inhibit growth was significantly less than that of normal spleen cells or of spleen cells taken later in the course of tumor growth.

As measured in this system, blocking appears to depend both on the killer spleen cell and the blocking sera. For example, day 6 sera cannot block regardless of the day of tumor growth of the spleen cell donor, whereas normal sera can block only those spleen cells taken after the tumor mass becomes large.

With this system, it is feasible to titrate the blocking activity; we plan to do so in future experiments. The blocking factor in normal sera may be (a) at a lower concentration or (b) a different material from that which develops as the tumor mass increases.

### Summary

We have developed a rapid assay for measuring cell-mediated immunity in the mouse melanoma system. Here we report how we measured the inhibition of $^3$H-thymidine incorporation during a 1-hour pulse by B16 mouse melanoma cells co-cultured for 24 h with normal cells or spleen cells from tumor-bearing animals during tumor growth. We also describe how the spleen cell inhibition of $^3$H-thymidine incorporation by the tumor cells is blocked. The immunity measured depends on both the cell component and the sera component.

### References

1  Hu, F. and Lesney, P. F.: The isolation and cytology of two pigment cell strains from B-16 mouse melanoma. Cancer Res. *24:* 1634 (1964).
2  Knudsen, R. C.; Ahmed, A. A., and Sell, K. W.: An *in vitro* microassay for lymphotoxin using microplates and the multiple automated sample harvester. J. Immunol. Meth. *5:* 55 (1974).
3  Peter, J. B.; Cardin, C., and Stempel, K. E.: Lysis of L cells in spinner culture by lymphocyte produced cytotoxin (human lymphotoxin). Cell. Immunol. *9:* 328 (1973).
4  Strong, D.; Ahmed, A. A.; Thurman, G. B., and Sell, K. W.: *In vitro* stimulation of murine spleen cells using a microculture system and a multiple automated sample harvester. J. Immunol. Meth. *2:* 279 (1973).

B. J. Wilson, PhD, Oregon Regional Primate Research Center, 505 N.W. 185th Avenue, *Beaverton, OR 97005* (USA)

Pigment Cell, vol. 2, pp. 140–149 (Karger, Basel 1976)

# Melanosome Antigens from B16 Melanoma

PHILIP DOEZEMA

Division of Biology, Kansas State University, Manhattan, Kans.

## Introduction

The results of this study demonstrate production of antibodies against a purified preparation of melanosomes. Results of an agglutination assay indicate that the melanosome fraction contains at least two classes of antigens: One class has been found only in the melanosome fraction, the other class of antigen(s) is shared with nonpigmented tissues. Evidence indicates that both classes of antigens are very stable and appear to be firmly bound to the particles of the melanosome fraction.

## Materials and Methods

Melanosomes were obtained from B16 mouse melanoma as previously described [4]. Melanosomes were counted with a Petroff-Hausser chamber and $8 \times 10^{11}$ particles together with Freund's adjuvant were used for a single immunizing injection. The criterion for antibody production was an agglutination assay consisting of 40 $\mu$l of antiserum mixed with an equal volume of a melanosome suspension containing $6 \times 10^{10}$ particles per ml of distilled water. The reagents were mixed on a depression slide and examined under a dissecting microscope.

Homogenates of tissues from C57Bl/6J mice (host strain for the B16 melanoma) were used to absorb antisera and for use in specificity testing. Liver, spleen, muscle, and brain were homogenized in borate-saline buffer (1 g tissue: 1 ml) and centrifuged at 10,000 $g$, retaining the supernatant. Liver homogenate was added by drops to antimelanosome serum until cross reaction to liver was completely absorbed as indicated by absence of a precipitin line in the Ouchterlony gel diffusion test [3].

*Results*

The Agglutination Assay

Rabbits injected with melanosomes at 30- to 40-day intervals developed agglutinating antibody shortly after the second injection (table I). First indications of agglutination usually appear within 2 min and the reaction progresses forming large aggregates visible to the unaided eye within 10–20 min (fig. 1).

The interaction between melanosomes and antiserum was quantified by recording the time required for first appearance of aggregates at 10X magnification. Agglutination time was linearly related to antibody concentration in serum and melanosome concentration in the reaction mixture (fig. 2 and 3). Preimmune serum and serum from an uninjected rabbit failed to agglutinate melanosomes (table II). Agglutination could be abolished by absorbing antiserum with melanosomes (table II).

Tests for Specificity

A mitochondrial particulate fraction from liver (10,000 $g$ pellet) containing approximately $6 \times 10^{10}$ particles per ml was used in place of melanosomes in the agglutination assay; no agglutination was observed.

A concentrated liver homogenate when tested against antimelanosome serum by the Ouchterlony gel diffusion assay showed one or more lines of cross reaction (fig. 4). Spleen, muscle, and brain homogenates also showed precipitin lines against antimelanosome serum, but brain and muscle homogenates reacted weakly (fig. 5). When antimelanosome serum was absorbed with liver homogenate, cross reaction to all four tissues was removed concurrently (fig. 5).

Antimelanosome serum which had been absorbed with liver to eliminate reactions with nonspecific antigens from unpigmented tissues was now tested against melanosomes in the agglutination assay. The results in figure 1b indicate that absorbed serum does agglutinate melanosomes, but the rate of agglutination is reduced to approximately that of a 1:5 dilution of unabsorbed antiserum (table III). This increase in agglutination time cannot be attributed to dilution by absorbent since only about 300 $\mu$l of homogenate were added per ml of antiserum.

Stability of Particulate Antigens

Melanosomes were suspended in 2% sodium dodecyl sulfate (SDS), heated, cooled, washed in 2% SDS, washed several times in distilled wa-

*Table I.* Sample data from rabbit No. 1

| Serum sample | Agglutination time, min |
|---|---|
| Day 0 (preinjection) | no agglutination |
| Day 38 (second injection) | no data |
| Day 54 | <0.2 |
| Day 68 | 0.2±0.03 |
| Day 98 | <0.2 |
| Day 158 (third injection) | no data |
| Day 188 | 0.4±0.03 |
| Day 218 | 1.3±0.03 |
| Day 258 | 1.5±0.05 |
| Day 332 | 1.4±0.07 |

*Table II.* Agglutination time for antiserum absorbed with melanosomes

| Serum type | Agglutination time, min |
|---|---|
| Preimmune serum | no agglutination |
| Serum from uninjected rabbit | no agglutination |
| Unabsorbed antiserum[a] | 0.4±0.03 |
| Antiserum[a] absorbed with $6 \times 10^{10}$ melanosomes/ml | 3.9±0.4 |
| Antiserum[a] absorbed with $12 \times 10^{10}$ melanosomes/ml | 10.1±0.6 |
| Unabsorbed antiserum[b] | 1.9±0.1 |
| Antiserum[b] absorbed with $6 \times 10^{10}$ melanosomes/ml | no agglutination |

[a] Antiserum from rabbit No. 1 bled 30 days after the 3rd injection.
[b] Antiserum from rabbit No. 1 bled 45 days after the 3rd injection.

*Table III.* Agglutination time for antiserum absorbed with liver homogenate

| Melanosome concentration, particles/ml | Serum type | Serum dilution | Agglutination time, min |
|---|---|---|---|
| $6 \times 10^{10}$ | preimmune | no dilution | no agglutination |
| $6 \times 10^{10}$ | serum from an uninjected rabbit | no dilution | no agglutination |
| $6 \times 10^{10}$ | unabsorbed antiserum | no dilution | 1.9±0.1 |
| $6 \times 10^{10}$ | unabsorbed antiserum | 1:5 | 8.2±0.5 |
| $6 \times 10^{10}$ | antiserum absorbed with liver homog. | no dilution | 7.5±0.3 |

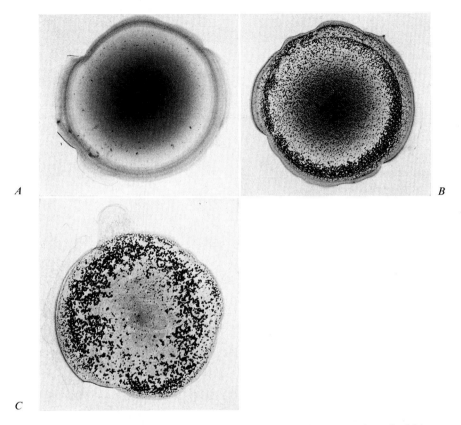

*Fig. 1.* The appearance of the agglutination reaction after approximately 1.5 h. × 2.4. *A* Control – preimmune serum plus melanosomes: melanosomes remain as a finely divided suspension. *B* Liver-absorbed antiserum plus melanosomes: the first indication of agglutination appeared at about 7.5 min under the dissecting microscope and aggregates of melanosomes are clearly visible to the unaided eye at 1.5 h. *C* Unabsorbed antiserum plus melanosomes: the first indication of agglutination was at 1.9 min, aggregates visible to the unaided eye appear within 10–15 min and after 1 h nearly all melanosomes are incorporated into floculent clumps up to 0.5 mm in diameter.

ter, and reconstituted to $6 \times 10^{10}$ particles per ml in distilled water. In the case of two successive treatments, the second was in fresh SDS. Even after boiling, recovery of the particles was 100%. The results in table IV show that 5 min at 100 °C or 2 h at 60 °C in SDS have little or no effect on the agglutination time. Only after two treatments at 100 °C is there a slight increase in agglutination time (table IV).

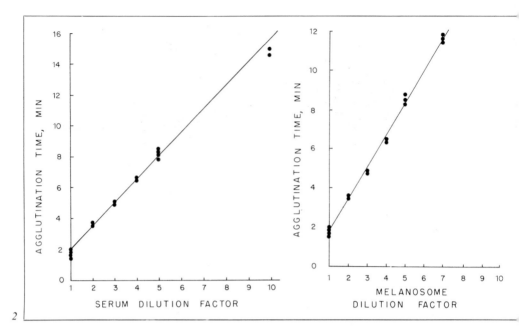

*Fig. 2.* The linear relationship between time of first melanosome agglutination and antibody concentration in serum. Undiluted serum agglutinated melanosomes in 1.9 min. Serum from an uninjected rabbit was used to dilute the antiserum and the results indicate a quantitative relationship between rate of agglutination and dilution factor. A melanosome suspension containing $6 \times 10^{10}$ particles/ml was mixed 1:1 with serum.

*Fig. 3.* The linear relationship between time of first melanosome agglutination and melanosome concentration in the agglutination assay. The undiluted melanosome suspension contained $6 \times 10^{10}$ particles/ml and the first aggregates appeared in 1.9 min when mixed with an equal volume of antiserum. Dilution of the melanosome suspension resulted in a corresponding linear increase in agglutination time.

Treatment of melanosomes with fungal protease (Sigma type IV from *S. griseus*, 1 mg/ml) had no effect on agglutination time, but was effective in eliminating agglutination after melanosomes had been pretreated with SDS at 100 °C (table IV).

*Soluble Melanosome Antigen(s)*

Melanosomes were suspended in a 1% Triton-X-100 solution. Soluble material was recovered from the supernatant after centrifugation by

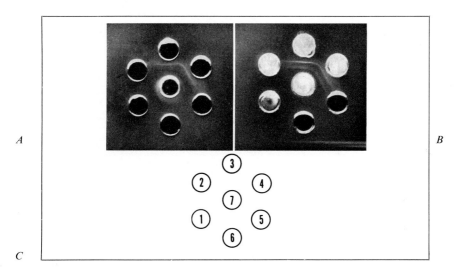

Fig. 4. Cross-reaction of liver homogenate (center well) with antimelanosome serum and elimination of this cross reaction by absorption. *A* Well No. 1, preimmune serum as control; well No. 2, antimelanosome serum absorbed with liver homogenate; wells No. 3 and No. 4, unabsorbed antimelanosome serum; the center well No. 7 contains liver homogenate. *B* Contents of the wells are identical to those in *A*. The result indicates that occasionally more than one precipitin line appears between liver homogenate and antimelanosome serum. *C* Indicates the numbering of the wells.

dialysis and lyophilization. The residue was dissolved in borate-saline and tested against liver-absorbed and unabsorbed antiserum in the Ouchterlony gel diffusion assay. The result in figure 6B shows that the soluble antigen from melanosomes reacts with antimelanosome serum from which cross-reactivity to liver, spleen, muscle, and brain had been absorbed.

## Discussion

Previous attempts to obtain antibodies against melanosomes, melanin and melanoprotein have been reported. BLOIS [1] and WASSERMAN and VAN DER WALT [10] were unsuccessful. LANGHOFF *et al.* [7] claim to have detected antibody against melanin in melanoma patients as well as in rabbits injected with subcellular fractions from melanomas. However, questions about the specificity of these antibodies have been raised [10].

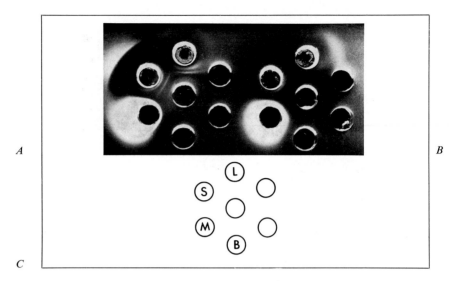

*Fig. 5.* Cross reaction of liver, spleen, muscle, and brain homogenates (outer wells) with antimelanosome serum and elimination of cross reaction by absorption with liver. *A* Organ homogenates distributed as indicated in the diagram; the center well contains unabsorbed antiserum against melanosomes. The result shows a clear cross reaction of antiserum with liver and spleen. The reaction against brain and muscle homogenates is very weak. *B* Organ homogenates distributed as indicated in the diagram. The center well contains antiserum against melanosomes which has been absorbed with liver. The result indicates that absorption of antimelanosome serum with liver eliminates cross reaction to spleen, brain and muscle as well.

The results reported in this paper indicate that when a given quantity of the melanosome fraction, purified by two successive density-gradient centrifugations, is injected into rabbits together with adjuvant, an agglutinating antibody is produced. This procedure has been applied to three different rabbits and all three produced detectable agglutinating activity.

Since the melanosome fraction does contain small amounts of particulate impurities [4] several experiments were done in an attempt to assess the specificity of the antiserum. Antiserum against the melanosome fraction does not exhibit any evidence of clumping activity against a crude particulate fraction from liver cells. This is evidence that the overt aggregation of the melanosome fraction by antiserum is due to particles specific to pigment cells presumably melanosomes.

When antisera absorbed with liver homogenate were tested against melanosomes, the ability to agglutinate was retained but the velocity of

*Table IV.* Effect of melanosome treatment on agglutination time

| Treatment of melanosomes | Agglutination time unabsorbed antiserum | Agglutination time in liver-absorbed antiserum |
|---|---|---|
| Untreated control | 1.9±0.1 | 7.5±0.3 |
| SDS, 2% solution at 100°C for 5 min | 1.7±0.3 | 7.4±0.2 |
| SDS, 2% solution at 60°C for 2 h | 1.7±0.2 | |
| SDS, 2% solution at 100°C for 5 min, two successive treatments | 3.5±0.4 | |
| Triton-X-100, 1% solution overnight at 4°C | 2.0±0.3 | |
| 0.2 M Carbonate at pH 10 4°C overnight | 1.6±0.2 | |
| Protease, 37°C, 8–10 h | 1.7±0.4 | |
| Protease as above after pretreatment with SDS at 100°C | no agglutination in three experiments | |

the agglutination reaction was reduced. This indicates that the particles in the melanosome fraction bear two classes of antigens: those in common with liver and spleen as well as a class of antigen(s) unique to the pigment cell at least to the extent that they are not found in liver, spleen, muscle, or brain homogenates.

Antigens in the melanosome fraction held in common with liver and spleen could be explained by any one of several hypotheses: These common antigens could be membranous contaminants of the melanosome fraction or they could be integral components of the melanosome which are not unique to pigment cells. If the first hypothesis is correct, one would expect to wash the melanosome particles free of casually adhering membrane particulates by detergents. Conversely, if these common antigens, as well as the relatively specific antigens, are integral components of the melanosomal structure, one might expect them to be resistant to mild solubilizing agents.

Since the detergent SDS is an effective general protein solvent as well as a solvent for hydrophobic proteins and membranes [5, 6, 8], one

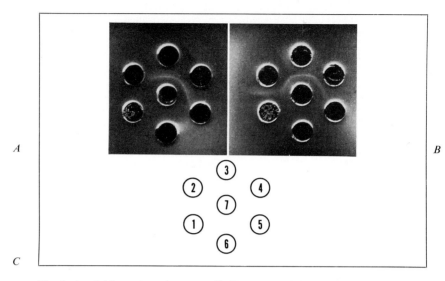

*Fig. 6.* A soluble antigen (center well, B) recovered from melanosomes by the non-ionic detergent Triton-X-100. *A* is similar to figure 4, showing that absorbed antiserum in well No. 2 no longer cross-reacts with liver homogenate. Well No. 1, control serum; well No. 2, antiserum absorbed with liver homogenate; wells No. 3 and No. 4, unabsorbed antiserum; the center well, No. 7, contains liver homogenate. *B* Contents of the outer wells 1 through 4 are identical to those in *A*. However, the center well contains soluble melanosome antigen(s). The detergent-soluble melanosome antigen(s) form a precipitin line with absorbed serum in well No. 2, indicating that the center well contains antigen(s) from the melanosome fraction not found in liver, spleen, brain or muscle cells.

would expect SDS to dissolve a significant portion of membrane fragments and nonspecifically adhering proteins which may contaminate the melanosome fraction. Since SDS seems to be relatively ineffective in destroying the antigenicity of particles in the melanosome fraction, the results indicate that both the specific and nonspecific antigens may be firmly bound to polymerized melanin. The fact that fungal protease does abolish agglutination is evidence that the antigen(s) are protein or associated with protein.

Evidence about the linkage between protein and melanin indicates that a thioether bond may be formed between cysteine and dopa during melanogenesis. Covalent bonding of this type between melanin and cysteine in protein would partially explain the observations that melanosome antigens are stable to detergents [2, 9, 11].

*References*

1 BLOIS, M. S.: Random polymers as a matrix for chemical evolution; in FOX Origins of prebiological systems, pp. 19–38 (Academic Press, New York 1965).

2 BRUMBAUGH, J. A. and FROILAND, T. G.: Dopa and cysteine incorporation into premelanosomes. Effects of cyclohexamide and gene substitution. J. invest. Derm. *60:* 172–178 (1973).

3 CAMPBELL, D. H.; GARVEY, J. S.; CREMER, N. E., and SUSSDORF, D. E.: Methods in immunology (Benjamin, New York 1964).

4 DOEZEMA, P.: Proteins from melanosomes of mouse and chick pigment cells. J. cell. Physiol. *82:* 65–73 (1973).

5 FAIRBANKS, G.; STECK, T. L., and WALLACH, D. F. H.: Electrophoretic analysis of the major polypeptides of the human erythrocyte membrane. Biochem. *10:* 2606–2616 (1971).

6 LAEMMLI, U. K.: Cleavage of structural proteins during assembly of the head of bacteriophage T4. Nature, Lond. *227:* 680–685 (1970).

7 LANGHOFF, H. VON; FEUERSTEIN, M. und SCHABINSKI, G.: Melanin Antikörperbildung bei Vitiligo. Hautarzt *16:* 209–212 (1965).

8 MAIZEL, J. V., jr.: Acrylamide gel electrophoresis of proteins and nucleic acids; in HABEL and SALTZMAN Fundamental techniques in virology, pp. 334–372 (Academic Press, New York 1969).

9 PROTA, G.: Structure and biogenesis of phaeomelanins; in RILEY Pigmentation: its genesis and biologic control, pp. 615–630 (Appleton Century Crofts, New York 1972).

10 WASSERMAN, H. P. and WALT, J. J. VAN DER: Antibodies against melanin: The significance of negative results. S. Afr. med. J. *47:* 7–9 (1973).

11 WHITTAKER, J. R.: Biosynthesis of a thiouracil pheomelanin in embryonic pigment cells exposed to thiouracil. J. biol. Chem. *246:* 6217–6226 (1971).

Dr. P. DOEZEMA, Division of Biology, Kansas State University, *Manhattan, KS 66506* (USA)

Pigment Cell, vol. 2, pp. 150–155 (Karger, Basel 1976)

# Allograft-Induced Antitumor Protection in the S91A Mouse Melanoma-DBA/2 Host System[1]

G. M. GORRIN and M. FOSTER

Mammalian Genetics Center, Department of Zoology,
The University of Michigan, Ann Arbor, Mich.

## Introduction

The pioneering studies of MacDowell et al. [7, 8] established that the antitumor (antileukemic) immunity of a susceptible mouse strain (C58) could be augmented by the administration of either sublethal doses of malignant cells or allogeneic tissue (minced fetal skin and/or viscera) prior to lethal tumor challenge. These studies were confirmed and extended, using the same tumor-host system, by HAN et al. [4]. In the latter study, allograft pretreatments consisted of homogenized adult liver, lymph node, thymus, or spleen, leading to augmented resistance to subsequently administered leukemic cells. This protective type of allograft pretreatment (using adult liver, spleen or, in our case, allogeneic B16 melanoma) was successfully extended to a solid tumor, namely the transplantable Harding-Passey melanoma growing in the susceptible BALB/c mouse strain [2, 3]. The study reported in this paper was pursued in an attempt to establish, by extension to another tumor-host system, the potentially general strategy of allograft-induced antitumor protection.

The basis of allograft-induced antitumor protection is still unclear. It could involve a general immune stimulus somehow leading to heightened host responsiveness to different tumor-associated antigens ('adjuvant effect'). It might also be due to cross reactions involving similar allograft and tumor antigens, in which case the augmented host's antitumor immunity might be essentially similar to a secondary graft rejection response. In contrast to these host-versus-graft reactions, the augmented antitumor re-

1 Work supported in part by grants from The University of Michigan Cancer Research Institute and Project FRR-967.

sponse might be initiated by allogeneic lymphocytes as graft-versus-host reactions, causing stimulated host antitumor defenses ('allogeneic effect' [5]. While our current study was not initially designed to discriminate among these *a priori* possibilities, our subsequent discussion will indicate that, in at least some instances, the elevated antitumor responses are likely to be cases of the host-versus-graft type.

## Materials and Methods

*Tumors and mice.* A transplantable amelanotic variant of mouse melanoma S91 ('S91A') was obtained from Microbiological Associates, Bethesda, Md., in the form of subcutaneous implants borne by strain DBA/2 ($H$-$2^d$) mice. This tumor presumably differs antigenically from the S91 melanoma grown in DBA/1J ($H$-$2^q$) mice. Preliminary screening tests of histocompatibility relations indicate that the 'S91A' almost invariably grows in DBA/2 graft recipients and in about 60% (24/39) of challenged BALB/c ($H$-$2^d$) graft recipients. It has not yet grown in such strains as DBA/1J ($H$-$2^q$; 0/2 takes), C57Bl/10 ($H$-$2^b$; 0/3 takes), and A/J ($H$-$2^a$; 0/5 takes). It is not clear whether the 'S91A' melanoma is completely syngeneic with DBA/2 cells, or whether it shares the major $H$-$2$ antigenic complement with normal DBA/2 cells, but differs from normal DBA/2 cells at one or more weak non-$H$-$2$ gene loci.

*Preimmunization.* One donor spleen was minced in 0.2 ml of Tissue Culture Medium 199 (Difco), drawn into a syringe and implanted subcutaneously into a tumor susceptible recipient. The same donor's liver (without the gallbladder), providing three to four preimmunizing doses, was minced in 0.4 ml of Medium 199 before subcutaneous implantation into recipients.

Following the lead of MacDowell *et al.* [8], we tested the protective effect of minced fetuses, prepared as follows: Female donors near term were sacrificed and both uteri were removed whole. In a sterile Petri dish, the fetuses were dissected out and the midsection (distal to the pectoral girdle and proximal to the pelvic girdle) of each fetus was removed and placed in a separate Petri dish. These were then minced in an approximately equal volume of TC Medium 199 until fine enough to be drawn into a syringe; 0.1 or 0.2 ml of this preparation was injected subcutaneously into each recipient.

*Tumor challenge.* Melanoma minces were prepared without any added material. Subcutaneous implants of 0.03 or 0.06 ml minced tumor resulted in nearly 100% takes in untreated DBA/2 hosts. Hosts pretreated with normal tissue implants were challenged contralaterally one week later. Untreated controls were challenged at the same time and on the same side with similar tumor implants. The challenge dosage was estimated to be of the order of $10^6$ viable tumor cells, as counted by dye exclusion in a 1:200 dilution of 0.2% trypan blue in TC Medium 199 (Difco).

*Treatment effects.* Tumor size was estimated by the product of externally measured greatest and least diameters (in mm$_2$). Complete tumor rejection was concluded when no recurrence was noted 2–4 weeks after disappearance of all external signs of tumor presence. Tumor growth retardation was scored when the tumors of

*Table I.* Tests of allograft protection of DBA/2 mice ($H$-$2^d$) challenged by S91A melanoma

| Treatment | No protection | | Protection | | Total |
|---|---|---|---|---|---|
| | takes, like controls | takes retarded | obvious rejection | rejection, 'no take' | |
| 1. Untreated DBA/2 controls (pooled) | 45 | – | 3 | – | 48 |
| 2. DBA/2 tumor propagators | 25 | – | – | – | 25 |
| 3. A/J ($H$-$2^a$) liver | 4 | 1 | 2 | 2 | 9 |
|     A/J spleen | 3 | 4 | 5 | 2 | 14 |
|     A/J fetus | 1 | 4 | – | 3 | 8 |
| 4. C57BL/10 ($H$-$2^b$) liver | 10 | – | 3 | – | 13 |
|     C57BL/10 spleen | 1 | – | 1 | – | 2 |
| 5. B10.D2 ($H$-$2^d$) liver | 6 | – | – | – | 6 |
|     B10.D2 spleen | 1 | – | – | – | 1 |
| 6. BALB/c ($H$-$2^d$) liver | 2 | – | – | – | 2 |
|     BALB/c spleen | – | 1 | – | – | 1 |
| 7. C3H ($H$-$2^k$) liver | 3 | – | – | – | 3 |
|     C3H spleen | – | – | 1 | – | 1 |
| 8. D2.GD ($H$-$2^g$) liver | 3 | – | – | – | 3 |
|     D2.GD spleen | 1 | – | – | – | 1 |
| 9. Lyophilized A/J liver | 4 | – | – | – | 4 |

the pretreated experimental host animals exhibited at least a 3-week delay in achieving progressive growth when compared with the slowest growing tumors in the corresponding control groups.

In a single pretreatment group (A/J allografts, table I), several instances of 'no take' were scored. In these cases, no early tiny tumor lump was observed one week after tumor implantation. In these cases, it seemed reasonable to conclude that these tumor challenges had been rejected sooner than usual after implantation. They were therefore classified as rejections, since other more obvious indications of antitumor protection had also been amply demonstrated in the same experimental pretreatment group.

## Results

The experimental results are summarized in table I and the following points can be made: (1) Significant antitumor protection was provided by

A/J (*H-2ª*) allografts. The pooled data, including cases of growth retardation, indicate a protection rate of more than 70⁰/₀ (23/31 protected). (2) Protection was also provided by C57Bl/10 (*H-2ᵇ*) allografts, but not by B10.D2 (*H-2ᵈ*) or BALB/c (also *H-2ᵈ*). In these cases, allografts differing from the DBA/2 (*H-2ᵈ*) hosts at *both H-2* and non-*H-2* gene loci were necessary for antitumor protection. When allografts were identical for the *H-2* complex, but differed from the DBA/2 recipients at only the weaker (non-*H-2*) gene loci, no significant antitumor protection was observed. (3) The data for protection by C3H (*H-2ᵏ*) allografts are meager, but suggestive. In any event, more data are required. Allografts from the *H-2* recombinant strain D2.GD also seemed to provide no protection. (4) Finally, despite the small sample size, there is an indication that lyophilized A/J liver fails to provide anti-S91A protection, in contrast with the better than 50⁰/₀ protection rate afforded by minced fresh liver. Presumably the lyophilization leads to sufficient alteration of cell-surface antigens so that the stimulus leading to antitumor protection is lacking.


*Discussion*

Our current and previous results [3, 4], together with those of Mac-Dowell *et al.* [7, 8] and Han *et al.* [4] indicate the emerging generality of allograft-induced antitumor protection as at least a feasible prophylactic strategy. It is clear, however, that the allograft stimulus must be a strong one, due to a major single histocompatibility gene difference (i.e. *H-2* in the mouse) and/or to the summation effect of a number of weaker histocompatibility gene differences (i.e. non-*H-2* differences in the mouse). The latter possibility was not demonstrated in our current study, but it has been shown to be effective in our laboratory by Mr. Larry Pease [10]. He implanted $F_1$ hybrid spleen or liver allografts from the *H-2ᵈ* identical parental strains BALB/c × DBA/2 into BALB/c recipients, followed by contralateral lethal dose challenges with Harding-Passey melanoma implants. Three of 4 $F_1$ spleen and 4 of 5 $F_1$ liver-pretreated mice rejected subsequent tumor challenges.

Because viable donor lymphocytes are present in the allogeneic tissue graft, two related reactions are possible: graft lymphocytes reacting against host tissues (GVH or graft-versus-host) and host lymphocytes rejecting graft tissue (HVG or host-versus-graft). In both cases, there may be nonspecific activation of lymphocytes, some of which are capable of antitumor activity. The data presented do not distinguish between these reactions, and it seems possible that both may play a role. The work of PEASE [10] indicates that HVG alone may be sufficient for inducing tumor immunity. This further supports the successful use of a similar strategy by MacDOWELL et al. [8] who transplanted $F_1$ hybrid fetal cells to protect susceptible parental strain recipients (C58) against lethal dose challenges of leukemic cells. In addition, the work of KATZ et al. [6] and ELLMAN et al. [1] show that GVH alone (the 'allogeneic effect') is sufficient to cause protection against leukemia in guinea pigs. Experiments have been initiated in our laboratory which may through the use of $F_1$ hybrids help decide whether either one or both of these reactions are important in our current study.

The question of possible cross-reactivity involving similar allograft and challenge tumor antigens appears to defy definitive resolution. MURPHY [9] has demonstrated cross-reactivity between the products of the K and the D portions of the *H-2* region of the mouse. Specifically, anti-*H-2K*$^k$ cross-reacts with *H-2D*$^d$. It seems likely, however, that this mechanism is not instrumental in the antitumor protection demonstrated here, primarily because there is no *H-2* difference between the tumor and host tissues. One would not expect the host to respond against his own antigenic specificities. If this were the case, then an autoimmune syndrome would be manifested, and there has been no evidence of such a response for at least several months after the rejection of both allograft pretreatment and challenge tumor grafts. Any cross-reactivity in a syngeneic tumor-host system must therefore be specifically limited to similarities between allograft and tumor-associated antigens. In contrast to the *H-2* situation, it is impossible to rule out cross-reactivity between these lesser but nonetheless important histocompatibility alleles (non-*H-2*), because of the extremely complex antigenic nature of the allograft.

The data presented do not distinguish among HVG, GVH, or cross-reactivity. Any one or any combination could account for the augmentation of the host's ability to reject transplanted syngeneic tumor grafts when preimmunized with living allogeneic tissue.

*Summary*

1. Allografts consisting of subcutaneously administered minced spleen, liver or fetuses from donor strains A/J (*H-2*$^a$) or C57Bl/10 (*H-2*$^b$) resulted in significant

protection of DBA/2 (*H-2*ᵈ) recipients when contralaterally challenged subcutaneously (one week later) by mouse melanoma S91.

2. No protection was observed when allograft donor strains differed from the DBA/2 recipients at only weaker non-*H-2* gene loci (i.e. *H-2*ᵈ strains BALB/c and B10.D2).

3. Lyophilized A/J liver provided no antitumor protection, in contrast with the protective effects of live A/J liver allografts.

## *References*

1   ELLMAN, L.; KATZ, D.; GREEN, I.; PAUL, W. E., and BENACERRAF, B.: Mechanisms involved in the antileukemic effect of immunocompetent allogeneic lymphoid cell transfer. Cancer Res. *32:* 141–148 (1972).

2   FOSTER, M.; HERMAN, J., and THOMSON, L.: Genetic and immunologic approaches to transplantable mouse melanomas; in RILEY Pigment Cell, vol. 1, pp. 390–398 (Karger, Basel 1973).

3   FOSTER, M.; HERMAN, J.; THOMSON, L., and EITZEN, L.: Induced melanoma rejection. Yale J. Biol. Med. *46:* 655–660 (1973).

4   HAN, I. H.; JOHNSON, A. G., and MURPHY, W. H.: Protection of C58 mice by normal murine tissues against transplantable leukemia, Line I_b. J. natn. Cancer Inst. *42:* 815–824 (1969).

5   KATZ, D. H.: The allogeneic effect on immune responses. Model for regulatory influences of T lymphocytes on the immune system. Transplantn Rev. *12:* 141–179 (1972).

6   KATZ, D. H.; ELLMAN, L.; PAUL, W. E.; GREEN, I., and BENACERRAF, B.: Resistance of guinea pigs to leukemia following transfer of immunocompetent allogeneic lymphoid cells. Cancer Res. *32:* 133–140 (1972).

7   MacDowell, E. C.; TAYLOR, M. J., and POTTER, J. S.: Immunization of mice naturally susceptible to a transplantable leukemia. Proc. Soc. exp. Biol. Med. *32:* 84–86 (1934).

8   MacDowell, E. C.; TAYLOR, M. J., and POTTER, J. S.: The dependence of protection against a transplantable mouse leukemia upon the genetic constitution of the immunizing tissue. Proc. natn. Acad. Sci. USA *21:* 507–508 (1935).

9   MURPHY, D. B.: Cross-reactivity between *H-2K* and *H-2D* products; PhD dissertation, Ann. Arbor (1974).

10  PEASE, L. R.: Personal commun. (1974).

Dr. G. M. GORRIN, Mammalian Genetics Center, Department of Zoology, The University of Michigan, *Ann Arbor, MI 48104* (USA)

Pigment Cell, vol. 2, pp. 156–162 (Karger, Basel 1976)

# Nature of Antigens Associated with Murine Melanoma

J.-C. Bystryn[1]

Department of Dermatology, New York University School of Medicine, New York, N.Y.

The identification and characterization of tumor antigens has progressed furthest when sensitive and quantitative assays have been available, such as the radioimmunoassays for carcinoembryonic antigen and some viral proteins. In the case of melanoma, where such assays are not generally available, progress in antigen purification has been slow. Jehn et al. [8] fractionated the fluid of a cystic melanoma by starch gel electrophoresis. An antigenic fraction, identified by lymphocyte stimulation, was found to have the mobility of a $\beta$-globulin and a molecular weight of 40,000. Char et al. [6] partially purified antigenic material, identified by delayed skin testing, from the sonicates of membranes of melanoma cells. The material had a molecular weight of 28,000 by Sephadex G-200 chromatography. In both cases, some specificity was demonstrated by lack of reactions in normal subjects or normal lymphocytes.

We have recently [4, 5] developed methods of radiolabeling and identifying tumor antigens which are sensitive and quantitative and which can be applied to the study of most cellular antigens. These methods have enabled us to identify and partially characterize some antigens associated with murine B16 melanoma.

### Methods and Results

*Radiolabeling, solubilization and assay of melanoma-associated antigens (MAA).* Cellular proteins (cytoplasmic and cell surface) of B16 me-

1   Supported by Public Health Service research Grants CA-13844-03 and CA-13662-03 and the Chernow Foundation.

lanoma or syngeneic fibroblast cells in tissue culture were radiolabeled with $^3$H-leucine and solubilized with detergent, or recovered directly from culture medium [4]. MAA were identified by an antigen-binding assay based on the co-precipitation by anti-IgG of complexes of radiolabeled MAA formed with an excess of antimelanoma IgG. Antimelanoma IgG was isolated from sera of syngeneic mice hyperimmunized to this tumor, and control IgG from normal mouse sera. Specific binding of MAA was calculated by subtracting radioactivity bound by normal IgG from that bound by an equimolar amount of antimelanoma IgG. MAA accounted for 0.5–2% of acid precipitable radioactivity in $^3$H-leucine-labeled cell lysates and for 1.6–3.7% of acid precipitable radioactivity in the corresponding culture medium.

*Partial purification and characterization of MAA.* Radiolabeled solubilized B16 melanoma proteins were precipitated by 52% ammonium sulfate and fractionated on Sephadex G-200. Three radioactive peaks were eluted after the exclusion volume. MAA were identified in only one of the peaks. In this fraction, as much as 48 times more radiolabeled material was bound by antimelanoma IgG than by equimolar amounts of normal IgG. The molecular weight of the MAA was estimated to be 150,000–200,000 daltons. The antigenic material was further fractionated by column chromatography on DEAE-Sephadex (A-25). Elution with NaCl in 0.01 M Tris buffer at pH 8.0 in discrete steps (0.1, 0.2 and 0.5 M) gave two peaks, both of which contained MAA. A number of different proteins was present in each peak, as shown by the presence of 2–3 bands in each peak obtained by acrylamide gel electrophoresis.

To obtain information on the chemical nature of Sephadex G-200 purified MAA, its *in vitro* antigenicity was determined from the proportion of radiolabeled material bound specifically by antimelanoma IgG, following treatment with proteolytic enzymes, neuraminidase, acid, base and heat. As can be seen in figure 1, antigenicity of MAA was markedly increased by neuraminidase, and decreased by proteolytic enzymes, heat, acid and base. These findings, together with the UV absorption spectrum of the material, allow tentative identification of MAA as glycoproteins.

*Specificity of MAA.* Specificity of Sephadex G-200 purified MAA was studied by:

1) Quantitative serum absorption: Serum of rabbits immunized to B16 melanoma was absorbed exhaustively with normal syngeneic murine tissue. Following absorption, rabbit antimelanoma serum bound approximately 10 times more radiolabeled MAA than did normal rabbit serum or

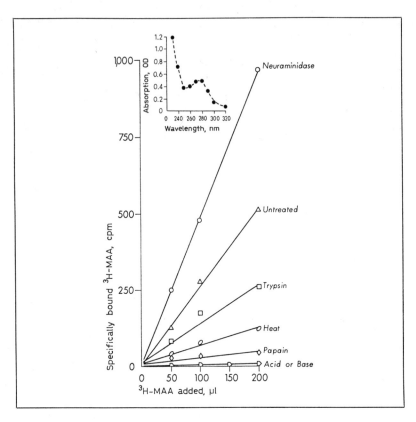

*Fig. 1.* Specific binding by antimelanoma IgG of ³H-leucine-labeled MAA (partially purified by G-200 chromatography) after treatment with proteolytic enzymes, heat, cold, or neuraminidase. Insert shows UV absorption spectra typical of a protein.

serum of rabbits immunized to normal syngeneic murine tissue absorbed in a similar manner. As can be seen in figure 2, further absorption of antimelanoma serum with normal syngeneic tissues (liver, kidney, brain, spleen or muscle) or allogeneic tissues prepared from a panel of mice carrying 23 of the 25 known murine transplantation antigens did not significantly decrease its ability to bind radiolabeled MAA. Absorption with unrelated syngeneic tumors (BW 10232 mammary adenocarcinoma or ESR 586 preputial carcinoma) or allogeneic melanoma (S91 melanoma) reduced binding of MAA by approximately 45 and 55%, respectively. By

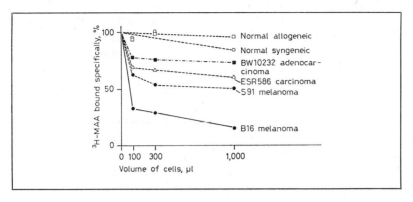

*Fig. 2.* Specific binding of ³H-leucine-labeled, partially purified MAA by rabbit antimelanoma serum following absorption with increasing volume of normal or malignant murine tissues. Specific binding was calculated by subtracting from cpm bound by rabbit antimelanoma serum, that bound by normal rabbit serum absorbed with an equal volume of cells.

*Table I.* Antibodies to MAA in immunized mice

| Immunizing antigen | Antibody to MAA, cpm |
|---|---|
| MAA in Freund's adjuvant | 342 |
| Freund's adjuvant | 24 |
| PBS | 25 |

1 Expressed as cpm of ³H-MAA (purified by G-200 chromatography; input cpm: 3,300) bound specifically by mouse serum. Specific binding was calculated by subtracting cpm bound by 10 µl of normal mouse serum from cpm bound by 10 µl of test serum.

contrast, absorption with B16 melanoma decreased binding of MAA by 80%.

2) Specific binding of radiolabeled syngeneic fibroblast materials: The ability of murine antimelanoma serum to specifically bind radiolabeled material in lysate or culture medium of syngeneic fibroblasts was determined. Parallel experiments were performed with melanoma cells. Murine antimelanoma serum bound specifically some radiolabeled material in fibroblast lysate in 4 of 7 experiments, and in culture medium in 1 of 8 experiments. By contrast, specific binding of radiolabeled material in

melanoma lysate and culture medium was present in every case. In every instance, the proportion of specifically bound acid precipitable radioactivity in melanoma preparations was 2–15 times greater than that in corresponding fibroblast preparations.

*Immunogenicity of MAA.* MAA, partially purified by Sephadex G-200 chromatography, were found to be immunogenic in syngeneic mice. Groups of 10 C57BL/6 mice were immunized by 3 weekly injections in the foot pad of 0.1 mg of MAA in complete Freund's adjuvant. Serum from each group was collected and pooled one week later. Antibodies to MAA were measured by a recently described double antibody antigen-binding assay [5]. As can be seen in table I, antibodies to MAA were present in mice immunized to this material, but not in mice immunized with Freund's adjuvant alone or PBS.


## Discussion

Our results indicate that murine B16 melanoma has antigens which are quantitatively and/or qualitatively different from those in normal allogeneic and syngeneic tissues and unrelated syngeneic malignancies and allogeneic melanoma. These antigens appear to be glycoproteins with a MW of approximately 150,000. The *in vitro* antigenicity of these antigens is markedly increased by treatment with neuraminidase. These MAA are immunogenic in syngeneic mice.

The innovative aspects of this study are: (1) The labeling of tumor-associated antigens by incubating viable tumor cells with radioactive precursors. This approach provides a generally applicable method of labeling tumor associated antigens, and may prove useful in attempts to isolate antigens from human melanoma and other cancer. (2) The isolation of tumor antigens from culture media. These findings suggest that 'shedding' or active secretion of tumor antigens by tumor cells may occur.

In earlier studies, we have shown that B16 melanoma is immunogenic in syngeneic mice and that mice can be partially protected from otherwise lethal doses of this cancer by active immunization with irradiated or sublethal doses of melanoma cells [3]. Our current observation that partially purified MAA are immunogenic in syngeneic mice suggests they may play a role in the immune response to this tumor. In this respect, it is particularly significant that *in vitro* antigenicity of MAA was markedly augmented by treatment with neuraminidase. Treatment of purified tumor antigens with this enzyme may enhance their potential effectiveness as immunotherapeutic agents. It has already been found that treatment of whole tumor cells with neuraminidase increases their ability to induce active specific immunity to a variety of animal tumors.

Our observations also support the growing evidence that some antigens may be shared by normal and malignant tissues. Thus, in mice, type C viral group-specific antigens may be present in normal and leukemic cells [10]. In man, embryonic antigens may be present in gastrointestinal malignancies and in small amounts in normal tissues [9]. Shared antigens between human melanoma and normal tissue is suggested by various autoantibodies to normal tissue in patients with melanoma [2, 12], of specifically sensitized lymphocytes [7] and antimelanoma antibodies [11] in normal black persons, and of fetal antigens on melanoma cell surfaces [1].

## Summary

Antigens associated with murine B16 melanoma were radiolabeled and partially purified by ammonium sulfate precipitation and Sephadex G-200 chromatography. They appear to be glycoproteins with MW of approximately 150,000. These antigens are quantitatively and/or qualitatively different from antigens in normal syngeneic and allogeneic tissues and in unrelated syngeneic malignancies and allogeneic melanoma. The antigenicity of these antigens was markedly increased by treatment with neuraminidase and they induced antibodies in syngeneic mice.

## References

1   Avis, P. and Lewis, M. G.: Brief communication: tumor-associated fetal antigens in human tumors. J. natn. Cancer Inst. 51: 1063–1066 (1973).
2   Bystryn, J.-C.; Abel, E., and Weidman, A.: Antibodies against the cytoplasm of human epidermal cells. Archs Derm. 108: 241–244 (1973).
3   Bystryn, J.-C.; Bart, R. S.; Livingston, P., and Kopf, A. W.: Growth and immunogenicity of B16 melanoma. J. invest. Derm. 63: 369–373 (1974).
4   Bystryn, J.-C.; Schenkein, I.; Baur, S., and Uhr, J. W.: Partial isolation and characterization of antigen(s) associated with murine melanoma. J. natn. Cancer Inst. 52: 1263–1269 (1974).
5   Bystryn, J.-C.; Schenkein, I., and Uhr, J. W.: Double-antibody radioimmunoassay for B16 melanoma antibodies. J. natn. Cancer Inst. 52: 911–915 (1974).
6   Char, D. H.; Hollingshead, A.; Cogan, D. G., et al.: Cutaneous delayed hy-

persensitivity reactions to soluble melanoma antigen in patients with ocular malignant melanoma. New Engl. J. Med. *291:* 274–277 (1974).

7    HELLSTRÖM, I.; HELLSTRÖM, K. E.; SJÖGREN, H. O., *et al.:* Destruction of cultivated melanoma cells by lymphocytes from healthy black (North American Negro) donors. Int. J. Cancer *11:* 116–122 (1973).

8    JEHN, U. W.; NATHANSON, L.; SCHWARTZ, R. S., *et al.: In vitro* lymphocyte stimulation by a soluble antigen from malignant melanoma. New Engl. J. Med. *283:* 329–333 (1970).

9    LO GERFO, P. and HESTER, F.: Demonstration of tumor-associated antigen in normal colon and lung. J. surg. Oncol. *4:* 1–7 (1972).

10   PARKS, W. P.; LIVINGSTON, D. M.; TODARO, G. J., *et al.:* Radioimmunoassay of mammalian type C viral proteins. III. Detection of viral antigen in normal murine cells and tissues. J. exp. Med. *137:* 622–635 (1970).

11   WHITEHEAD, R. H. and HUGHES, L. E.: Fluorescent antibody studies in malignant melanoma. Br. J. Cancer *28:* 525 (1973).

12   WHITEHOUSE, J. M. A.: Circulating antibodies in human malignant disease. Br. J. Cancer *28:* suppl. 1, p. 170 (1973).

Dr. J.-C. BYSTRYN, Room H-307, Department of Dermatology, New York University Medical Center, 550 First Avenue, *New York, NY 10016* (USA)

Pigment Cell, vol. 2, pp. 163–173 (Karger, Basel 1976)

# Melanoma Enhancement by Viral-Induced Stress[1]

VERNON RILEY and DARREL SPACKMAN

Pacific Northwest Research Foundation and Fred Hutchinson Cancer Research Center, Seattle, Wash.

## Introduction

Melanomas have a reputation for unpredictable clinical behavior [1, 2]. Cumulative data suggest that certain melanomas may generate an immunological response in the host that occasionally results in a temporary or permanent regression of the malignant lesions [3, 4]. It thus seems that such tumors are either capable of eliciting a specially vigorous host immunological response or, as an alternative, they may exist in a more fragile histocompatible equilibrium, and are thus more susceptible to an ordinary immune response by the host.

For comparative experimental purposes, we have carried in continuous transplant a nonpigmented variant of the B-16 mouse melanoma. The growth rate of this tumor is significantly less than its pigmented counterpart, and its tendency to undergo spontaneous regression also distinguishes it from the more syngeneic pigmented parent. This suppressible nonpigmented melanoma is thus a suitable experimental model for testing the influence of subtle immunological modifiers.

The lactate dehydrogenase-elevating virus (LDH-virus) is a useful benign biological device for inducing moderate immunological alterations in either a normal or tumor-bearing mouse [5–8]. The following data will illustrate the capabilities of this ubiquitous virus in enhancing neoplastic behavior when the tumor-host relationship is sufficiently tenuous that

1   These studies were partially supported by National Cancer Institute grants CA 12188 and CA 16308; and by the National Science Foundation, the Leukemia Research Foundation, and the Eagles Cancer Fund. Valuable assistance was provided by HEATHER MCCLANAHAN, MARY DENNIS, JOAN BLOOM, M. A. FITZMAURICE, and Dr. G. A. SANTISTEBAN.

small shifts in immunological competence can determine the course of the malignancy and the subsequent fate of the host. The LDH-virus appears to function as an immunosuppressant and tumor-enchancing agent through its adverse effects upon T and B cells [5–8]. The destruction of T cells and thymus tissue by the virus is apparently caused indirectly through a typical stress response that includes an elevation in plasma corticosterone, which is known to attack lymphatic cells and tissues [9, 10].

## Materials and Methods

### Mice

Two mouse strains were employed in these studies. These were female $F_1$ hybrid C57BL/6 × DBA/2 (referred to as BDF), and inbred C3H/Hef mice, all between 8 and 12 weeks of age, and weighing 18–22 g. These mice were obtained from commercial breeders at approximately 5 weeks of age. Upon arrival in our laboratory they were randomly segregated into groups of ten, and housed in standard plastic holding cages. These cage groupings were maintained throughout the experimental period. Female BDF mice were used both for routine passage of the B-16 melanomas and for the experiments utilizing these tumors. The Gardner tumor was implanted into C3H/Hef females for both serial passage and experiments.

### Animal Environment

Standard plastic cages, 11.5×7×5 inches, containing 0.5–0.75 inches of San-I-Cel ground corncob bedding, were used to house ten mice. In our experience, plastic cages are superior to metal cages in terms of insulation, resistance to temperature changes, and thus minimization of sound and thermal stress factors. Inasmuch as endocrine and other diurnal effects are related to light and dark exposures, the plastic cages are also preferable for controlling admittance of light to the animals. Standard 12-hour intervals of light and dark were controlled by automatic clock switches.

### Tumors

Without special processing, most transplantable tumors carry the LDH-virus as a perpetual contamination [5, 8]. Since the hazards that this virus may cause in the interpretation of data have been demonstrated [12, 13], all tumors utilized in these studies were processed to remove this virus. For experimental purposes, the virus was intentionally reintroduced into specific mouse groups as appropriate. Such infected mice and noninfected controls were housed and handled so as to avoid cross-contamination. Critical monitoring for absence of the virus in controls was a standard procedure.

The B-16 pigmented and nonpigmented mouse melanomas have been maintained in our laboratory for about 8 years by intermittent passage in BDF female mice, or stored at –80 °C. For nonmelanoma comparative purposes, the 6C3HED-OG Gardner lymphosarcoma was employed.

### Protection from Stress

All animals, including both stock and experimental groups, were protected by a special barrier housing system consisting of ventilated enclosed shelves. Fresh, tempered air was provided using a single pass, filtered, laminar airflow that is vented outside of the building following contact with the mice and their generated aerosols, odors, and pheromones [14]. These housing facilities minimize uncontrolled stress-inducing stimuli that are of importance in studies concerned with adrenal cortical and related stress responses [15]. In order to minimize the stress known to be involved in handling mice, the animals were not numbered until death or autopsy, and were not subjected to any other manipulations not essential to the experimental procedures.

### Mouse Diet and Sanitation

The mouse diet consisted of Wayne Lab Blox pellets supplied through the cage-top hopper. This nutritionally complete diet was available at all times, as was clean water provided by pint glass bottles and stainless steel drinking tubes. High standards of sanitation were employed in the routine changing and sterilization of drinking bottles, tubes, and cages.

### DMS Injections

Dexamethasone (DMS) was administered intraperitoneally as a freshly prepared saline suspension. Because of limited solubility, the DMS diffused slowly to give a long-lasting effect from a single dose of 50 mg/kg.

### LDH-Virus

The LDH-virus was administered intraperitoneally to appropriate groups, usually at the time of tumor implantation. A 0.1 ml dose of 1:100 dilution of pooled mouse plasma having an original titer of $10^{10}$ infectious U/ml ($ID_{50}$) was used. Characterization of the LDH-virus and a description of assay methods have been previously reported [5].

### Organ Weights

The thymus weight responses of intact mice to infection with the LDH-virus were compared with those of animals adrenalectomized 24 h prior to inoculation with the virus. Noninfected mice were sham-injected with saline and used as controls. At autopsy the weights of the thymus, spleen, and pooled inguinal and axillary lymph nodes were determined for each animal. Similar measurements were made following administration of DMS or of any other stress-inducing procedure such as rotational-induced anxiety [19].

### Tumor Implantation and Measurements

The B-16 melanomas and the Gardner lymphosarcoma (6C3HED) grow as solid tumor masses when implanted intramuscularly or subcutaneously. The donor tumors were harvested aseptically and injected into recipient mice as a 20–50% suspension of free cells and small fragments of tumor tissue in 0.9% NaCl solution [5]. In order to follow the tumor growth and regression quantitatively, the tumor mass was measured in three dimensions by calipers [5].

*Assay for Plasma Corticosterone in Mice*

The microfluorimetric assay was developed in our laboratories [15, 16] and is based on the procedure described by GLICK *et al.* [17]. Our assays use 50 $\mu$l of plasma and thus duplicate assays can be performed on the 100–120 $\mu$l of plasma obtained from each mouse by the nonharmful orbital bleeding procedure [18].

## Results

Figure 1 illustrates the differential influence of LDH-virus infection upon the growth of the pigmented B-16 melanoma, as compared with the slower growing nonpigmented B-16 melanoma. Apparently, transformation from the pigmented to nonpigmented neoplastic state results, in this case at least, in a tumor with less histocompatibility than the original pigmented tumor. As a consequence, a striking difference in the growth rate and of the percentage of lethal tumors developing has been observed. This may be interpreted to indicate that the pigmented tumor is more syngeneic than the nonpigmented variant. Thus, under these circumstances the presence of the virus, which has a moderate modulating effect upon the immunocompetence of the host, is unable to exhibit any tangible influence upon the rapidly growing pigmented tumor. This is in contrast to the increased growth rate observed in LDH-virus-infected animals bearing the nonpigmented tumor.

Figure 2b indicates that the LDH-virus has a similar enhancing effect upon the Gardner lymphosarcoma, whose degree of syngeneity is also questionable. Again, in this instance, the presence of the virus enhances tumor growth rate and increases the percentage of lethal tumor takes following transplantation. Thus at 30 days following tumor cell implantation, 5 of 10 tumors in the nonvirus mice had completely regressed, while in the virus-infected group, only 1 out of 10 had regressed. In respect to survival, 9 out of 10 of the nonvirus mice were alive, but only 3 out of 10 of the virus-infected animals.

Figure 2a shows the hormonal-mediated enhancement of tumor growth that was produced by the direct administration of DMS. This synthetic corticoid functions in a manner similar to the elevated corticosterone that results from infection by the LDH-virus. Thus the actions of an infectious biological entity and of a biochemical hormone both produced a significant tumor growth enhancement. These results are consistent with the working hypothesis that the stresses resulting from each of these phy-

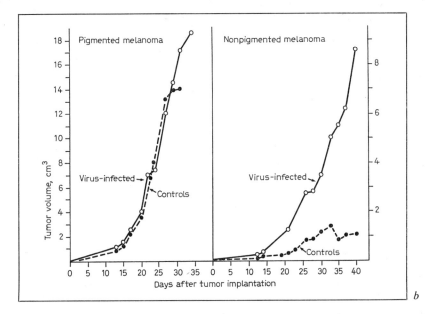

Fig. 1. Comparison of the influence of an LDH-virus infection on a rapidly growing pigmented B-16 mouse melanoma (a), with a slower growing, suppressed nonpigmented variant of B-16 origin (b). Similar tumor suspensions were implanted in all groups using BDF females between 10 and 14 weeks of age. Tumor growth was determined by three-dimensional caliper measurements.

siological activities have similar damaging effects, namely an adverse influence upon the immunological competence of the tumor-bearing host.

This hypothesis is further supported by the data shown in figure 3 which illustrate the influence of three distinct stress factors on the induction of thymus involution. Figure 3a shows the effect of the LDH virus on loss of thymus weight as a function of time following infection, whereas figure 3b indicates that a similar effect can be induced by the administration of a single dose of dexamethasone. In figure 3c similar effects were obtained by the induction of anxiety stress through the slow rotation of mice at 45 rpm. This nontraumatic stress causes an increase in plasma corticosterone, which is followed by thymus involution and lymphocytopenia, as well as by a loss in weight of other lymphatic tissues such as lymph nodes and spleen [19].

The LDH-virus-infected groups were inoculated with $10^7$ ($ID_{50}$) infectious units per mouse. All groups were autopsied at 24, 48 and 96 h

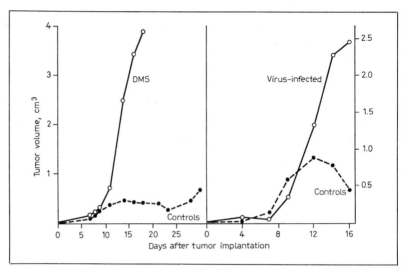

*a*

*b*

*Fig. 2.* Demonstration of the tumor-enhancing effects of two varieties of stress on the Gardner lymphosarcoma. *a* The consequences of synthetic corticoid elevation following the administration of a single dose of a long-acting preparation of DMS. This chart shows the tumor enhancement which presumably occurs as the result of impairment of the host immunological apparatus, as indicated by T cell lymphocytopenia, and partial destruction of thymus tissue, peripheral nodes and spleen. *b* A similar tumor enhancement may be observed following the intentional inoculation of a benign murine virus (LDH-virus). It has been established that the LDH-virus is also capable of causing an impairment of the immunocompetence of normal or tumor-bearing mice as evidenced by lymphocytopenia and thymus involution. Both DMS and the LDH-virus were inoculated on day 0, which was the day of the 6C3HED Gardner lymphosarcoma implantation.

after virus inoculation or sham injection. These intervals were chosen to coincide with the early peak in LDH-virus titers, and with the lymphocytopenia that has been shown to occur following inoculation with the LDH-virus.

## Discussion

As a consequence of several interrelated developments, it has been established that experiments using mouse models for the study of immunological and neoplastic problems are undoubtedly complicated, and in

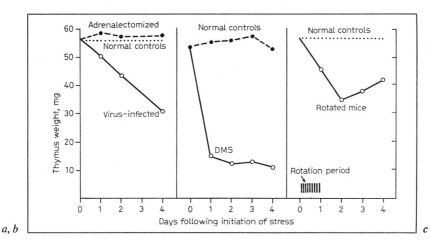

*Fig. 3.* Thymus involution variously produced by an infectious agent (the LDH-virus), a biochemical substance (DMS, a synthetic corticoid), and anxiety-stress associated with the disorienting effects of slow rotation of an entire cage of mice following their removal from protective storage. *a* $10^7$ infectious units of the LDH-virus were injected on day 0 into both intact and adrenalectomized female BAF mice. The regression line of the thymus weights of the virus-infected mice were fitted by the method of least squares; its difference from the response of the virus-infected adrenalectomized mice, or the normal controls, was highly significant statistically ($p<0.001$). *b* The thymus involution produced by a single injection of an insoluble suspension of DMS, providing a total dose of 50 mg/kg which was absorbed over an extended period. *c* The thymus destruction which results from stress associated with cage rotation at 45 rpm for 10 min out of each hour for a 24-hour period. During this mild stress period the plasma corticosterone was elevated approximately 5-fold.

some cases compromised, by the inadvertent and unappreciated stress that is present in mice maintained in conventional housing facilities and handled in the usual manner. The anxiety-stress of such mice is readily demonstrated by a determination of their plasma corticosterone. The quiescent corticosterone level of unstressed animals in our protective animal rooms is 30–50 ng/ml during the morning hours, whereas in mice housed in conventional animal rooms, the plasma corticosterone levels are usually elevated and have been shown to be in the range of 150–500 ng/ml for those tested.

The physiological consequences of such stress is readily demonstrable only if the investigator has access to protective animal housing facilities, and is alert to the special requirements for handling and bleeding the experimental animals. When the foregoing basic conditions are met, the following hormonal, cellular and organ alterations can be shown to occur in stressed mice: a 5- to 10-fold increase in plasma corticosterone, a substantial lymphocytopenia (largely T cells), involution or weight loss in lymphatic organs including the thymus, peripheral lymph nodes, and spleen. These biochemical and physical alterations produce an animal that is not suitable for most critical experimental purposes. The importance and potency of these stress-induced or stress-mediated effects can be further demonstrated by controlled studies with certain neoplastic processes. By selection of an appropriate tumor, as shown in figures 1 and 2, striking changes of enhanced tumor growth can be shown to occur in variously stressed mice as compared with nonstressed controls. Such stresses can unknowingly be present in mice, resulting either from most types of conventional animal housing, or from the ubiquitous presence of the LDH-virus perpetuated in serial tumor passages [5, 8].

In order to clearly demonstrate these important biological phenomena, which have obvious significance to animal studies, the following experimental requirements are either desirable, or mandatory: suitable protective, stress-free animal housing facilities; animals that are environmentally adjusted and in social equilibrium; modified animal handling techniques designed to minimize or to eliminate stress; and access to experimental tumors that are free of the LDH-virus. Techniques that are desirable for such studies include the use of a rapid bleeding technique, such as the retro-orbital procedure [18], which will permit 10 mice to be bled in 3.5 min; mastery of a sensitive microassay for plasma corticosterone utilizing 50-$\mu$l samples of plasma; a controlled, nontraumatic means for intentionally inducing quantitative and reproducible anxiety-stress that can be automatically programmed for intensity and periodicity [19], and laboratory personnel capable of reliably performing sophisticated techniques in endocrinology, immunology, biochemistry, surgery, and animal handling.

We do not ascribe the differential tumor growth effects observed to the presence or absence of pigment or melanin. The enhancement of tumor growth, or incidence, by factors that impair the immunocompetence of the host, probably could only be observed where the host is able to exert a controlling influence on either the establishment or subsequent growth rate of the tumor. Our limited observations imply that no tumor enhancement would be produced by the LDH-virus, by DMS, or any oth-

*Table I.* Influence of pregnancy and psychosocial stress on plasma corticosterone in female C3H mice

| Experimental conditions | Plasma corticosterone, ng/ml | |
|---|---|---|
| | exp. 1 | exp. 2 |
| Controls (nonstressed) | 38 | 42 |
| Population cage females (not pregnant) | 190 | 197 |
| Population cage females (pregnant) | 1,040 | 1,085 |

The plasma corticosterone values in each experiment were determined from pooled plasma from 4 mice for each group. Duplicate determinations on each pool provided the average values shown for each experiment.

er immunosuppressant, when the tumor is not under the partial control of the host. It is the disruption of such control that permits stress, DMS, or the LDH-virus to produce an enhancing effect. Thus, the potential hazards of stress-inducing circumstances, in neoplasia or other diseases, reside primarily where a controlled equipoise exists between the host and a malignant or incipient pathological process.

Pregnancy has been shown in some instances to be an additional risk in women with melanoma [21–23], and is thus frequently terminated to avoid exacerbation of quiescent or limited disease. Similar risks apply to the potential course of other pathologies such as ocular histoplasmosis. These observations carry two relevant implications: (1) such disease processes are restrained by the normal defense mechanisms of the host, and (2) pregnancy tends to impair optimum defense. A further extension of these observations would predict that pregnancy would only be capable of a detrimental effect if the host were exerting partial control over the growth or extension of the malignancy. While a variety of physiological and hormonal alterations occur during pregnancy, only minimal attention has been given to the increase of corticosteroids and their potential effects. Table I demonstrates the striking increase that occurs in the plasma corticosterone of pregnant mice maintained in a stressful population cage. Since such corticoid elevations have an adverse effect on both the thymus and T cells, impairment of cell-mediated immunity is a logical consequence. Thus any increase in adrenal corticoids to the level where T cell populations are compromised carries a risk of neoplastic enhancement.

## Summary

The influence of biological stress in promoting the enhancement of tumor growth in a nonpigmented melanoma is demonstrated and analyzed. Similar effects were obtained with other stress-associated stimuli. Biological stress was imposed by infecting the tumor-bearing mice with a relatively benign murine agent, the LDH-virus, which is capable of causing a temporary increase in plasma corticosterone, followed by thymus involution and T cell destruction. Tumor growth enhancement and thymus involution were also produced by the direct administration of a synthetic corticoid, dexamethasone, or by imposing a controlled anxiety-stress.. The implications of these observations for the basic technical requirements in experiments that require a controlled or defined immunological status are discussed. The possible role of pregnancy in the exacerbation of certain neoplastic and other pathological processes is correlated with striking elevations in plasma corticosterone.

## References

1 IKONOPISOV, R. L.: Morphologic patterns of spontaneously regressing malignant melanoma in relation to host immune reactions; in McGOVERN and RUSSELL Pigment cell – mechanisms in pigmentation, vol. 1, pp. 402–409 (Karger, Basel 1973).

2 VERONESI, U.; TURRI, M., and CASCINELLI, N.: Prognostic factors in malignant melanoma; in PORTA and MUHLBOCK Structure and control of the melanocyte, pp. 319–324 (Springer, Berlin 1966).

3 WHITE, L. P.: The role of natural resistance in the prognosis of human melanoma. Ann. N. Y. Acad. Sci. 100: 115–122 (1963).

4 CLARK, D. A. and NATHANSON, L.: Cellular immunity in malignant melanoma; in McGOVERN and RUSSELL Pigment cell – mechanisms in pigmentation, vol. 1, pp. 350–359 (Karger, Basel 1973).

5 RILEY, V.: Lactate dehydrogenase in the normal and malignant state in mice and the influence of a benign enzyme-elevating virus; in BUSCH Methods in cancer research, vol. 4, pp. 493–619 (Academic Press, New York 1968).

6 RILEY, V.; SPACKMAN, D., and FITZMAURICE, M. A.: Critical influence of an enzyme-elevating virus upon long-term remissions of mouse leukemia following asparaginase therapy. Recent Results Cancer Res. 33: 81–101 (1970).

7 SANTISTEBAN, G. A.; RILEY, V., and FITZMAURICE, M. A.: Thymolytic and adrenal cortical responses to the LDH-elevating virus. Proc. Soc. exp. Biol. Med. 139: 202–206 (1972).

8 RILEY, V.: Persistence and other characteristics of the lactate dehydrogenase elevating virus (LDH-virus); in MELNICK Progress in medical virology: slow virus diseases, vol. 13, pp. 198–213 (Karger, Basel 1974).

9 SANTISTEBAN, G. and RILEY, V.: Thymo-lymphatic organ response to the LDH-virus. Proc. Am. Ass. Cancer Res. 14: 112 (1973).

10 SPACKMAN, D. and RILEY, V.: The modification of cancer by stress: effects of

plasma corticosterone elevations on immunological system components in mice. Fed. Proc. Fed. Am. Socs exp. Biol. *35:* 1693 (1976).

11   RILEY, V.; SPACKMAN, D.; MCCLANAHAN, H., and SANTISTEBAN, G.: The role of stress in malignancy. Abstracts. 3rd Int. Symp. on Cancer Detection and Prevention, New York 1976, No. 67.

12   RILEY, V.: Erroneous interpretation of valid experimental observations through interference by the LDH-virus. J. natn. Cancer Inst. *52:* 1673–1677 (1974).

13   RILEY, V.: Biological contaminants and scientific misinterpretations. Cancer Res. *34:* 1752–1754 (1974).

14   RILEY, V.: Protective ventilated shelves for experimental animal storage. Proc. 23rd annu. Session Am. Ass. for Laboratory Animal Science, St. Louis 1972, No. 113A.

15   RILEY, V. and SPACKMAN, D.: Modifying effects of a benign virus on the malignant process and the role of physiological stress on tumor incidence. Fogarty International Center Proceedings, No. 28 (US Government Printing Office, Washington, in press, 1976).

16   SPACKMAN, D. and RILEY, V.: Manuscript in preparation.

17   GLICK, D.; VON REDLICH, D., and LEVINE, S.: Fluorometric determination of corticosterone and cortisol in 0.02–0.05 milliliters of plasma or submilligram samples of adrenal tissue. Endocrinology *74:* 653–655 (1964).

18   RILEY, V.: Adaption of orbital bleeding technique to rapid serial blood studies. Proc. Soc. exp. Biol. Med. *104:* 751–754 (1960).

19   RILEY, V. and SPACKMAN, D.: Manuscript in preparation.

20   RILEY, V.; BRAUN, W.; ISHIZUKA, M., and SPACKMAN, D.: Antibody-producing cells: virus-induced alteration of response to antigen. Proc. natn. Acad. Sci. USA *73:* 1707–1711 (1976).

21   SUMMER, W. C.: Spontaneous regression of melanoma: report of a case. Cancer *6:* 1040–1043 (1953).

22   ALLEN, E. P.: Malignant melanoma: spontaneous regression after pregnancy. Br. med. J. *ii:* 1067 (1955).

23   STEWART, H.: Case of malignant melanoma and pregnancy. Br. med. J. *i:* 647 (1955).

    Dr. V. RILEY, Chairman, Department of Microbiology, Pacific Northwest Research Foundation, 1102 Columbia Street, *Seattle, WA 98104* (USA)

Pigment Cell, vol. 2, pp. 174–181 (Karger, Basel 1976)

# The Relationship of Nucleolar Antigens in Malignant Melanoma Cells to Disease Prognosis

J. M. Bowen, C. M. McBride, M. F. Miller and L. Dmochowski

Departments of Virology and Surgery, The University of Texas System Cancer Center, M.D. Anderson Hospital and Tumor Institute, Houston, Tex.

A number of investigators have reported the presence of one or more kinds of antigens associated with cells of human malignant melanoma [2, 4–7, 10, 11]. These antigens, detected by a variety of techniques, have been either cytoplasmic, cell surface, or both. We have reported observation in sera of some patients with melanoma of antibody to antigens associated with the nucleoli of their own and homologous melanoma cells [1, 9]. We will describe the results of experiments carried out in an attempt to characterize the nucleolar antigen, to analyze its distribution, and to correlate its presence in tumor cells with the clinical status of the patients.

The methodology used in testing melanoma cells and sera for the presence of nucleolar antigen has been described in detail elsewhere [1]. Briefly, frozen sections of resected tumor tissue or cover slip preparations of cultured melanoma cells were fixed in acetone or methanol and tested against autologous or homologous sera by the indirect immunofluorescence test. The fluorescein-conjugated reagent used to develop the reaction was goat antihuman IgG serum.

Selected tumor cell-serum combinations were also tested by the indirect immuno-peroxidase test [3b]. These studies showed that cells of a number of frozen sections of melanoma tissue tested against autologous sera had brightly stained nucleoli. The nucleolus was subsequently confirmed as the site of the positive reaction by comparison with hematoxylin-eosin stained material from the same tumor specimen and by electron microscopy after application of the indirect immuno-peroxidase test.

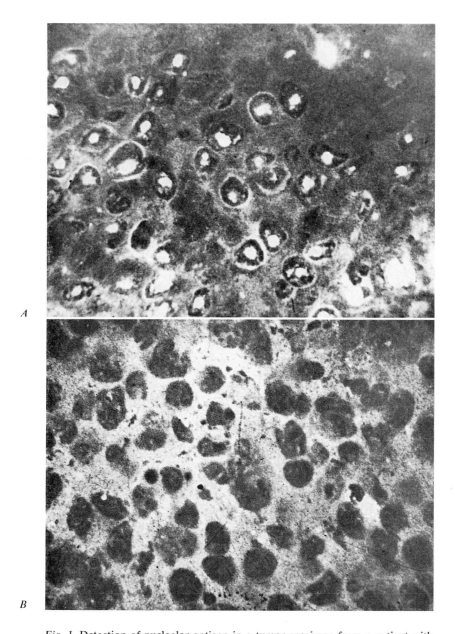

*Fig. 1.* Detection of nucleolar antigen in a tumor specimen from a patient with melanoma. Frozen sections of a melanoma specimen treated with either autologous serum (A) or serum of a healthy laboratory worker (B), then with fluorescein-conjugated goat antiserum against human IgG. The specimens were examined in a Zeiss fluorescence microscope and photographed using high-speed Ektachrome film, from which black-and-white negatives were prepared. × 1,140.

*Table I.* Results of immunofluorescence tests of melanomas for nucleolar antigen

| Number of patients positive with: | | | Number negative | Total |
|---|---|---|---|---|
| autologous serum | homologous serum | control serum | | |
| 33 (19%) | 63 (45%) | 0 | 79 | 175 |

Frozen sections were fixed in acetone, treated first with test or control serum, and then with fluorescein-conjugated goat antihuman IgG serum. Preparations were examined by UV illumination in a Zeiss fluorescence microscope. Control sera used were from two healthy laboratory workers with no history of cancer. In every case, diagnosis of melanoma was histologically confirmed.

Panel A of figure 1 illustrates a typical nucleolar reaction of a melanoma specimen reacted with autologous serum, compared with a section from the same specimen treated with normal control human serum. Note the characteristic brightly stained nucleolus. The intense staining of virtually every tumor cell nucleolus has been a striking feature of most positive cases. Only the nucleoli of tumor cells were stained. Nontumor cells could be found in every section, but the nucleoli of such cells were never stained.

Table I presents a summary of a study involving 175 melanoma patients. Frozen sections of each melanoma specimen were tested against autologous serum and against one or more sera from patients found positive in autologous tests. Autologous serum-cell combinations from 33 patients, or 19%, were found positive for the nucleolar reaction. Use of homologous positive sera revealed the presence of nucleolar antigen in a total of 63 patients, or 45%. The remaining 79 patients were negative for both antigen and antibody. It should be noted that cytoplasmic fluorescence was also observed in a number of the combinations (about 8%). Cytoplasmic reactions did not correlate with nucleolar reactions and will not be considered in this report.

Frozen sections from 8 patients positive in autologous tests were tested against a total of 52 sera from normal blood bank donors and healthy laboratory workers. All were negative, suggesting that normal individuals do not contain antibodies against the melanoma nucleolar antigen. Sera of melanoma patients reactive with melanoma nucleoli did not react with nucleoli of cells of a variety of laboratory cell lines, including HeLa, KB,

HEp-2, human embryonic kidney, lung, trachea, or skin, whole human embryo, or adult human skin. This observation was in contrast to the results of tests with sera of individuals with scleroderma, which reacted with nucleoli of all human cells tested.

In an effort to determine whether the nucleolar antigens were melanoma-specific, similar studies were done on a total of 42 other tumors of widely varying histological types. Of these, 5 have given detectable nucleolar reactions. These included one carcinoma of the ovary, 2 adenocarcinoma of the colon, 1 osteosarcoma, and 1 advanced Hodgkin's disease. These data suggest that the nucleolar antigen is not melanoma-specific. Our studies have principally involved melanoma patients, however, and no definite conclusions can be drawn about the nucleolar reaction in other types of tumors. The results of blocking antibody tests indicated that the sera of all positive melanoma patients are detecting the same antigen in melanoma cells. Similar blocking tests must be done with other types of tumors.

Cells of melanomas positive for nucleolar antigen have remained positive after growth in tissue culture. With one exception, cells of negative melanomas have remained negative during growth in tissue culture. The exceptional culture converted after more than 50 subcultures. The factors controlling expression of the nucleolar antigen are unknown and require much further study. Pigmentation of the cells did not correlate with the presence or absence of the nucleolar antigen, since the antigen was found in both melanotic and amelanotic cells.

Results of studies done to characterize the nucleolar antigen have shown that it is a ribonucleoprotein which is destroyed by ribonuclease or proteases, but it is unaffected by deoxyribonuclease. Neither nucleoli nor nucleolar antigen could be detected in cultured melanoma cells treated with actinomycin D at 0.1 $\mu$g/ml. Removal of drug resulted in reappearance of typical antigen-positive nucleoli over a 6- to 9-hour period. Dissociation of nucleoli with actinomycin D, followed by removal of actinomycin D and addition of 6-azauridine at 100–500 $\mu$g/ml resulted in reformation of structurally aberrant, antigen-negative nucleoli. These data suggested that RNA synthesis was necessary to regenerate the antigen.

There was no relationship between the presence of the nucleolar antigen or antibody and the age, sex, blood group, or transfusion history of the patients.

However, a striking aspect of the association of the nucleolar antigen with melanoma cells of some patients was the correlation between the

*Table II.* Relationship of nucleolar antigen to survival time of stage III and stage IV melanoma patients during a 13-month observation period

| Clinical stage of patient | Patients surviving at the end of the observation period | | Patients dying during the observation period | |
|---|---|---|---|---|
| | positive, % | negative, % | positive, % | negative, % |
| III | 21[1] | 79[2] | 66 | 34 |
| IV | 25[1] | 75[2] | 43 | 57 |

1 The majority of these patients had progressive tumor at the end of the observation period.
2 Patients who did not demonstrate the nucleolar antigen survived significantly longer ($\chi^2 = 12.0120$ and $p < 0.01$) than those with the antigen.

presence of the antigen in the tumor cells and the clinical status of the patient. In a comparison of the relationship of the presence of nucleolar antigen to the clinical stage of the disease, it was observed that 91% of the positive patients were in clinical stages III (57%) or IV (34%) (clinical staging of patients is described by McBride and Clark [8]). Patients in stages I and II accounted for only 9% of the total positive patients. More importantly, there was a marked inverse correlation between the presence of nucleolar antigen in the melanoma cells and the prognosis of the patient's disease. Table II shows a comparison of the survival of stages III and IV melanoma patients with the detection of nucleolar antigen in their tumor cells. The observation period was 13 months; 66% of the patients who died during this period had nucleolar antigen in their melanoma cells and 34% were negative for the antigen. In stage IV patients dying during this period, 43% of the patients were positive and 57% were negative. Only 21% of surviving stage III patients and 25% of surviving stage IV patients were positive for nucleolar antigen. Most of these patients had rapidly progressing tumor at the time of data compilation. The lower figures observed with stage IV patients probably represent an artifact, since only patients for whom palliative surgical therapy was indicated could be studied. Stage IV patients considered inoperable therefore were excluded, a situation which would reduce the stage IV figures.

The correlation between the presence of nucleolar antigen and the clinical status of the patient was also observed with several patients who were followed throughout the course of their disease. Four patients whose tumor cells were negative on initial testing became positive as the disease progressed. One patient whose melanoma was positive on initial testing became negative during a period of relative quiescence of her tumor. However, her tumor cells again became positive when tumor progression resumed and they remained positive until her death.

In conclusion, some patients with melanoma have serum antibodies to a ribonucleoprotein antigen associated with the nucleoli of their own and homologous melanoma cells. The presence of the nucleolar antigen in the tumor cells, whether detected by autologous or homologous antibody, signals rapidly progressing tumor, poor disease prognosis, and shortened survival, as compared with patients of the same clinical stage, but whose tumor cells are negative for the antigen. The nucleolar antigen and its antibody were also observed with several different types of tumors other than melanoma. Whether the nucleolar antigen present in cells of other tumors is the same as the melanoma nucleolar antigen and whether there is a similar correlation between the presence of the antigen and disease prognosis has not yet been determined and requires further study.

Detection of the nucleolar antigen may eventually serve as an aid in following tumor progression and planning the mode and time of therapy.

## Summary

We have described an antigen associated with the nucleoli of melanoma cells of some patients. The purpose of the present study has been to characterize the nature, distribution, and significance of the nucleolar antigen (NA) associated with melanoma cells.

Sera of 20% of more than 200 melanoma patients studied had antibodies to (NA) autologous melanoma cells as detected by direct immunofluorescence tests. Sera from patients selected for high autologous anti-NA antibody titers detected the same antigen in melanomas of 45% of patients whose sera were negative for antibody.

Sera from melanoma patients positive for NA in melanoma cells did not react with nucleoli of cells from human embryo, from a variety of laboratory cell lines, or from nontumor cells from the same patients. The NA was detected in some tumors other than melanoma.

Cytochemical and immunoelectron microscopy studies revealed that the NA was a ribonucleoprotein associated with the nucleolonema of the tumor cells. Inhibitors of RNA synthesis reversibly blocked formation of the antigen in melanoma cell culture. The presence of the NA in melanoma cells could be correlated with rapid tumor growth and poor progress. Survival of patients whose tumor cells did not contain NA was higher than those whose melanomas were positive. The presence of NA did not correlate with the presence or absence of cytoplasmic or other melanoma cell-associated antigens.

The possible application of monitoring of the NA in tumor cells of melanoma patients to management of the neoplasm is discussed.

## Acknowledgements

The authors acknowledge excellent technical assistance of Ms. JOHANNA ANGERMANN and the preparation of frozen sections by the technicians of the Department of Anatomical Pathology. Two of the melanoma tissue cultures used in this study were kindly provided by Dr. EVAN HERSH of the Department of Developmental Therapeutics.

This research was supported in part by Contract No. 1 CP 33304, within the Virus Cancer Program of the National Cancer Institute and Grant RR05511 from the Division of Research Resources, USPHS.

## References

1   BOWEN, J. M.; MCBRIDE, C. M.; HERSH, E.; MILLER, M. F., and DMOCHOWSKI, L.: Tumor associated changes in nucleolar antigens. Immunological aspects of neoplasia (abstr.). 26th Annual Symposium on Fundamental Cancer Research of the University of Texas at Houston, M. D. Anderson Hospital and Tumor Institute, Houston, Texas, March 1973).

2   CURRIE, G. A.; LEUJEUNE, F., and FAIRLEY, G. H.: Immunization with irradiated tumour cells and specific lymphocyte cytotoxicity in malignant melanoma. Br. med. J. *ii:* 305–310 (1971).

3   GRAHAM, R. C. and KARNOVSKY, M. J.: The early stages of absorption of injected horseradish peroxidase in the proximal tubule of the mouse kidney. Ultrastructural cytochemistry by a new technique. J. Histochem. Cytochem. *14:* 291–302 (1966).

4   HELLSTRÖM, K. E. and HELLSTRÖM, I.: Immunity to neuroblastomas and melanomas. A. Rev. Med. *23:* 19–38 (1965).

5   HELLSTRÖM, I.; SJÖGREN, H. O.; WARNER, G. A., and HELLSTRÖM, K. E.: Blocking of cell-mediated tumor immunity by sera from patients with growing neoplasms. Int. J. Cancer *7:* 226–237 (1971).

6   LEWIS, M. G.: Possible immunological factors in human malignant melanoma in Uganda. Lancet *ii:* 921–922 (1967).

7   LEWIS, M. G.; IKONOPISOV, R. L.; NAIRN, R. C.; PHILLIPS, T. M.; FAIRLEY, G. H.; BODENHAM, D. C., and ALEXANDER, P.: Tumour-specific antibodies in human malignant melanoma and their relationship to the extent of the disease. Br. med. J. *iii:* 547–552 (1969).

8   MCBRIDE, C. M. and CLARK, R. L.: Experience with *l*-phenylalanine mustard

dihydrochloride in isolation-perfusion of extremities for malignant melanoma. Cancer 28: 1293–1296 (1971).

9   McBRIDE, C. M.; BOWEN, J. M., and DMOCHOWSKI, L.: Antinucleolar antibodies in sera from patients with malignant melanoma. Surg. Forum 23: 92–93 (1972).

10  MORTON, D. L.; MALMGREN, R. A.; HOLMES, E. C., and KETCHAM, A. S.: Demonstration of antibodies against human malignant melanoma by immunofluorescence. 29th Ann. Meet. Society of University of Surgeons, New York, New York. Surgery 64: 233–240 (1968).

11  MUNA, N. M.; MARCUS, S., and SMART, C.: Detection by immunofluorescence of antibodies specific for human malignant melanoma cells. 68th Ann Meet. American Society for Microbiology, Detroit. Cancer 23: 88–93 (1968).

Dr. J. M. BOWEN, Department of Virology, The University of Texas System Cancer Center, M. D. Anderson Hospital and Tumor Institute, 6723 Bertner Avenue, Houston, TX 77030 (USA)

Pigment Cell, vol. 2, pp. 182–190 (Karger, Basel 1976)

# Studies of the Immunology of Melanoma Patients

A. J. Cochran, R. M. Mackie, C. E. Ross, D. E. Hoyle, L. Ogg and R. M. Grant

The University Departments of Pathology and Dermatology,
The Western Infirmary, Glasgow

*Introduction*

Studies of patients with malignant melanoma during the past decade provide evidence of relatively specific tumor-directed humoral [1–3] and cell-mediated [4–8] immune responses. The significance of these responses to the clinical progress of the disease remains unclear and it is not certain that they are not simply epiphenomena, concomitants of the disease process, perhaps akin to some of the antibodies present in organ-specific autoimmune disease. Tumor-directed antibodies and specifically sensitized cells are best detected in patients with early disease, but it is not known whether the stage-related decline of these phenomena precedes or is simply a sequel of disease extension.

Another matter of interest is whether the cancer patient has immunological defects which precede and perhaps lead to the development of cancer. The concept of immunological surveillance [9, 10] remains attractive, but the evidence which supports it remains incomplete and there are observations [11] which suggest that the theory will require modification to allow its continued acceptance. Apart from certain rare conditions, such as the inherited immunological deficiencies and the imposed immunological deficiences of organ transplantation, the individual immunological abnormalities demonstrated in patients with premalignant conditions or with early cancer are slight in relation to the disastrous events of tumor development, spread, and metastases which are alleged to result from them.

We have therefore undertaken a study of several aspects of the immune response and have assessed them simultaneously in a group of cancer patients and control individuals with nonmalignant diseases. We have attempted to relate these findings to demonstrable tumor-directed cell-mediated immunity assessed by the leukocyte migration technique. We have published the results of previous studies of patients with malignant melanoma [7, 8, 12] and breast carcinoma [8, 12, 13] using the leukocyte migration technique. During these studies, it became apparent that while this technique identified a majority of individuals with the type of cancer appropriate to the antigen employed, there were problems inherent in the technique as then performed using tumor extract as antigen. The tumor extract was heterogeneous and the components of the tumor cells which caused the observed inhibitions were not known. The inhibition of migration observed was relatively small (20–30% relative to migration in the medium alone) and it was not possible consistently to demonstrate dose-response curves. We did not find these preparations toxic, except at high protein concentrations, but this possibility has to be excluded with each extract and WOLBERG [14] has recorded problems of this nature.

We have now developed a method which employs formalin-fixed single tumor cells as antigen in migration studies [15, 16] and appears to solve some of the problems cited above. This technique was employed during the present study.

## Patients

All melanoma patients attended Canniesburn Hospital, The Western Infirmary, or Gartnavel General Hospital, and the diagnosis was confirmed in each case by histology. Donors of control leukocytes were patients attending the above hospitals with diseases other than melanoma and normal disease-free individuals.

## Materials and Methods

*Reagents.* 10% buffered formalin: pH 7.2. 100 ml 40% formaldehyde, 4 g $NaH_2PO_4H_2O$ and 6.5 g $Na_2HPO_4$ were made up to 1 liter.

*Cell preparation.* Fresh tumor tissue, freed as far as possible from fat and stroma, was dispersed by finely chopping in physiological saline. The suspension was then filtered through 49-gauge stainless steel mesh. The resulting cells were washed with 0,85% NaCl solution and spun at $400 g$ for 15 min. 25 volumes of 10% buffered formalin were added to the packed cells which were resuspended and left at room temperature (approximately 20 °C) for at least 12 h. The cells were washed twice with 0,85% NaCl solution and stored at 4° C until required.

*Leukocyte migration inhibition technique.* Human peripheral blood leukocytes, prepared as previously described [8] were added to the formalinized cells at ratios of 100:1, 200:1 and 500:1 (leukocytes:tumor cells). Capillaries were filled with the cell mixture, sealed at one end with inert clay and spun at 200 *g* for 5 min. The cell buttons were cut with a diamond at the cell-fluid interface and mounted horizontally in a spot of silicone grease on the base of disposable tissue culture plates. The wells were filled with Eagle's medium + 10% FCS, closed with a cover slip and the completed plates incubated in air at 37 °C for 18–24 h. Four capillaries were prepared for each leukocyte-tumor cell combination. The areas of cell migration were drawn using a drawing tube attached to a light microscope and measured by planimetry. The migration index was calculated by dividing the mean area of migration of test leukocytes plus tumor cells by the mean area migration of leukocytes alone or of leukocytes mixed with tumor cells of a histogenetically different type to that of the leukocyte donors. Significance at the 5% level was assessed by the Mann-Whitney-Wilcoxon U test of ranking.

## Results

### Migration Studies (tables I and II)

The leukocytes of 105 melanoma patients were tested against between 1 and 10 preparations of formalinized homologous melanoma cells; migration inhibition was seen with the leukocytes of 79 patients (75%) and enhancement with 8 (8%). Autologous combinations of leukocytes and tumor cells showed migration inhibition in 11/15 tests (73%) and enhancement in 1/15 (7%).

Migration inhibition was most frequently seen with leukocytes from patients with relatively localized disease; the leukocytes of patients with a primary tumor being inhibited in 15/19 tests (79%), those of patients with nodal metastases in 19/21 tests (90%), and those of patients with local recurrences in 7/7 tests. The situation with patients who had visceral metastases varied in relation to whether they were receiving immunotherapy (BCG or BCG plus irradiated autologous tumor cells) or not. Migration inhibition was seen with the leukocytes of 5 of 9 patients with visceral metastases who were not receiving immunotherapy (56%) and with the leukocytes of 10 of 12 patients on immunotherapy (83%). Enhancement was not seen in the visceral metastasis group without immunotherapy, but was seen with 2 of 12 patients receiving immunotherapy. Migration inhibition was seen with the leukocytes of all three patients examined when tumor deposits were regressing.

We examined patients attending purely for follow-up who were all

*Table I.* The frequency of leukocyte migration inhibition and enhancement by formalin-fixed melanoma cells in different categories of leukocyte donors

| Leukocyte donors | Migration | | |
|---|---|---|---|
| | number | inhibited | enhanced |
| *I. Melanoma patients* | | | |
| All stages – homologous | 105 | 79 (75) | 8 (8) |
| Autologous | 15 | 11 (73) | 1 (7) |
| Primary tumor | 19 | 15 (79) | 1 (5) |
| Nodal metastases | 21 | 19 (90) | 2 (10) |
| Visceral metastases – *no* immunotherapy | 9 | 5 (56) | 0 |
| Visceral metastases – immunotherapy | 12 | 10 (83) | 2 (17) |
| Local recurrences | 7 | 7 (100) | 0 |
| Regressing tumors | 3 | 3 (100) | 0 |
| Tumor-free after surgery | | | |
| Less than 2 years | 9 | 7 (78) | 1 (11) |
| More than 2 years | 26 | 14 (54) | 2 (8) |
| *II. Control donors* | | | |
| Nonmalignant disease | 31 | 4 (13) | 0 |
| Breast carcinoma | 30 | 5 (17) | 0 |
| Total | 61 | 9 (15) | 0 |

Percentages are given in parentheses.

*Table II.* The frequency of inhibition of migration of melanoma patients' leukocytes by formalin-fixed cells from various sources

| Source of formalinized cells | Patients' leukocytes | | |
|---|---|---|---|
| | tested | inhibited | % |
| Human melanomas (6) | 105 | 79 | 72 |
| Mouse melanomas (2)[1] | 8 | 2 | 25 |
| Human breast carcinomas (5) | 25 | 8 | 32 |
| Normal human liver cells | 10 | 2 | 20 |

1 Melanomas B16 and S91.

cised less than two years before had a high frequency of reactions – 7 of 9, (78%) showing inhibition and 1 of 9 (11%) enhancement. By contrast, of 26 individuals who had had their surgery more than two years before, only 14 showed migration inhibition (54%) and 2, enhancement (8%). ostensibly tumor-free after surgery. Patients who had had their tumor ex-

We tested melanoma patients' leukocytes against a variety of formalin-fixed cells. Cells from mouse melanomas B16 and S91 inhibited the migration of the leukocytes of 2 of 8 melanoma patients (25%). Formalinized cell suspensions from 5 human breast carcinomas inhibited the migration of leukocytes from 8 of 25 melanoma patients (32%). Formalinized liver cells from normal human autopsy inhibited the migration of the leukocytes of 2 of 10 melanoma patients.

## Assessment of the Immune Status of Melanoma Patients (table III)

It is not the purpose of this paper to analyze in detail the results of this continuing study. However, it is of interest to give some general indication of the results available at this time.

The study at present comprises 52 melanoma patients and 51 control donors. The distribution by age is very similar (melanoma patients $53.5 \pm 3$ years, control donors $53.9 \pm 2$ years). The melanoma patients

*Table III.* Studies performed simultaneously as an assessment of the immune status of melanoma patients

| | |
|---|---|
| 1. | Differential white cell count on peripheral blood |
| 2. | Intradermal skin testing with, PPD (1/1,000), Candida (Bencard), *T. rubrum* (Bencard), mumps (Eli Lilly) and streptokinase-streptodornase |
| 3. | Leukocyte migration inhibition with formalinized melanoma cells |
| 4. | Lymphocyte transformation to PHA and PPD |
| 5. | Lymphocyte cytotoxicity to melanoma target cells and blocking effect of lymphocyte donor serum |
| 6. | Quantitation of complement components |
| 7. | Anticomplementary activity of serum |
| 8. | IgG, A, and M quantification in serum |
| 9. | Quantitation of T, activated T and B cells |
| 10. | Cytoplasmic and membrane immunofluorescence |
| 11. | Immune adherence technique |

comprize 8 males and 34 females, the control group 27 males and 24 females.

Abnormalities of hematological findings were rare and those which did occur were not consistent. The absolute frequency and relative proportion of T and B lymphocytes and of activated T cells were found within normal limits in the majority of melanoma patients and in all controls. However, 2 patients were identified, both with advanced disease, in whom there was a major reduction in the T cell count. Skin testing with PPD antigens indicated a small but significant decrease in the frequency with which melanoma patients were Mantoux-positive. Reactions to streptokinase and streptodornase were similar in control and melanoma groups and, surprisingly, reactions to mumps antigen were more frequent in the melanoma group. Reactions to all 'recall' antigens were less frequent in patients with advanced melanoma. Migration studies employing formalinized cells confirmed our earlier results. Transformation of lymphocytes by PHA and PPD was within the normal range in both the melanoma patients and in the control group. However, patients receiving BCG immunotherapy were found to have a high level of transformation to both these stimulants. Lymphocytotoxicity studies have encountered the same lack of specificity encountered by other workers. However, a general correlation between positivity or negativity in the migration studies and the cytotoxicity studies has become apparent. Serum IgG and IgM were significantly raised in the melanoma patients. Tumor-directed membrane-specific antibodies were detected in the serum of 66% of the melanoma patients and 18% of the control donors by membrane immunofluorescence studies. Such antibodies were most frequently detected in patients with localized melanoma or patients with visceral metastases receiving immunotherapy. By contrast, patients with visceral metastases not receiving immunotherapy infrequently had detectable antibodies. Abnormalities of the individual complement components were found in 7 of 13 melanoma patients who were examined and anticomplementary activity was identified in serum of 2 of 12 melanoma patients.

## Discussion

These results confirm our previously published experience with the leukocyte migration inhibition test using tumor extracts as antigen [7, 8, 12, 13]. Thus, a majority of melanoma patients react with materials derived from their own tumors and from the tumors of other patients. Patients reacted significantly less often with mouse melanoma cells, normal liver cells and the cells of breast carcinoma. Sensitization was less frequently demonstrable in patients with visceral metastases, but the administration of BCG to such patients frequently causes the return of demonstrable migration inhibition. Patients with locally recurrent disease but no evidence of other metastases, patients with ipsilateral nodal secondaries and those whose tumors showed clinical evidence of regression demonstrated migration inhibition as frequently as patients with primary tumors only. This suggests that loss of detectable sensitization occurs only in patients with either a large volume of tumor or widely disseminated tumor deposits.

Patients remaining tumor-free after surgery show sensitization with decreasing frequency as the time interval between surgery and testing lengthens. This finding is similar to that reported by O'TOOLE *et al.* [17] and in our view indicates a decline of cells capable of reacting with tumor cell antigens below the level detectable by the relatively crude techniques presently available.

The advantages of the formalinized cells are that they are simple to prepare, simple to store, and allow repeated testing of patients' leukocytes with their own tumor cells over a long period of time. The cells produce strong inhibition of leukocyte migration and dose-response curves are consistently obtainable. Disadvantages are that the cell preparations at high concentrations inhibit the migration of control leukocytes and that the technique performed in this way is less discriminatory than when tumor extracts are employed. Minor differences in detectable sensitization, such as were shown previously between patients with nodal metastases and patients with primary tumors only, were not detected in the present study.

The initial results of our study of multiple immunological tests performed simultaneously on melanoma patients and controls suggest this to be a worthwhile approach. Abnormalities of several different tests were detected even in patients with relatively early disease, but the significance of these abnormalities and correlations between different test *in vivo* and *in vitro* must await final analysis of the study groups. However, it seems likely that serial studies employing several approaches simultaneously, for instance, skin testing, the leukocyte migration test, lymphocyte transformation techniques and assays of tumor-directed antibodies will be necessary to evaluate further the immunology of melanoma patients.

## Summary

We have examined leukocytes from 105 melanoma patients and 61 control donors by a modified leukocyte migration technique, and find that a majority of patients (75%) react to autologous and homologous tumor cells while relatively few control donors (15%) so react. Reactions were less frequent in patients with visceral metastases (56%) and those who had been tumor-free for more than 2 years (54%). Patients with visceral metastases who were receiving BCG therapy had a high level of reactivity (83%).

We report the early results of a study of melanoma patients by several immunological tests performed simultaneously.

## Acknowledgements

These studies were performed with the aid of a grant from the Secretary of State for Scotland and the McMillan Research Fund of the University of Glasgow. We are grateful to surgical colleagues at the West of Scotland Regional Plastic Surgery Service, Canniesburn Hospital, the Western Infirmary, and Gartnavel General Hospital for the opportunity to study patients under their care.

## References

1 MORTON, D. L.; MALMGREN, R. A.; HOLMES, E. C., and KETCHAM, A. S.: Demonstration of antibodies against human malignant melanoma by immunofluorescence. Surgery, St Louis *64:* 233–240 (1968).

2 LEWIS, M. G.; IKONOPISOV, R. L.; NAIRN, R. C.; PHILLIPS, T. M.; FAIRLEY, G. H.; BODENHAM, D. C., and ALEXANDER, P.: Tumour-specific antibodies in human malignant disease and their relationship to the extent of the disease. Br. med. J. *iii:* 547–552 (1969).

3 ROMSDAHL, M. M. and COX, I. S.: Human malignant melanoma antibodies demonstrated by immunofluorescence. Archs Surg., Lond. *100:* 491–497 (1970).

4 JEHN, U. W.; NATHANSON, L.; SCHWARTZ, R. S., and SKINNER, M.: *In vitro* lymphocyte stimulation by a soluble antigen from malignant melanoma. New Engl. J. Med. *283:* 329–333 (1970).

5 FOSSATI, G.; COLNAGHI, M. I.; DELLA PORTA, G.; CASCINELLI, N., and VERONESI, U.: Cellular and humoral immunity against human malignant melanoma. Int. J. Cancer *8:* 344–351 (1971).

6 CURRIE, G. A.; LEJEUNE, F., and FAIRLEY, G. H.: Immunisation with irradiated tumour cells and specific lymphocyte cytotoxicity in malignant melanoma. Br. med. J. *2:* 305–310 (1971).

7 COCHRAN, A. J.; JEHN, U. W., and GOTHOSKAR, B. P.: Cell mediated immunity in malignant melanoma. Lancet *i:* 1340–1341 (1972).

8   COCHRAN, A. J.; SPILG, W. G. S.; MACKIE, R. M., and THOMAS, C. E.: Post-operative depression of tumour-directed cell-mediated immunity in patients with malignant disease. Br. med. J. *iv:* 67–70 (1972).

9   THOMAS, L.: in LAWRENCE Cellular and humoral aspects of the hypersensitive state, p. 529 (Hoeber, New York 1959).

10  BURNET, F. M.: in Prog. exp. Tumor Res., vol. 13, pp. 1–27 (Karger, Basel 1970).

11  PREHN, R. T. and LAOPE, M. A.: An immunostimulation theory of tumor development. Transplantn Rev. *7:* 26–54 (1971).

12  COCHRAN, A. J.; MACKIE, R. M.; THOMAS, C. E.; GRANT, R. M.; CAMERON-MOWAT, D. E., and SPILG, W. G. S.: Cellular immunity to breast carcinomas and malignant melanoma. Br. J. Cancer *28:* suppl. 1, pp. 77–82 (1973).

13  COCHRAN, A. J.; GRANT, R. M.; SPILG, W. G. S.; MACKIE, R. M.; ROSS, C. E.; HOYLE, D. E., and RUSSELL, J. M.: Sensitisation to tumour-associated antigens in human breast carcinoma. Int. J. Cancer *14:* 19–25 (1974).

14  WOLBERG, W. H.: Inhibition of migration of human autogenous and allogeneic leukocytes by extracts of patients' cancer. Cancer Res. *31:* 798–802 (1971).

15  ROSS, C. E. and COCHRAN, A. J.: Formalin-fixed tumour cells in the leucocyte migration test. Lancet *ii:* 1087 (1973).

16  ROSS, C. E.; COCHRAN, A. J.; HOYLE, D. E.; GRANT, R. M., and MACKIE, R. M.: Formalinised tumour cells in the leucocyte migration inhibition test. Clin. exp. Immunol. *22:* 126–129 (1975).

17  O'TOOLE, C.; UNSGAARD, B.; ALMGÅRD, L. E., and JOHANSSON, B.: The cellular immune response to carcinoma of the urinary bladder. Correlation to clinical stage and treatment. Br. J. Cancer *28:* suppl. 1, pp. 266–275 (1973).

Dr. A. J. COCHRAN, The University Departments of Pathology and Dermatology, The Western Infirmary, *Glasgow G11 6NT* (Scotland)

Pigment Cell, vol. 2, pp. 191–200 (Karger, Basel 1976)

# Effector Cells and Specificity of Cell-Mediated Cytotoxicity against Human Melanoma Cell Lines

P. Hersey, A. E. Edwards, J. Edwards, D. S. Nelson and G. W. Milton

Immunology Unit, Department of Bacteriology and Medicine, University of Sydney, and Melanoma Unit, Sydney Hospital, Sydney

## Introduction

Since the introduction of *in vitro* cell-mediated cytotoxic tests to human tumor immunology 6–7 years ago, there has been consistent concern regarding the tumor specificity of the cytotoxic reaction detected. Specificity in these assays is usually accepted when it can be shown that effector cells from patients have selective cytotoxicity to autologous tumor or to tumor cells bearing tumor antigens cross-reactive with their own tumor. An essential corollary is that similar cell populations from nontumor-bearing subjects are nonreactive to both the relevant tumor cell and unrelated target cells.

A number of studies in human subjects do appear to have detected at least partial tumor specificity when assessed by these criteria. Prominent among these in melanoma subjects have been those of Fossati *et al.* [6], Currie *et al.* [2], De Vries *et al.* [3], Hellström *et al.* [7], and Romsdahl and Cox [19]. A number of more recent studies utilizing similar assays produced no evidence for tumor specificity. Takasugi *et al.* [24] in extensive studies against a variety of primary and long-term carcinoma cell lines found that effectors from normal people were as reactive as those from tumor-bearing subjects. Similar reports have appeared by a number of other authors [4, 14, 17, 18]. The problem is not confined to carcinoma or sarcoma cell lines, as shown by similar findings against lymphoid cell lines [20].

A simple explanation for the divergent results is not readily apparent from these studies. When such variables as the assay system, tumor-cell type and the effector cell separation methods are examined, there appears to be no consistent differences which would adequately account for the divergence noted in the reports.

Our own results from cytotoxic assays on a large number of melanoma subjects reported herein are among those showing no tumor specificity. We therefore have examined more closely the effector cells responsible for the cytotoxicity in our assays using cell separation methods based on red cell rosette formation. The evidence from these studies suggests that cytotoxicity is largely mediated by cells having the characteristics of activated thymus ('T') lymphocytes. Their specificity appears to be directed broadly to cells with abnormal membranes rather than to particular antigens on the membrane. Some understanding of the different reports regarding specificity can be offered from these results. Their major value may be toward the rational development of assays of cell-mediated cytotoxicity which give meaningful results of value in the management of tumor-bearing subjects.

## Materials and Methods

### Patients

All patients with melanoma were in attendance at the University of Sydney Melanoma Clinic at the Sydney Hospital. Normal subjects were either laboratory volunteers or hospital staff personnel.

### Target Cells

The melanoma cell lines MM200 and MM96 were obtained from Dr. J. Pope of the Queensland Institute of Medical Research. They were grown in Dulbecco's modified Eagles medium (DEM) supplemented with 20% heat-inactivated fetal bovine serum (FBS) (Australian Laboratory Services, Sydney). Mycoplasma contamination was kept at minimal levels by culturing the cells 1 week in every 4 in an antibiotic mixture consisting of tetracycline, chloramphenicol, and kanamycin at recommended dosage levels. Chang liver cells (Commonwealth Serum Laboratories, Melbourne) were grown in minimal essential medium (MEM) for suspension cultures supplemented with 10% FBS. Melanoma cells were harvested by trypsinization (0.25% for 30 min). Chang cells were obtained in suspension by vigorous agitation of the tissue culture vessel.

### Inhibitor Cells

Lymphoid cell lines Raji, Wil, and MOLT-4 were obtained from Dr. J. Pope as above and grown in RPMI 1640 (Gibco) supplemented with 10% FBS. Allogeneic melanoma cells were from cells stored in liquid nitrogen from 2 subjects. Viability of recovered cells ranged from 50 to 80%. Allogeneic carcinoma cells were from primary cultures established from breast and endometrium. Amnion cells were collected by trypsinization of fresh amnion for 2–3 h. Xenogeneic mouse target cells were B16 mouse melanoma and $H_1$ mouse fibrosarcoma cells grown in culture.

## Effector Cells

Mononuclear cells were separated from defibrinated peripheral blood by the method of BoyÜM using a Hypaque:Ficoll (H:F) mixture at SG 1.078. Monocytes were removed by incubation on 2-mm glass beads for 30 min at 37 °C in RPMI 1640+50% autologous serum at a concentration of $5 \times 10^6$/ml. Further fractionation of the nonglass adherent cells was carried out by formation of rosettes with SRBC on the basis of surface receptors for the Fc portion of IgG (EA rosettes), complement (EAC rosettes), and SRBCs (E rosettes). These methods are described in detail elsewhere [9]. The rosetted cells were separated from the nonrosetted cells by centrifuging the cell suspension on H:F (SG 1.078) for 30 min at 400 g. Cell fractions remaining at the interface of the H:F are referred to as EA top, EAC top, and E top, respectively, and then passing through the H:F as EA bottom, EAC bottom, and E bottom, respectively. The identity of cells in these fractions has been described elsewhere [9].

## $^{51}$Cr Release Assay

Target cells were labeled with $^{51}$Cr by incubation of $1–2 \times 10^6$ cells in 1 ml of DEM 10% FBS with 100 $\mu$Ci of $Na_2$ $^{51}$Cr $O_4$ for 2 h. They were washed twice in 30 ml of MEM and resuspended in DEM 10% FBS at a cell concentration of $6 \times 10^3$/ml prior to use. Target cells (0.5 ml) and effector cells (0.5 ml) were added to round-bottomed $3 \times 1/2''$ polystyrene tubes to give ratios of 100, 30, and 10:1. The tubes were capped and incubated overnight for 16 h at 37 °C. $^{51}$Cr release was assessed by centrifuging the tubes at 400 g for 5 min and removing 0.5 ml of the culture medium with an Eppendorf pipette. The percentage of $^{51}$Cr release was assessed as follows:

$$\frac{(\text{Radioactivity in 0.5 ml supernatant-background}) \times 2}{(\text{Total radioactivity in both supernatant and cell sediment-bkg})} \times 100.$$

## Target Cell Inhibition Assay

The procedure was adapted from previously described methods [8, 16]. Glass-absorbed effector cells from normal or melanoma subjects were cultured with $^{51}$Cr-labeled MM200 target cells at a ratio of 100:1. Unlabeled inhibitor MM200 cells (MM200 inhib.) and other inhibitor target cells (inhib. TC) described above were added at cell numbers $10^5$, $3 \times 10^4$, and $10^4$ in 0.5 ml. Inhibition of % $^{51}$Cr release produced by MM200 served as a reference to measure the degree of inhibition produced by other target cells.

Relative inhibition =

$$\frac{\% \ ^{51}\text{Cr release no inhib.TC} - \% \ ^{51}\text{Cr release} + \text{inhib.TC}}{\% \ ^{51}\text{Cr release no inhib.TC} - \% \ ^{51}\text{Cr release} + \text{MM200 inhib.}} \times 100.$$

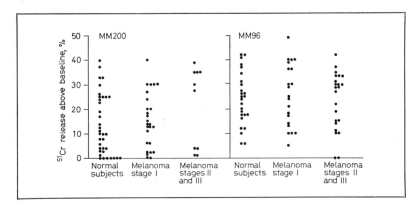

*Fig. 1.* Cytotoxicity against two melanoma cell lines in terms of $^{51}$Cr release above baseline at a ratio of 30:1 H:F-separated blood mononuclear cells to target cells.

## Results

### Comparison of Cell-mediated Cytotoxicity by Melanoma and Normal Subjects

In figure 1, the cytotoxicity of H:F separated mononuclear cells from normal and melanoma subjects at a ratio of 30:1 is illustrated against MM96 and MM200 cells. No difference in the degree of cytotoxicity is seen between the two groups. This applied to patients with both primary melanoma (stage I) and to those with more advanced disease (stages II and III). The cytotoxicity was lower against the control Chang liver cells, reflecting the lower sensitivity of this cell, but again no significant differences between normal or patient groups were seen.

### Cytotoxicity by Subfractions of Mononuclear Cells

H:F-separated mononuclear cells were tested for their cytotoxicity both before and after glass absorption and after the glass absorbed cells had been further fractionated on the basis of surface receptors for the Fc portion of IgG and for SRBC as described under Methods. Figure 2 illustrates the cytotoxicity against MM200 at a ratio of 30:1 for all subfractions from 7 normal subjects and 16 patients. (Seldom was it possible to obtain sufficient blood from patients to carry out all separation procedures; therefore, mononuclear cells from patients were submitted to either

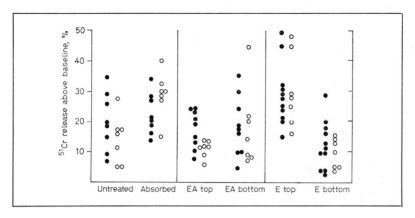

*Fig. 2.* Cytotoxicity by subfractions of blood mononuclear cells at a ratio of 30:1. ● Patients. ○ Control normal subjects.

EA rosetting or E rosetting after glass absorption.) Attention is drawn to the following observations from the data: (1) As noted previously [8, 9], glass absorption of H:F-separated cells resulted in an increase in cytotoxicity rather than a decrease. (2) Cytotoxicity by the T cell-enriched fractions (EA top and E bottom) was low and comparable to each other (mean values for % $^{51}$Cr release above baseline for EA top, patients = 17.8; controls = 11; E bottom, patients – 12.6; control = 9,4). (3) Some differences between the patient and control groups appeared evident with the EA top and to a lesser extent the E bottom population. These differences did not reach statistical significance with the numbers available, but we believe the difference seen may be meaningful because no differences in the same populations were seen against the control Chang cell. (Mean % $^{51}$Cr release above baseline EA top, patients = 7.0; controls = 8.6; E bottom, patients = 3.0; controls = 5.0). (4) Cytotoxicity by both patient and control groups separate largely in the E top fraction.

Identity of Cytotoxic Cells in the T Top Fraction

Whereas EA top and E bottom fractions are almost entirely T cells, the E top fraction is heterogenous consisting of 25–50% 'B' lymphocytes, 30–50% T cells, and variable numbers of K cells and other unidentified cells [9]. To more closely identify the cytotoxic cell, the E top fraction was therefore further fractionated after formation of EA and EAC ro-

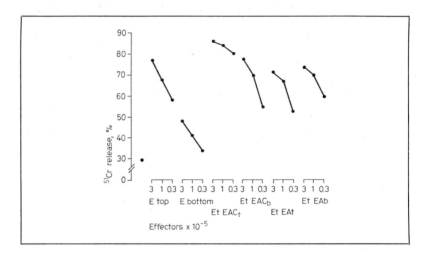

*Fig. 3.* Identification of cytotoxic cells in the non-E rosetting fraction of a normal subject.

settes. Figure 3 illustrates the result of 1 of 3 experiments of this nature for the E top fraction from normal subjects. In all cases, removal of complement receptor-bearing cells resulted in an increase in cytotoxicity rather than a decrease. Removal of Fc receptor cells did not enrich for cytotoxicity, but resulted in some decrease. The converse changes were observed in the EAC-enriched and EA-enriched (bottom) fractions.

Measurement of tritiated thymidine ($^3$HT) uptake by the cell fractions showed that the E top fraction had a high spontaneous $^3$HT uptake, suggesting that the cells were activated into cell division. It was also found that there was a good correlation between spontaneous $^3$HT uptake and the cytotoxicity of the E top subfractions.

Antigenic Specificity of the Cytotoxicity towards
MM200 Target Cells

In a series of experiments (results in table I), unlabeled target cells were added to effector cells from normal or melanoma subjects, as described, to see if they carried antigens cross-reacting with those on the MM200 cells. Control Chang cells, allogeneic carcinoma cells, and the $H_1$ mouse fibrosarcoma were found to produce as much inhibition as the unlabeled MM200 cells. The amnion cells from 3 individuals all inhibited poorly. The B16 mouse melanoma gave partial inhibition and allogeneic melanoma cells from one subject also inhibited poorly. This latter result

*Table I.* Target cell inhibition of cell-mediated cytotoxicity to MM200 cells

| Subject | Reduction in % $^{51}$Cr release by $10^5$ MM200 | Relative inhibition[1] by | | | | | |
|---|---|---|---|---|---|---|---|
| | | Chang cells | allogeneic melanoma | allogeneic carcinoma | amnion cells | lymphoid cell line | xenogeneic cells |
| N.H. | 16 | 100 | | | | 20,0 | |
| H. | 13 | 106 | | | | 0,0 | |
| A.E. | 18 | 100 | 50 | | 40 | 0,0 | |
| G.H. | 30 | 90 | 66 | | 16 | | |
| T. | 30 | 100 | 56 | | 37 | | |
| B. | 18 | | 96, 30 | | | | 70 |
| C. | 23 | | 80, 50 | | | | 66 |
| U. | 25 | | | 100, 100 | 40 | | 71, 100 |
| J. | 21 | | | 100, 100 | 25 | | 56, 100 |

1 Values recorded were obtained by expressing reduction in % $^{51}$Cr release with target cells indicated, relative to reduction in % $^{51}$Cr release with equivalent number of MM200 cells.

may reflect the poor viability of this preparation after storage in liquid nitrogen.

## Discussion

Some emphasis has been given in previous studies in cell-mediated cytotoxic assays to activated macrophages as the effector cells responsible for nonspecific killing. There is substantial evidence for this mechanism in animal models [5, 11, 12, 15], but it appears unsatisfactory as the major explanation in our studies with melanoma subjects. Depletion of macrophages by glass absorption resulted in an increase in cytotoxicity rather than a decrease. Removal of complement receptor-bearing cells from the most actively cytotoxic cell fraction resulted in an increase in cytotoxic activity rather than a decrease. Macrophages are known to bear complement receptors on their surface, so it appears most unlikely that this cell is responsible for the nonspecific killing of melanoma cells that we have observed.

Our data suggest instead that the cells responsible are activated T cells. The activated nature of the cell is indicated by the high spontaneous $^3$HT uptake of the most actively cytotoxic cell fractions (E top). Their T-cell nature is suggested by previous studies [9] using a goat anti-T cell serum showing that approximately 50% of the actively cytotoxic E top fraction were T cells. Further separation of this fraction by complement rosetting methods enriched for T cells and cytotoxic activity. Also, no correlation existed between immunoglobulin-bearing cells and the cytotoxic activity of the various cell fractions.

The separation of T cells in the non-SRBC rosetting E top fraction of cells appears confusing in that adherence to SRBC is widely accepted as a marker of T cells. The explanation for this phenomenon is suggested by a series of experiments reported elsewhere [10], showing that E rosetting T cells on stimulation by PPD or in mixed lymphocyte culture became cytotoxic to a wide range of cells and that the actively cytotoxic fraction separated largely in the nonrosetting E top fraction. It was found also that such cells acquired Fc receptors detectable by aggregated human IgG, which would explain why removal of Fc rosetting cells has generally resulted in a decrease in cytotoxic activity against the melanoma cells in the current studies.

The specificity of the cytotoxic cells is not entirely clear. We were unable to obtain evidence by target cell inhibition studies that there were clones of cytotoxic lymphocytes with specificity to melanoma tumor antigens. The cytotoxicity against melanoma cells could be inhibited completely by nonmelanoma cells and no consistent difference could be seen in the degree of inhibition produced against effector cells from normal or tumor-bearing subjects. Normal amnion cells produced only slight inhibition, and this is against the specificity being mainly directed to alloantigens on the target cells. It appears instead that the cytotoxicity is directed broadly toward cells with abnormal membranes, as suggested by HIBBS et al. [12] for activated macrophages.

Nonspecific killing by activated lymphocytes, presumably T lymphocytes, has been described by a number of authors [1, 13, 21–23]. Our suggestion that they are present in the circulation of patients and normal subjects is new but perhaps not unexpected if it is accepted that the normal human environment presents a frequent source of antigenic stimuli to the immune system. If the above suggestions are correct, it would appear that a prerequisite to development of specific cell-mediated cytotoxic assays will be the selective removal of these cells from the effector cell populations. When this is done, development of specific melanoma cytotoxicity may be seen as suggested by our data with the Fc receptor cell depleted populations. Previous authors reporting specificity may have fortuitously achieved this by the particular effector cell preparation method that they used.

## Summary

The reasons for nonspecificity of cell-mediated cytotoxicity against melanoma cell lines have been examined in the $^{51}$Cr release assay system. Effector cells were defined by use of rosette formation and separation of nonrosetting from rosetting cells by centrifugation on Hypaque:Ficoll mixtures. The findings suggest that nonspecificity results from killing by a cell in the non-SRBC rosetting fraction which has a wide range of cytotoxic specificity to cells with abnormal membranes. The cytotoxic cell appears to be activated into cell division and does not possess receptors for complement. Additional evidence is presented, suggesting that the cell is an activated T cell.

## Acknowledgements

This work was supported by grants from the University of Sydney Cancer Research Fund. We would like to thank Sisters CHALMERS and COX for collection of clinical samples and the Bill White Fund for donations to the study.

## References

1   BUTTERWORTH, A. E.: Non specific cytotoxic effects of antigen transformed lymphocytes. Kinetics cell-requirements and the role of recruitment. Cell. Immunol. 7: 357–369 (1973).

2   CURRIE, G. A.; LEJEUNE, F., and FAIRLEY, G. H.: Immunization with irradiated tumour cells and specific lymphocyte cytotoxicity in malignant melanoma. Br. med. J. ii: 305–310 (1971).

3   DE VRIES, J. E.; CORNAIN, S., and RÜMPKE, P.: Humoral and cellular immunity in melanoma patients. Cytotoxic effects of E and EAC rosette-forming cells 'T' and 'B' on plated melanoma cells. Behring Inst. Mitt. 56: 148–156 (1975).

4   DE VRIES, J. E.; RÜMPKE, P., and BERNHEIM, J. L.: Cytotoxic lymphocytes in melanoma patients. Int. J. Cancer. 9: 567–577 (1972).

5   EVANS, R. and ALEXANDER, P.: Mechanism of immunologically specific killing of tumour cells by macrophages. Nature, Lond. 236: 168–170 (1972).

6   FOSSATI, G.; COLNAGHI, M. I.; DELLA PORTA, G.; CASCINELLI, N., and VERONESI, U.: Cellular and humoral immunity against human malignant melanoma. Int. J. Cancer 8: 344–350 (1971).

7   HELLSTRÖM, I.; WARNER, G. A.; HELLSTRÖM, K. E., and SJÖGREN, H. O.: Sequential studies on cell-mediated tumor immunity and blocking serum activity in ten patients with malignant melanoma. Int. J. Cancer 11: 280–292 (1973).

8   HERSEY, P.: Thymus-dependent cytotoxic lymphocytes in the rat. Eur. J. Immunol. 3: 748–754 (1973).

9   HERSEY, P.; EDWARDS, A. E., and EDWARDS, J.: Characterization of effector cells in human blood. Clin. Exp. Immunol. 23: 104–113 (1976).

10  HERSEY, P.; EDWARDS, J., and CHIA, E.: Generation of non-SRBC adherent cytotoxic T cells with Fc receptors from SRBC rosetting T cells (submitted).

11  HIBBS, J. B.; LAMBERT, L. H., and REMINGTON, J. S.: Possible role of macrophage mediated nonspecific cytotoxicity in tumour resistance. Nature new Biol. *235:* 48–50 (1972).

12  HIBBS, J. B.; LAMBERT, L. H., jr., and REMINGTON, J. S.: Control of carcinogenesis. A possible role for the activated macrophage. Science *177:* 998–1000 (1972).

13  HOLM, G. and PERLMANN, P.: Cytotoxic potential of stimulated human lymphocytes. J. exp. Med. *125:* 721–736 (1967).

14  KAY, D. H. and SINKOVICS, J. G.: Cytotoxic lymphocytes from normal donors. Lancet *ii:* 296–297 (1974).

15  LOHMANN-MATHES, M. and FISCHER, H.: T cell cytotoxicity and amplification of the cytotoxic reaction by macrophages. Transplantn Rev. *17:* 150–186 (1973).

16  ORTIZ-LANDAZURI, M. and HERBERMAN, R. B.: Specificity of cellular immune reactivity to virus-induced tumours. Nature new Biol. *238:* 18–21 (1972).

17  PETER, H. H.; DIEHL, V.; KALDEN, J. R.; SEELAND, P., and ECKERT, G.: Cell and serum-mediated cytotoxicity *in vitro* against allogeneic and autologous human melanoma cells. Behring Inst. Mitt. *56:* 167–177 (1975).

18  RIEHMÜLLER, G.; SAAL, J.; RIEBER, E. P., and FRANK, F.: *In vitro* destruction of melanoma tumour cells by isolated lymphocytes and monocytes from tumour bearing patients and healthy donors. Behring Inst. Mitt. *56:* 177–183 (1975).

19  ROMSDAHL, M. M. and COX, I. S.: Immunological studies on malignant melanomas of man. Yale J. Biol. Med. *46:* 693–701 (1973).

20  ROSENBERG, E. B.; MCCOY, J. L.; GREEN, S. S.; DONNELLY, F. C.; SIWARSKI, D. F.; LEVINE, P. A., and HERBERMAN, R. B.: Destruction of human lymphoid tissue culture cell lines by human peripheral lymphocytes in [51]Cr release cellular cytotoxicity assays. J. natn. Cancer Inst. *52:* 345–353 (1974).

21  STEEL, C. M.; HARDY, D. A.; LING, N. R., and ALUDER, I. J.: The interaction of normal lymphocytes and cells from lymphoid cell lines. VI. Line-directed cytotoxic specificity of lymphocytes activated by autochthonous or allogeneic LCL cells. Immunology *26:* 1013–1023 (1974).

22  STEJSKAL, V.; HOLM, G., and PERLMANN, P.: Differential cytotoxicity of activated lymphocytes on allogeneic and xenogeneic target cells. I. Activation by tuberculin and by Staphylococcus filtrate. Cell. Immunol. *8:* 71–81 (1973).

23  SVEDMYR, E. A.; DEINHARDT, F., and KLEIN, G.: Sensitivity of different target cells to the killing action of peripheral lymphocytes stimulated by autologous lymphoblastoid cell lines. Int. J. Cancer *13:* 891–903 (1974).

24  TAKASUGI, M.; MICKEY, M. R., and TERASAKI, P. I.: Reactivity of lymphocytes from normal persons on cultured tumor cells. Cancer Res. *33:* 2898–2902 (1973).

Dr. P. HERSEY, Medical Research Unit, Kanematsu Institute, Sydney Hospital, *Sydney, NSW 2006* (Australia)

Pigment Cell, vol. 2, pp. 201–209 (Karger, Basel 1976)

# Immune Stimulation of Patients with Advanced Malignant Melanoma Using BCG
## A Clinical Study of 18 Cases

R. M. MACKIE, R. M. GRANT, A. J. COCHRAN, E. L. MURRAY and C. E. ROSS

University Departments of Dermatology and Pathology,
Western Infirmary, Glasgow

## Introduction

In view of the poor prognosis of melanoma patients with stage II or III disease, the use of immune stimulation as an addition to established surgical management is currently under trial and some reports show encouraging results [2, 11]. We here report on continuing studies using BCG as a nonspecific immune stimulant and, in some cases, irradiated autologous tumor cells.

## Materials and Methods

Glaxo percutaneous BCG (approximately $10^8$ live organisms per ml) was administered by scarification. The contents of 1 vial were reconstituted in 0.3 ml distilled water, applied to upper arm or thigh, and the area scarified in a gridiron pattern. This was repeated weekly until a brisk erythematous response was obtained, then fortnightly, and finally at monthly intervals. BCG was also injected directly into accessible (usually subcutaneous) tumor nodules (250–500 $\mu$g in 0.1 ml diluent). BCG was also combined with autologous irradiated (12,500 rad) tumor cells where such cells were available, and the mixture injected intramuscularly or subcutaneously. Heterologous antiserum in association with chlorambucil was prepared according to the method of GHOSE and NIGAM [5] and administered intravenously in 4 cases.

Investigations carried out prior to and during therapy were: (1) full blood count including differential white cell count and platelet count[1]; (2) serum urea, electrolytes[1]; (3) liver function studies; (4) quantitation of circulating IgG, IgA and

---

[1] These procedures were repeated at monthly intervals or more frequently throughout therapy.

Table I. Patients showing regression of tumor

| Patient No. | Age | Sex | Primary site | Stage at start of therapy | Therapy[1] | Response | Outcome | Complications |
|---|---|---|---|---|---|---|---|---|
| 1 | 63 | M | back | multiple subcutaneous metastases | 1, 2, 3 | disappearance of all injected nodules | died of myocardial infarction | BCG infection, splenomegaly |
| 2 | 70 | F | nasal | extensive local recurrence | 1, 2, 3, 4 R | regression of all tumor | alive, tumor-free, 18/12 | none |
| 3 | 83 | F | vaginal | local recurrence | 1, 2 R | regression | alive, some residual tumor, 12/12 | pyrexia; elevated transaminase levels |
| 4 | 38 | F | lower leg | pulmonary metastases | 1, 3, 4 | shrinkage of metastases 4/12 | died of melanoma, 7/12 | pyrexia, lethargy splenomegaly |
| 5 | 50 | F | nasal | extensive local recurrence | 1, 3 | shrinkage of tumor 1/12 | died of melanoma, 3/12 | pyrexia, tachycardia |
| 6 | 81 | F | upper limb | pulmonary metastases | 1 | shrinkage of metastases | alive and well, 12/12 | none |
| 7 | 25 | F | ear | cutaneous metastases | 1, 2, 3 | resolution of 6 injected + 2 uninjected metastases | alive, 10/12 | elevated transaminase levels |
| 8 | 76 | F | lower leg | massive local recurrence | 1 R | shrinkage of tumor mass | died at 3/12, cause of death unknown | none |

1 Therapies: (1) BCG by scarification; (2) BCG+intradermal injection into tumor mass; (3) BCG+autologous irradiated tumor cells; (4) antitumor antibody+chlorambucil; R=concomitant radiotherapy; C=concomitant chemotherapy.

IgM (Mancini technique); (5) leukocyte migration inhibition to melanoma-associated antigens [3, 13]; (6) lymphocyte transformation in response to PHA (modified from COULSEN and CHALMERS [4]); (7) estimation of circulating T and B lymphocytes by rosetting techniques [14]; (8) cytotoxic effect of lymphocytes on melanoma target cells *in vitro* [15]; (9) intradermal skin testing to Mantoux 1/1000, Candida (Bencard), *T. rubrum* (Bencard), mumps (Eli Lilly) and streptokinase-streptodornase (Lederle); (10) chest X-ray[2], and (11) sensitization to dinitrochlorobenzene.

## *Results*

Details of immune stimulation and clinical changes observed are given in tables I–III. In eight patients (table I) there was significant regression of tumor mass, the most striking being case 1 in whom over 70 injected tumor nodules underwent regression. No uninjected nodules were observed to regress in this case, but regression of two uninjected nodules was seen in case 7. One of these nodules was on the lower limb at a site distal to all other nodules, and thus not in an area through which lymphatics draining a BCG-treated lesion were passing. Six of the eight patients in this group received BCG in combination with autologous irradiated cells in addition to other treatment.

Of the four patients detailed in table II, showing temporary arrest of tumor growth, only one received autologous cells as part of the immune stimulation program.

The third group, comprising six patients in whom no response was noted, included four patients with visceral metastases (table III). Three of these patients died rapidly of their tumor, and three who are still alive showed some response only after combined chemoimmunotherapy. This comprised a seven-day course of vincristine, BCNU, and DTIC.

### Complications

These are also detailed in tables I–III. Several patients had pyrexia (up to 40 °C), tachycardia and lethargy after BCG, The symptoms developed within 24 h of treatment, and lasted for 48–72 h. Four patients showed elevation of transaminase levels, and all responded to therapy with INAH 150 mg daily. BCG was thereafter continued and no further disturbances in liver function tests observed. Six patients developed clinically detectable splenomegaly. Patient No. 14, who had a past history of

2    These procedures were repeated at monthly intervals or more frequently throughout therapy.

*Table II.* Patients showing arrest of tumor growth

| Patient No. | Age | Sex | Primary site | Stage at start of therapy | Therapy | Response | Outcome | Complications |
|---|---|---|---|---|---|---|---|---|
| 9 | 19 | M | unidentified | cerebral metastases | 1 R | regression all symptoms 5/12 | died of melanoma 10/12 | elevated transaminase levels |
| 10 | 43 | M | back | multiple cutaneous deposits | 1, 2, 3, 4 | no new tumor lesions 2/12 | died of melanoma 5/12 | pyrexia, lethargy, splenomegaly |
| 11 | 63 | F | subungual | local recurrence | 1 | no new lesions | alive and well 5/12 | none |
| 12 | 57 | F | upper limb | local recurrence, one skeletal metastasis | 1 | no new lesions | alive and well 6/12 | none |

*Table III.* Patients showing no response

| Patient No. | Age | Sex | Primary site | Stage at start of therapy | Therapy | Outcome | Complications |
|---|---|---|---|---|---|---|---|
| 13 | 40 | F | lower limb | local recurrence skeletal metastases | 1, 2 | died 1/12 | pyrexia, splenomegaly |
| 14 | 29 | M | back | pulmonary metastases | 1, 4 | died 3/12 | splenomegaly, anaphylactic shock |
| 15 | 56 | F | nasal | pulmonary metastases | 1, 3 | died 3/12 | none |
| 16 | 57 | F | back | involvement of draining lymph nodes | 1 C | alive, pulmonary metastases 3/12 | none |
| 17 | 23 | F | upper limb | extensive local recurrence | 1, 3 C | alive – lesions static after chemotherapy | pyrexia, nausea |
| 18 | 62 | M | nasal | local recurrence | 1, 3 C | alive, visceral metastases 8/12 | elevated transaminases, persistent draining sinuses |

atopic dermatitis, developed acute anaphylaxis from which he was resuscitated during his first administration of chlorambucil-associated rabbit antiserum.

The most serious complication encountered was in patient 1 who developed persistent pyrexia and cough 2 weeks prior to death from myocardial infarction. Chest X-ray showed diffuse mottling more suggestive of infection than tumor, and he was therefore given both antibiotics and antituberculous therapy. No mycobacteria were cultured from sputum samples at any time, although these were sought on several occasions.

## Autopsy Findings

Autopsies were performed on five patients. Strikingly small quantities of residual tumor were found in cases 1 and 10. Follicular granulomata were observed in multiple organs in case 1, in the lymph nodes of case 10 and in the liver and spleen of case 13. These three patients had all received BCG by the intralesional route, and in cases 1 and 13 alcohol/acid-fast bacilli were identified in small numbers in the granulomata. All five patients had splenomegaly, and two (cases 10 and 15) had tumor deposits in the spleen. Histological examination of BCG-injected tumors from two patients showed extensive replacement of tumor tissue by lymphocytes, macrophages and giant cell-containing follicular granulomata with no identifiable intact tumor cells. Alcohol/acid-fast mycobacteria were again found in these lesions.

## In vitro and in vivo Immunological Investigations

Of the 15 patients who had Mantoux test (1/1,000 dilution) prior to therapy, ten were positive, and all of the remaining five became positive within 2 months of starting therapy. Skin test reactions to 'recall' antigens were not significantly different from a control population of similar age, and no 'anamnestic' conversion was observed during therapy. Three of six patients sensitized to DNCB were negative on challenge.

T and B lymphocyte proportions were normal in those patients tested, and showed no changes during immune stimulation. Peripheral blood lymphocytes from nine of ten patients tested killed homologous melanoma cells in vitro, and of these nine, three showed this phenomenon only after BCG stimulation. Leukocyte migration inhibition to autologous or homologous tumor extract was carried out in all patients, and prior to therapy, ten of the 18 showed inhibition. During stimulation, the remaining eight all became positive. Only one patient who gave a positive reac-

tion prior to testing became negative during stimulation (case 12). Leukocyte migration inhibition was maintained even at terminal stages of disease in contrast to untreated patients who show no inhibition at this stage.

Lymphocyte transformation studies were carried out in 15 patients
using both PHA and PPD as stimulants. Prior to BCG, 13 patients had
normal PHA responses and two low responses. During therapy, six patients showed an augmented PHA response. PPD induced transformation
was also increased during treatment in the six patients in whom this was
tested before and during therapy. Decline in responsiveness to both PHA
and PPD was noted terminally in five patients. Normal lymphocyte
counts were recorded in all cases except on two occasions in preterminal
cases.

## Discussion

These results are similar to other reports [7, 8, 9], and suggest that immune stimulation with BCG may be of value in patients with advanced
malignant melanoma. It is not yet clear whether specific or nonspecific
stimulation is the treatment of choice, but it is of interest in this study that
six of the eight regressors (table I) had irradiated autologous cells in conjunction with BCG. Of the ten patients who showed only arrest of tumor
growth or no response, four had received autologous cells. It is our present policy to give autologous cells whenever these are available, and pilot studies are in progress with irradiated allogeneic cells.

Side effects have been fairly common, and include minor problems
with transient pyrexia, rigors and nausea, all more commonly seen after
intralesional BCG than after scarification which was well tolerated. Although no liver biopsies have been carried out, the elevated transaminase
levels observed in four cases with prompt response to antituberculous
therapy would support the diagnosis of granulomatous hepatitis. Persistent drainage of pus containing viable BCG organisms from sites of injection of BCG and tumor cells may be a public health hazard [6].

In contrast to Hunt's study of BCG-associated granulomatous hepatitis, we have identified alcohol/acid-fast mycobacteria in the granulomas
of two patients, confirming that these lesions are infective rather than a
manifestation of hypersensitivity remote from the site of infection. Dissemination of organisms occurred rapidly in patient 13 who had hepatic
granulomas two weeks after initiation of therapy, despite normal liver

function tests. By contrast, patient 1 did not develop evidence of lung involvement until he had received BCG by scarification and intralesionally for three months. He too had granulomatous hepatitis without altered liver function. Two further patients, with breast cancer and thus not included in this report, while receiving BCG intralesionally, have shown evidence of early lung and liver disease which has responded promptly to antituberculous therapy. Close monitoring of liver function and lung radiography is clearly mandatory in all patients receiving BCG.

Autopsy findings of interest were granulomatous disease, the relatively small volume and limited distribution of metastases in patients 1, 4 and 13 and the presence of splenomegaly in all five patients who came to autopsy. Splenomegaly is in keeping with stimulation of the reticulo-endothelial system: however, lymphadenopathy was not seen. The spleens of two patients contained metastases. This organ is not a common site of secondary spread and consideration must be given to the possibility that immune stimulation renders the spleen more susceptible to tumor growth.

Opinions are divided on the value of tests of immunological function as a guide to selection of patients for BCG therapy, and as monitors of progress. Some workers describe a poor prognosis in patients anergic to PPD or DNCB [1, 10, 12], while others find no significant difference in prognosis. Our study would suggest that demonstrable tumor-associated immunity may be of value in the selection of patients, as six of the eight responders showed leukocyte migration inhibition prior to treatment. In this series, only three of these eight responders had a positive skin reaction to PPD prior to therapy, compared with 4 positive tests in the six nonresponders, suggesting that this may not be a good criterion for patient selection.

These results suggest that controlled use of BCG as an immune stimulant should continue, but that consideration should be given to potential hazards. Further studies are required to determine the dose, timing, and route of administration of BCG most likely to be of value. The identification of those patients most likely to benefit is also a matter for further study.

## Summary

18 patients with advanced or recurrent malignant melanoma have been treated with BCG as a form of immune stimulation in addition to surgery in all cases,

chemotherapy in 3 instances, and radiotherapy in 3 instances. BCG has been administered by scarification, by subcutaneous injection in combination with autologous irradiated tumor cells, and by direct injection into intradermal tumor deposits where these were present. Four patients also received antitumor antibody in association with chlorambucil by intravenous infusion.

Eight patients showed regression of tumor deposits, 4 showed arrest in rate of tumor growth and 6 patients showed no response.

Side effects included the development of multiple granulomata in 3 patients, in 2 of whom acid/alcohol-fast bacilli were identified.

## References

1 BAKER, M. A. and TAUB, R. N.: BCG in malignant melanoma. Lancet i: 1117–1118 (1973).

2 BLUMING, A. Z.; VOGEL, C. L.; ZIEGLER, J. L.; MODY, N., and KANYE, G.: Immunological effects of BCG in malignant melanoma. Two modes of administration compared. Ann. intern. Med. 76: 405–411 (1972).

3 COCHRAN, A. J.; SPILG, W. G. S.; MACKIE, R. M., and THOMAS, C. E.: Postoperative depression of tumour directed cell-mediated immunity in patients with malignant disease. Br. med. J. iv: 67–70 (1972).

4 COULSON, A. S. and CHALMERS, D. G.: Separation of viable lymphocytes from human blood. Lancet i: 468–491 (1964).

5 GHOSE, T. and NIGAM, S. P.: Antibody as carrier of chlorambucil. Cancer 29: 1398–1400 (1972).

6 GORMSEN, H.: On the occurrence of epithelioid cell granulomas in the organs of BCG vaccinated human beings. Acta path. microbiol. scand., suppl. 111: 117–120 (1955).

7 GRANT, R. M.; MACKIE, R. M.; COCHRAN, A. J.; MURRAY, E. L.; HOYLE, D. E., and ROSS, C. E.: Results of administering BCG to patients with melanoma. Lancet ii: 1096–1108 (1974).

8 GUTTERMANN, J. U.; MAVLIGIT, G.; MCBRIDE, C.; FREI, E.; FREIREICH, E. J., and HERSH, E. M.: Active immunotherapy with BCG for recurrent malignant melanoma. Lancet i: 1208–1212 (1973).

9 HUNT, J. S.; SILVERSTEIN, M. J.; SPARKS, F. C.; HASKELL, C. M.; PILCH, Y. H., and MORTON, D. L.: Granulomatous hepatitis. A complication of BCG immunotherapy. Lancet i: 820–821 (1973).

10 MORTON, D. L.; MALMGREN, R. A.; HOLMES, E. C., and KETCHAM, A. S.: Demonstration of antibodies against human malignant melanoma by immunofluorescence. Surgery, St Louis 64: 233–240 (1968).

11 MORTON, D. L.; EILBER, F. R.; MALMGREN, R. A., and WOOD, W. C.: Immunological factors which influence response to immunotherapy in malignant melanoma. Surgery, St Louis 68: 158–164 (1970).

12 MORTON, D. L.: in WELLS, KYLE and DUNPHY Scientific foundations of surgery, 2nd ed. (Heinemann Medical, London 1974).

13 Ross, C. E.; Cochran, A. J.; Hoyle, D. E.; Grant, R. M., and Mackie, R. M.: Formalin-fixed tumour cells in the leucocyte migration test. Lancet *ii:* 1087–1088 (1973).

14 Sandilands, G. P.; Gray, K.; Cooney, A.; Browning, J. D.; Grant, R. M.; Anderson, J. R.; Dagg, J. H., and Lucie, N.: Lymphocytes with T and B cell properties in a lymphoproliferative disorder. Lancet *i:* 903 (1974).

15 Takasugi, M. and Klein, E.: A microassay for cell mediated immunity. Transplantation *9:* 219–227 (1970).

Dr. R. M. Mackie, University Department of Dermatology and Pathology, Western Infirmary, *Glasgow G11 6NT* (Scotland)

Pigment Cell, vol. 2, pp. 210–215 (Karger, Basel 1976)

# Immunological Anergy in Melanoma [1]

R. C. Nairn, A. P. P. Nind, E. Pihl, J. M. Rolland and
N. Matthews

Department of Pathology and Immunology, Monash University, Melbourne

Autologous blood lymphocytes, obtained by simple glass-wool filtration of buffy layer of sedimented blood, are at the time of melanoma excision frequently cytotoxic for the cultured tumor cells.

## Methods and Results

Cytotoxicity is measured on primary 24-hour tumor cell cultures in Falcon 3034 microtitration chambers to which are added test or control lymphocytes: comparative counts are made on six replicate culture wells after a further 48-hour incubation. Positive results were obtained in 44% of 61 patients (table I). Such cytotoxic lymphocytes were also positive whenever tested (6 cases) against homologous melanoma cultures, but less often against other human carcinomas (in 3 of 8 cases studied). However, as also shown in table I, local lymphocytes from regional lymph nodes were nonreactive in 14 of 16 cases, half of which had cytotoxic blood lymphocytes. Furthermore, local lymphocytes from the tumor itself, studied in 5 cases by cell fractionation procedures on glass-bead columns, were also anergic as judged by failure of lymphocyte enrichment or depletion to affect tumor cultures [6].

Lymphocyte cytotoxicity was inhibited by the patients' sera in 4 of 9 positive cases tested. This serum reaction is attributed to effector lymphocyte inhibition rather than target tumor cell blockade because it

1 This work was supported by grants from the Anti-Cancer Council of Victoria and the National Health and Medical Research Council.

could be obtained by preincubating serum with the lymphocytes, but not with the tumor cells. The reaction was melanoma-specific in the few cross-reactivity tests with other tumors that could be made (tables II and III).

Serial testing was feasible in 4 patients, in one (fig. 1) over a year in association with immunotherapy by BCG plus irradiated autologous melanoma cells. This patient had had a melanoma of the left leg locally excised some five years before coming to our attention because of the development of metastases in left inguinal and iliac nodes. As shown in figure 1, autologous blood lymphocyte cytotoxicity for the cultured melanoma cells was then negative. One week after extensive resection of

Table I. Incidence of anti-melanoma reactivity by autologous blood, regional lymph node and intrinsic tumor lymphocytes

| Lymphocytes from: | Anti-melanoma cytotoxicity |
| --- | --- |
| Blood | 27/61 |
| Regional lymph node | 2/16 |
| Intrinsic tumor | 0/5 |

Table II. Specificity of serum inhibition of lymphocyte cytotoxicity for melanoma

| Serum[1] | Blocking of lymphocyte vs melanoma system |
| --- | --- |
| Autologous | 4/9 |
| Homologous melanoma | 2/2 |
| Homologous ca. colon | 0/3 |

1 From cytotoxicity-positive cases.

Table III. Specificity of serum inhibition in different lymphocyte-tumor systems

| Serum | Number tested | Homologous lymphocyte/tumor cell system (number studied) | | |
| --- | --- | --- | --- | --- |
| | | melanoma | ca. colon | ca. stomach |
| Melanoma | 2 | + (2) | − (2) | − (1) |
| Ca. colon | 3 | − (3) | + (3) | − (1) |

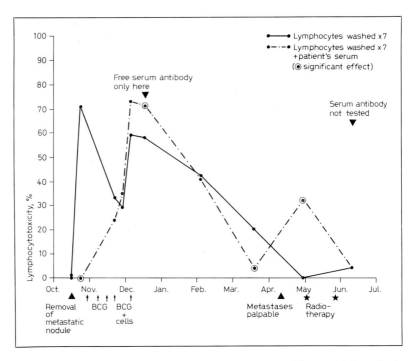

*Fig. 1.* Anti-tumor lymphocyte reactivity with and without added patient's serum in relation to clinical course and treatment in a case of melanoma.

the inguinal and iliac nodes, some of which contained metastatic tumor, the blood lymphocytes had become strongly cytotoxic. This reactivity declined on subsequent testing, and a course of immunotherapy was started 2 weeks after the groin dissection. Because very few autologous melanoma cells were available for irradiation and injection, the immunotherapy was initiated without cells by BCG (75 mg CSL) by Heaf gun successively at weekly intervals into the right leg, right arm and left arm. This was followed by intradermal inoculation of $10^7$ irradiated (10,000 rad) autologous melanoma cells plus 0.4 mg BCG into all three sites at two further weekly intervals. Lymphocyte cytotoxicity increased after these procedures. The serum which had been slightly inhibitory before the immunization became now potentiating. Perhaps we were obtaining 'K' cell activation at this stage in contrast to earlier 'T' cell effects, but unfortunately this could not be analyzed. Subsequently, lymphocyte reactivity declined, the serum again became inhibitory, and it was clear that the tumor had recurred even though clinical evidence was lacking until some few weeks later. A rapidly progressive groin nodule then appeared, and despite local radiotherapy with an accompanying return of minor reactivity by the lymphocytes, the downhill clinical course continued with signs of general dissemination. Death occurred 10 months after the first recurrence was diagnosed. The only other immunological data of note in the patient were the absence of serum antibodies reactive with melanoma cells as judged by serial immunofluorescence testing of the sera indicated in figure 1, except for the single positive finding of anti-tumor cell cytoplasm activity in December. During the course of the observations, the cytotoxicity of the lymphocytes was not shown to be significantly elevated by the extensive (sevenfold) washing used routinely for the figures in the chart; indeed, for the penultimate test, the washing significantly decreased cytotoxicity of unwashed lymphocytes.

## Discussion

In general, our data support the view that loss of lymphoid immunoreactivity is due to inhibition by tumor antigen of the effector cells, whether this be due to proximity of these cells to the tumor itself or to an abundance of antigen in the blood. There seems little doubt that such inhibition may be stabilized by complexing with humoral antibody, in antigen excess. Nevertheless, interpretation in individual cases will be greatly complicated by the likelihood of free serum antibody acting *inter alia* by (a) reactivating anergic lymphocytes, (b) reacting with any accessible target cells either to blockade T lymphocyte cytotoxicity or contrariwise to activate 'K' cell killing.

Variation and modulation of anti-melanoma immunoreactivity must take account of such equilibrium reactions between tumor antigen, serum antibody and their complexes binding to effector and target cells [2, 4]. For competent study of such effects, it will be necessary to analyze not only the effector immunocyte – T, B, K lymphocyte, macrophage [1, 3], but also their particular mode of reactivity (table IV), and moreover humoral antigens, antibodies and their complexes.

Not unexpectedly, our studies have confirmed that the most profound increase of lymphocyte immunoreactivity occurs after reduction of tumor mass, especially following radical surgical excision.

*Table IV*. Possible mechanisms of cell-mediated anti-tumor cytotoxicity

| Cell type | Other cells involved | Comments |
|---|---|---|
| T | – | specific or lymphotoxin |
| T | macrophages | ? SMAF |
| AFC | – | C′-dependent |
| AFC | macrophages | Ab determines specificity |
| AFC | K cell | Ab determines specificity |
| K | – | attached Ag-Ab complexes in Ab excess |
| Macrophage | – | nonspecific 'angry cell' e.g. by BCG |

SMAF = Specific macrophage-arming factor; AFC = antibody-forming cell.

## Summary

Anti-tumor blood lymphocyte cytotoxicity was detected in 44⁰/₀ of 61 melanoma patients tested by an *in vitro* micro-culture assay. Lymphocytes from regional lymph nodes or from the tumor itself were respectively much less often or never reactive. Experiments *in vitro* demonstrated reduction of lymphocyte cytotoxicity after incubation with certain melanoma patients' sera. In addition, serial testing of patients' blood lymphocytes showed an increase in cytotoxicity following tumor excision, and in one case after immunization with BCG and irradiated tumor cells. This patient also showed a progressive decrease in reactivity with tumor regrowth. These findings support the theory that the inhibitory factors are tumor-antigen or antigen-antibody complexes. Effects on anti-tumor reactivity will depend on local antigen and antibody concentration and on the nature of the effector cell.

## References

1   Matthews, N.; Chalmers, P. J.; Flannery, G. R., and Nairn, R. C.: Characterization of cytotoxic spleen cells and effects of serum factors in a syngeneic rat tumour system. Br. J. Cancer *33:* 279–289 (1976).

2   Matthews, N.; Kretser, T. de, and Nairn, R. C.: Use of the DASS system as a model for analysing possible mechanisms of inhibition-blockade of anti-tumour lymphocytotoxicity. Immunology *28:* 1081–1087 (1975).

3   Matthews, N.; Rolland, J. M., and Nairn, R. C.: Lymphoid cell fractionation by aggregated immunoglobulin-agarose columns. J. immunol. Methods *9:* 323–335 (1976).

4    NAIRN, R. C.: Immunological reactions in human cancer: (3) Carcinoma of
      colon, squamous cell carcinoma of skin and other tumours; in SYMINGTON and
      CARTER Scientific foundations of oncology (Heineman, London 1976).
5    NIND, A. P. P.; MATTHEWS, N.; PIHL, E. A. V.; ROLLAND, J. M., and NAIRN,
      R. C.: Analysis of inhibition of lymphocyte cytotoxicity in human colon car-
      cinoma. Br. J. Cancer *31:* 620–629 (1975).
6    NIND, A. P. P.; NAIRN, R. C.; ROLLAND, J. M.; GULI, E. P. G., and HUGHES,
      E. S. R.: Lymphocyte anergy in patients with carcinoma. Br. J. Cancer *28:*
      108–117 (1973).

Dr. R. C. NAIRN, Department of Pathology and Immunology, Monash University, *Melbourne* (Australia)

Pigment Cell, vol. 2, pp. 216–234 (Karger, Basel 1976)

# Fetal-Associated and Tumor-Specific Antigens of Cultured Malignant Melanoma Cells

## An Electron Microscope Immunocytochemical Study[1]

Geoffrey Rowden and Martin G. Lewis[2]

McGill University Cancer Research Unit, Montreal, Que.

## Introduction

It has been clearly demonstrated by immunofluorescent, cytotoxicity and immunodiffusion studies that a number of distinct antigens are expressed in human malignant melanoma cells [1–3]. These tumor-specific and tumor-associated antigens, which are not present in normal pigment cells, may stimulate the production of antibodies which appear in the circulation [4]. The appearance in the blood of the various antibodies against cytoplasmic or membrane-bound antigens appears to be related to the stage of development of the disease. In the early stages for example, when the melanoma is localized at a primary site, a highly patient-specific antibody against antigen(s) associated with cell membrane is often detectable [4]. Tumor-associated antigens such as the so-called embryonal or fetal antigens have also been detected on human malignant melanoma cells using xenoantisera raised in rabbits [5]. Recently, these fetal antigens have also been identified in certain non-malignant conditions as for example, in normal bone marrow [6] and in long-term cultured human skin [7].

Since it appears that studies of the antigens expressed by tumors may be important in understanding the nature of the patients' immune response, precise methods of localizing the antigens might prove extremely important in permitting a complete mapping of the various antigenic sites. De-

1   This research was supported by the National Cancer Institute of Canada.
2   We thank Miss C. Quirk, Miss L. Biddle, and Mr. E. Hedderson for excellent technical assistance.

tection of antigens by means of fluorescent antibodies has certain disadvantages, including variability in interpretation, particularly when differing reagents and filter systems are in use [8]. These have been circumvented by the development of methods for electron microscopy using ferritin [9] and, more recently, enzymes as markers for the specific antibodies [10–12]. The immunoenzyme methods have the advantage of application at both light and electron microscope levels. In addition, the problems of impermanence and bleaching of the label and difficulties of interpretation of morphology associated with fluorescent microscopy are obviated. The most important advantage, however, is the improved resolution of the final reaction product observed in the electron microscope [13]. Immunoenzyme techniques using peroxidase as a label have been reported to be somewhat more sensitive than the fluorescein methods [14, 15].

As a result of the institution of various immunotherapy programs for the treatment of malignant melanoma, in which cultured cell lines may prove important for testing of the various immunologic parameters and eventually, in immunization as well, an investigation was made of tumor antigens in a cultured human malignant melanoma cell line.

*Materials and Methods*

*1. Cells.* A human malignant melanoma cell line (M40) derived from a lymph node secondary has been maintained in culture for 3 years. A second human malignant melanoma cell line (M5) was obtained from Dr. P. DENT (McMaster University, Hamilton, Ont.) and maintained in our laboratory. Control cells included freshly obtained suspensions of adult and fetal (12- to 14-week-old) skin, fresh breast tumor suspensions, and normal choroidal melanocytes. All cell suspensions were prepared without the use of trypsin, i.e. by mechanical means, for initial seeding of cultures. Cells were harvested for immunocytochemical studies by means of a rubber policeman. Cells were maintained in TC 199 plus 10% fetal calf serum, penicillin, streptomycin, chlortetracycline, and Fungizone.

*2. Antisera.* An antiserum against the M40 cells was raised by hyperimmunizing goats with cultured cells. The immunoglobulins of the sera were obtained by ammonium sulphate precipitation and the IgG fractions obtained by means of Sephadex G-200 chromatography. This fraction was absorbed extensively with human liver, kidney, skin, and muscle powders. Specific antibodies were obtained by elutions from cyanogen bromide-Sepharose 4B columns with linked M40 cell antigen extracts [16]. The final preparation was concentrated by means of Amicon filters and the protein concentration determined. An antiserum was raised in rabbits against a perchloric acid extract of human fetal corpus tissues (12–14 weeks) [5].

The IgG fraction was absorbed extensively with human adult tissue powders and the specific antibodies obtained as above, with fetal extract linked to cyanogen bromide-Sepharose 4B columns. Specificity of both antisera was tested by immunodiffusion and immunoelectrophoresis prior to use for immunocytochemistry.

*3. Conjugation and immunocytochemistry.* For direct reactions, horseradish peroxidase (Sigma grade VI RZ –3.0) was conjugated to the IgG fraction by means of a two-step procedure involving glutaraldehyde [14]. Horse heart cytochrome *c* (Sigma grade VI) [17, 18] was conjugated by a single-step procedure using glutaraldehyde [19]. Horse spleen ferritin (Pentex, 6 times recrystallized, cadmium-free) was conjugated with glutaraldehyde also using a single-step method [20]. The antibody protein levels in the conjugates ranged from 5 to 8 mg/ml. Unconjugated antibodies were utilized for specific immune blocking experiments. For indirect reactions, the IgG fraction of rabbit anti-goat IgG coupled to horseradish peroxidase (Cappel Labs) or the IgG fraction of sheep anti-rabbit IgG coupled to horseradish peroxidase (Pasteur Institute) were used as the second reagents. Antibody protein levels in these reagents were adjusted to 5 mg/ml. Dilutions of from 0 to 1:50 were employed in both the direct and indirect reactions.

Cells were washed three times in PBS (phosphate-buffered saline) and incubated unfixed for 30 min to 1 h in the conjugated or unconjugated antibody. Incubations were carried out at 4 °C or room temperature. Some cells were initially fixed for 15 min in 1.25% paraformaldehyde in 0.1 M phosphate buffer pH 7.4, room temperature, prior to incubation as above. In the case of cells exposed to antibodies without prior fixation, morphology was stabilized after incubation by fixing for 15 min in $^1/_2$ strength Karnovsky fixative, room temperature. Cells were washed thoroughly in 0.1 M phosphate buffer pH 7.4, between exposure to the various antibody and cytochemical solutions. Peroxidase activity was demonstrated by 5–10 min incubation, room temperature, in the 3-3′-diaminobenzidine tetrahydrochloride (DAB) medium of Graham and Karnovsky [21, 22]. Cytochrome *c* was revealed by the same reagent, using the method of Karnovsky and Rice [23].

After osmication, cells were pelleted in capillary tubes in a hematocrit centrifuge [24] and subsequently processed as tissue blocks. Dehydration and embedding in either Epon or Spurr was by standard methods. Thin sections, cut with diamond knives using a Reichert OMU3 ultramicrotome, were observed with a Philips EM301 microscope. Thick sections either unstained or after toluidine blue staining were observed using a light microscope. Thin sections of the ferritin-treated material were contrasted with a solution of bismuth subnitrate [25]. Thin sections were only counterstained for photographic purposes with lead citrate and/or uranyl acetate after identification of the sites of immunostaining.

*4. Controls.* The following immunocytochemical controls were carried out: (a) Demonstration of endogenous peroxidase or cytochrome *c* activity by incubation of cells in the cytochemical substrates without any exposure to conjugates. (b) Non-specific absorption of free enzymes onto the cells. Cells incubated with free enzyme solutions (5 mg/ml), washed, then treated as above. (c) Specific immune blocking with unconjugated IgG prior to conjugated IgG. (d) Incubation in an unrelated antibody such as peroxidase-labeled rabbit IgG. (e) Incubation of the antisera with the antigen extracts used for immunization, before use in indirect tests. (f) Incubation of M5, breast tumor cells, normal choroidal melanocytes, human adult and fetal cell suspensions, as above.

The possibility that uptake of antigen from fetal calf serum in the culture medium [26] might influence the results with the antifetal antisera was checked by immunodiffusion and immunoelectrophoretic tests to determine lines of identity between the antifetal IgG and fetal calf serum; none were detected.

5. *Fluorescent microscopy.* Fluorescein isothiocyanate-labeled (FITC) anti-M40 and antifetal antisera were prepared [27] and used to compare the sensitivity of the two methods of localizing antigens. Membrane fluorescence with fresh cells and cytoplasmic fluorescence with snap-frozen cells were carried out [28]. The cells were observed under a Wild M20 microscope with an FITC interference filter and a BG 38/1 mm red stop for excitation, with an OG 0.5-mm barrier filter.

## Results

Figure 1 illustrates the typical appearance of the M40 cells utilized in the immunoenzyme investigations. The nuclei showed various irregularities, and the cytoplasm contained an abundance of small vacuoles and often lipid droplets. Melanin granules were detected only if the cultures were allowed to form a stationary phase with piling up of cells. Few premelanosomes were evident.

1. *Anti-M40 antiserum.* A summary of the staining reactions with the antitumor antiserum is presented in table I. Direct staining with either enzyme or ferritin label gave weaker reactions than the equivalent indirect reaction. The reaction product was in most cases continuous over the cell surface when enzyme labels were used (fig. 2). Some variations in staining intensity were noted both between cells and on different areas of individual cells (fig. 3). The intensity of the surface staining diminished with increasing dilution of the antisera. Unfixed cells always gave stronger staining reactions than did fixed cells stained for similar times. Ferritin-conjugated IgG gave a weak discontinuous distribution when used at the same antibody protein concentration as for the enzyme label, but gave a continuous labeling if used undiluted (fig. 4). No endogenous enzyme activity was noted on the cell surface for either peroxidase or cytochrome $c$, and the absorption controls were also negative. The specific immune blocking gave a significant decrease in the staining reaction, this being within the limits expected for an antibody-antigen reaction, where exchange of conjugated for unconjugated antibody might be expected to occur. Incubation of the antiserum with the M40 antigen extract, prior to its use in an indirect reaction, removed the activity against the cell membrane. Approxi-

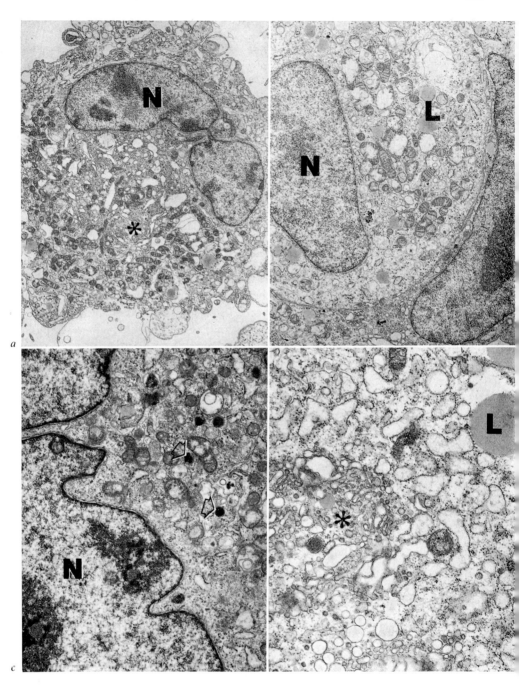

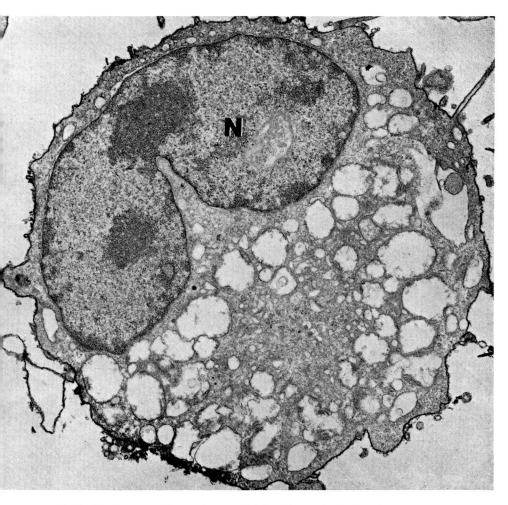

*Fig. 2.* Continuous surface staining of M40 cells. Unfixed cells, indirect staining with anti-M40 IgG. N = Nucleus. × 7,200.

*Fig. 1. a* Typical cultured M40 cell with an irregular nucleus (N) and an extensive Golgi complex (*). No melanin granules are evident. × 4,800. *b* M40 Cells in close association. L = Lipid droplets; N = nucleus. × 6,440. *c* M40 cell with melanin granule formation (arrows). N = Nucleus. × 9,700. *d* M40 cell cytoplasm with a prominent Golgi complex (*) and lipid droplets (L). × 21,000.

*Table I.* Cells reacted with antimelanoma antiserum

| Cells | | GAM40 –FITC (direct) | GAM40 –HRP (direct) | GAM40 –C (direct) | GAM40 –FER (direct) | GAM40⇢ RAG– HRP (indirect) | Specific immune blocking |
|---|---|---|---|---|---|---|---|
| M40 | (1) | + + + | + + | + + | + | + + + | – |
| (unfixed) | (2) | + | | | | | |
| M40 | (1) | NT | + | + | – | + + | – |
| (fixed) | (2) | NT | | | | | |
| M5 | (1) | + | – | NT | NT | + | NT |
| (unfixed) | (2) | – | | | | | |
| Breast tumor | (1) | – | – | NT | NT | – | NT |
| (unfixed) | (2) | – | | | | | |
| Choroidal melanocytes | (1) | – | – | NT | NT | – | NT |
| (unfixed) | (2) | – | | | | | |

GAM40 = IgG fraction goat anti-M40 cells; –HRP = conjugated to horseradish per-oxidase; –C = conjugated to cytochrome *c;* –FER = conjugated to ferritin; RAG = IgG fraction rabbit anti-goat IgG. (1) = Cytoplasmic fluorescence; (2) = membrane fluores-cence. NT = Not tested; – = negative reaction; +, + +, + + + = increasingly strong positive reaction.

*Table II.* Cells reacted with antifetal antisera

| Cells | RAF –FITC (direct) | RAF –HRP (direct) | RAF –FER (direct) | RAF⇢ SAR –HRP (indirect) | Specific immune blocking |
|---|---|---|---|---|---|
| M40 (unfixed) | + + +[1] | + + | + | + + + | – |
| M40 (fixed) | NT | + | – | + + | – |
| M5 (unfixed) | + + + | + + | NT | + + + | – |
| Fetal skin (unfixed) | + + + | + | NT | + + + | – |
| Adult skin (unfixed) | – | – | NT | – | – |
| Breast tumor (unfixed) | + | NT | NT | + | – |

RAF = IgG fraction rabbit antihuman fetal tissue extract; SAR = IgG fraction sheep anti-rabbit IgG. NT = Not tested; – = negative reaction; +, + +, + + + = increasingly strong positive reaction.
1 Membrane fluorescence.

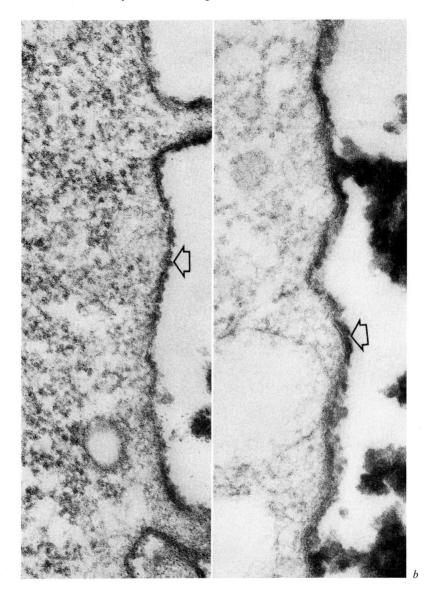

*Fig. 3. a* Surface staining of M40 cells. Fixed cells, direct staining with anti-M40 IgG-cytochrome *c.* × 85,000. *b* Areas of intense surface staining. × 100,000.

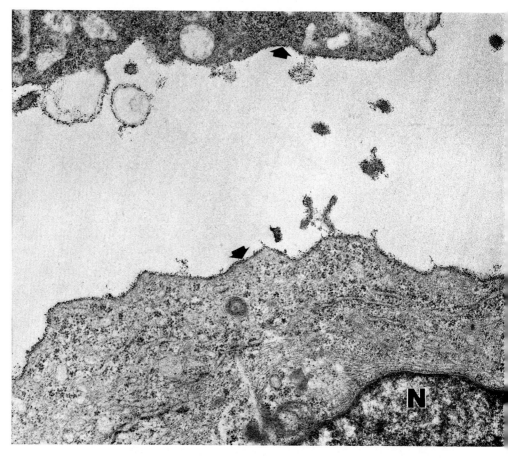

*Fig. 4.* Surface labeling with ferritin. M40 cells, unfixed and incubated with anti-M40 IgG-ferritin undiluted. N = nucleus. × 23,700.

*Fig. 5. a* Continuous surface staining of M40 cells. Fixed cells, indirect staining with antifetal IgG. N = Nucleus. × 7,900. *b* M40 cells, unfixed, stained directly with antifetal IgG-peroxidase undiluted. Penetration of the stain into the cytoplasm (arrows). N = Nucleus. × 12,200.

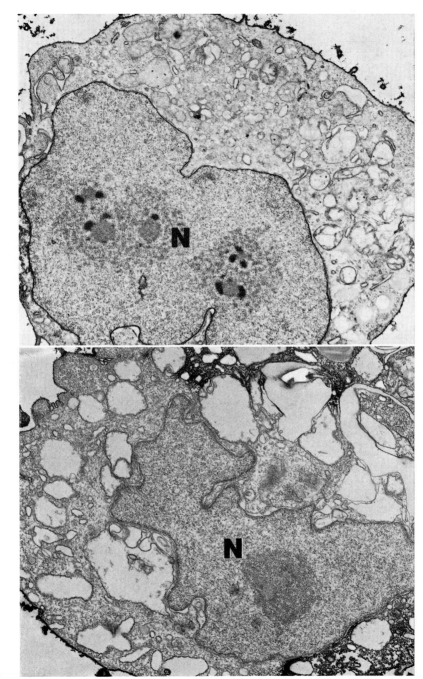

*a*

*b*

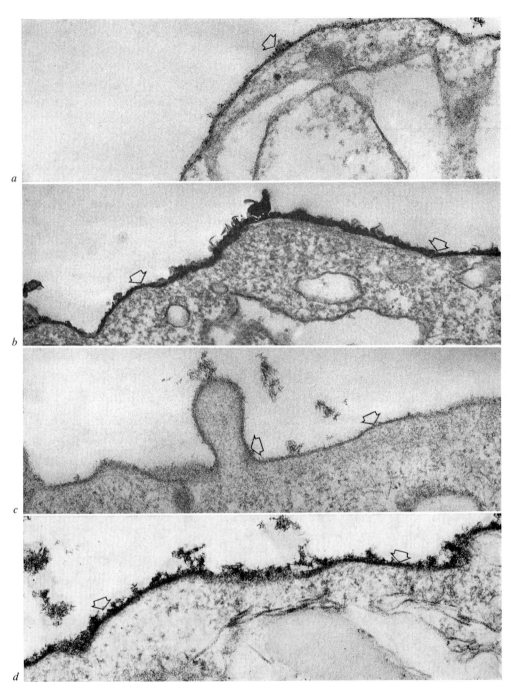

a

b

c

d

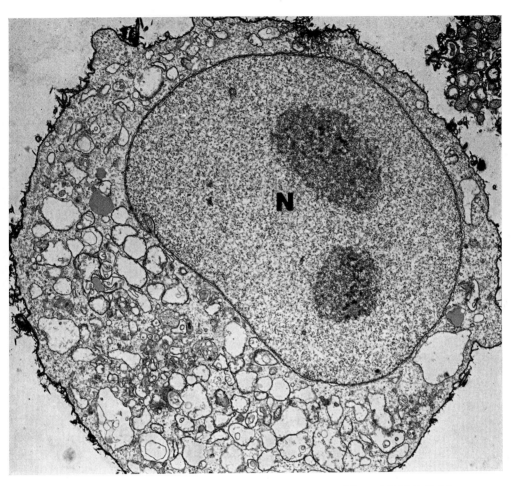

*Fig. 7.* Surface staining of M40 cells. Unfixed, incubated in anti-M40 IgG followed by indirect staining with antifetal IgG. N = Nucleus. × 7,200.

*Fig. 6. a* Surface staining of M40 cells. Fixed, direct staining with antifetal IgG-peroxidase, diluted 1:20. × 70,300. *b* As above, incubated in antifetal IgG-peroxidase undiluted. × 55,400. *c* Surface staining of M40 cells. Fixed, indirect staining with antifetal IgG, diluted 1:15. × 60,700. *d* As above, indirect technique with antifetal IgG, undiluted. × 63,000.

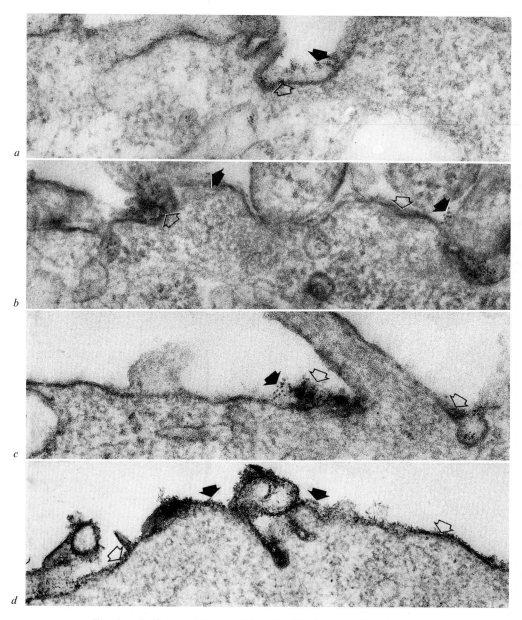

*Fig. 8. a* Surface staining of M40 cells. Unfixed, incubated concurrently with anti-M40 IgG-ferritin and antifetal IgG-peroxidase. Enzymic reaction product (open arrows), ferritin (solid arrows). × 93,000. *b* As above. × 133,600 *c* As above. × 105,000. *d* As above. × 70,300.

mately 30% of the cells bore no staining reaction on their surfaces with either the direct or indirect methods.

Other melanoma cell lines, such as M5, gave a negative result with the direct reaction and a weak surface staining in the indirect. Breast tumor cells and normal choroidal melanocytes were negative. The fluorescent antibody staining agreed with the immunoenzyme results, with respect to the membrane reaction. Surface staining was, however, rather weak. Specific immune blocking removed the surface staining completely. Cytoplasmic fluorescence was demonstrated in the snap-frozen M40 cells and the M5 cells showed some cross-reactivity with the M40 antiserum.

*2. Antifetal antiserum.* Table II presents the results of staining with the antifetal antiserum. As expected, strong surface reactions were noted with fetal skin but not with adult skin. As with the anti-M40 antiserum, unfixed cells gave more consistent results: however, continuous labeling of the cell surface was also achieved with fixed cells (fig. 5). Penetration of the labeled antibodies into the cytoplasm was noted in dead or damaged cells (fig. 5). The intensity of the reaction varied with the dilution of the antiserum (fig. 6). Ferritin, again, gave a weak, discontinuous surface pattern compared to enzymes as labels. The controls were negative and the specific immune blocking produced a striking reduction in surface staining.

M5 and breast tumor cells both gave positive surface staining similar to M40 cells, but of a lower intensity. As above, 20–30% of the cells were not stained in positive preparations. Fluorescent microscopy demonstrated strong membrane reactions against the melanoma cells (M40 and M5) as well as against fetal skin, and weak reactions against the breast tumor cells.

*3. Successive Incubations.* Prior incubation of unfixed M40 cells with goat anti-M40 IgG, prior to incubation with conjugated antifetal IgG, or vice versa, did not block the surface reactions with the second antibodies (fig. 7). Dual localization of the surface antigens was achieved only when ferritin-labeled antibodies were applied as the first reagent, followed by dilute (1:20 to 1:50) peroxidase-labeled antibodies (fig. 8). In this situation, the surface labeling was not continuous, as was the case when either antisera were used alone. The enzyme reaction product obscured the bound ferritin if more concentrated reagents were used, or if the incubation times for demonstration of the enzymes were extended beyond 10 min.

*4. Summary of results.* In all cases, the antibodies only attached to surface sites in viable cells. Penetration of a non-specific nature into the cytoplasm was noted when cells were obviously damaged or dead.

(a) Specific and distinct staining of antigenic sites on the surface of cultured melanoma cells was demonstrated by direct and indirect EM immunocytochemical methods using antimelanoma and antifetal antibodies.

(b) Blocking experiments demonstrated that staining reaction for anti-M40 antisera could not be blocked with the antifetal antiserum and vice versa. Thus, the melanoma antigen(s) did not have common determinants with the fetal antigen.

(c) Two distinct antigenic affinities were demonstrated by incubation with ferritin-labeled and enzyme-labeled antibodies.

(d) Immunoenzyme methods gave results that corresponded to the immunofluorescent staining. The staining reactions were, however, stronger and easier to interpret.

*Discussion*

The results confirm the finding of other investigators using immunocytochemical methods in a number of respects. Firstly, although it is possible to utilize briefly fixed cells for incubations, the reduced surface staining indicates some destruction or inhibition of antigenic expression, leading to reduced affinity for the specific antibodies [13]. Cells may, however, be incubated unfixed, without serious loss of morphology. The enzyme labels proved to be more satisfactory than the ferritin as has been demonstrated by studies in other systems [29]. In particular, the continuous labeling obtained with enzyme-conjugated antibodies versus the patchy distribution with ferritin as the label, agrees with the studies of Bretton *et al.* [29].

Clearly, the results indicate the usefulness of immunoenzyme techniques in mapping antigen distribution and also appears to resolve some disputes concerning the relationships between tumor-specific and fetal or embryonal antigens. Although it is clear that in certain experimental systems, it is possible to demonstrate a close relationship, if not identity, between the two types of antigens, the staining results presented here, together with the immunoelectrophoretic and immunodiffusion results, indicate that in the model studied they appear to be distinct and separate entities. Whereas it has been possible to demonstrate the effectiveness of immunization with fetal cells in retarding growth of SV-40 and adenovirus-induced tumors in animals [30], human malignant melanoma appears to be closer to the situation observed for chemically induced hepatomas and sarcomas in rats [31, 32] and for polyoma-virus-induced tumors [33], where the results indicate distinction between the tumor-specific and fetal antigens.

Investigations concerning the intracellular antigens previously identified in malignant melanoma by fluorescent microscopy are under way. Attempts to accomplish this at the electron microscope level have so far failed, owing to the lack of penetration of labeled antibodies into either fixed or unfixed cells. Further studies are in progress using Fab fragments produced by papain digestion of specific antibodies [34]. Labeling of the small fragments with heme octapeptide [35] or iodination and EM autoradiography with $^{125}$I [36] may permit the identification of the sites of intracytoplasmic antigen activity. Similarly, unlabelled antibody methods used on thin sections [37] will provide new information concerning the antigens characteristic of malignant melanoma, with a higher resolution than has previously been available with fluorescent antibody methods.

## Summary

The surface distribution of tumor-specific and tumor-associated antigens (embryonal or fetal) was investigated in a human amelanotic malignant melanoma cell line, by means of immuno-electron microscopy and xenoantisera. IgG fractions were employed for direct and indirect staining of the melanoma cells, with either ferritin or enzymes as antibody labels. Separate and distinct staining of the membrane sites for the tumor-specific and fetal antigens was achieved by successive incubations with ferritin and enzyme labels for the antibodies. The significance of these observations is discussed with respect to the results obtained with fluorescent antibody staining.

## References

1   MORTON, D. L.; MALMGREN, R. A.; HOLMES, E. C., and KETCHAM, A. S.: Demonstration of antibodies against human malignant melanoma by immunofluorescence. Surgery, St. Louis 64: 233–240 (1968).

2   LEWIS, M. G.; IKONOPISOV, R. L.; NAIRN, R. C.; PHILLIPS, T. M.; HAMILTON-FAIRLEY, G.; BODENHAM, D. C., and ALEXANDER, P.: Tumor-specific antibodies in human malignant melanoma and their relationship to the extent of the disease. Br. med. J. iii: 547–552 (1969).

3   CZAJOWSKI, N. P.; ROSENBLATT, M.; WOLF, P. L., and VASQUES, J.: A new

method for active immunization to autologous human tumor tissue. Lancet *ii:* 905 (1967).

4   Lewis, M. G. and Phillips, T. M.: The specificity of surface membrane immunofluorescence in human malignant melanoma. Int. J. Cancer *10:* 105–111 (1972).

5   Avis, P. G. J. and Lewis, M. G.: Tumour-associated fetal antigens in human tumours. J. natn. Cancer Inst. *51:* 1063–1066 (1973).

6   Lewis, M. G.; Sheikh, K. M. A.; Avis, P. G. J.; Whitehead, M., and Vera, C.: The identification of fetal antigens in human bone marrow cells. Differentiation *3:* 149–154 (1975).

7   Rowden, G.; Lewis, M. G.; Sheikh, K. M. A., and Summerlin, W. T.: Longterm organ culture of human skin. An ultrastructural and immunochemical study. J. Pathol. *117:* 139–149 (1975).

8   Lewis, M. G.: Technical and interpretative problems with immunofluorescence. Recent Results Cancer Res. *47:* 58–66 (1974).

9   Singer, S. J.: Preparation of an electron-dense antibody conjugate. Nature, Lond. *183:* 1523–1524 (1959).

10  Nakane, P. K. and Pierce, G. B., jr.: Enzyme labelled antibodies. Preparation and application for localization of antigens. J. Histochem. Cytochem. *14:* 929–931 (1966).

11  Sri Ram, J.; Nakane, P. K.; Rawlinson, E. G., and Pierce, G. B., jr.: Enzyme-labelled antibodies for ultrastructural studies. Fed. Am. Socs exp. Biol. *25:* 732 (1966).

12  Avrameas, S. et Uriel, J.: Méthode de marquage d'antigènes et d'anticorps avec des enzymes et son application en immunodiffusion. C. r. Acad. Sci. *262:* 2543–2545 (1966).

13  Avrameas, S.: Immunoenzyme techniques. Enzymes as markers for the localization of antigens and antibodies. Int. Rev. Cytol. *27:* 349–385 (1970).

14  Avrameas, S.: Coupling of enzymes to proteins with glutaraldehyde. Use of the conjugates for the detection of antigens and antibodies. Immunochemistry *6:* 43–52 (1969).

15  Davey, F. R. and Busch, C. J.: Immunohistochemistry of glomerulonephritis using HRP and fluorescein labelled antibody. A comparison of two techniques. Am. J. clin. Path. *53:* 531–536 (1970).

16  Axén, R.; Porath, J., and Ernback, S.: Chemical coupling of peptides and proteins to polysaccharides by means of cyanogen halides. Nature, Lond. *214:* 1302–1304 (1967).

17  Kraehenbuhl, J. P.; DeGrandi, P. B., and Campiche, M. A.: Ultrastructural localization of intracellular antigen using enzyme labelled antibody fragments. J. Cell Biol. *50:* 432–445 (1971).

18  DeGrandi, P. B.; Kraehenbuhl, J. P., and Campiche, M. A.: Ultrastructural localization of calcitonin in the parafollicular cells of pig thyroid gland with cytochrome *c*-labelled antibody fragments. J. Cell Biol. *50:* 446–456 (1971).

19  Avrameas, S. and Ternynck, T.: Peroxidase-labelled antibody and Fab conjugates with enhanced intracellular penetration. Immunochemistry *8:* 1175–1179 (1971).

20  NEAUPORT-SAUTES, C. and SILVESTRE, D.: Ferritin-antibody coupling with glu-taraldehyde. Transplantation 13: 536–540 (1972).

21  GRAHAM, R. C. and KARNOVSKY, M. J.: The early stages of absorption of in-jected horseradish peroxidase in proximal tubules of mouse kidney. Ultrastruc-tural cytochemistry by a new technique. J. Histochem. Cytochem. 14: 291–302 (1966).

22  AVRAMEAS, S.; TAUDOU, B., and TERNYNCK, T.: Specificity of antibodies syn-thesized by immunocytes as detected by immunoenzyme techniques. Int. Archs Allergy appl. Immun. 40: 161–170 (1971).

23  KARNOVSKY, M. J. and RICE, D. F.: Exogenous cytochrome c as an ultrastruc-tural tracer. J. Histochem. Cytochem. 17: 751–753 (1969).

24  DOANE, F. W.; ANDERSON, N.; CHAO, J., and NOONAN, A.: Two hour embed-ding procedure for intracellular detection of viruses by electron microscopy. Appl. Microbiol. 27: 407–410 (1974).

25  AINSWORTH, S. K. and KARNOVSKY, M. J.: An ultrastructural staining method for enhancing the size and electron opacity of ferritin in thin sections. J. Histo-chem. Cytochem. 20: 225–229 (1972).

26  IRIE, R. F.; IRIE, K., and MORTON, D. L.: Natural antibody in human serum to a neoantigen in human cultured cells grown in fetal bovine serum. J. natl. Cancer Inst. 52: 1051–1057 (1974).

27  CLARK, H. F. and SHEPARD, C. C.: A dialysis technique for preparing fluores-cent antibody. Virology 20: 642–644 (1963).

28  PHILLIPS, T. M. and LEWIS, M. G.: A system of immunofluorescence in the study of tumor cells. Revue eur. Etud. clin. biol. 15: 1016–1020 (1970).

29  BRETTON, R.; TERNYNCK, T., and AVRAMEAS, S.: Comparison of peroxidase and ferritin labelling of cell surface antigens. Expl. Cell Res. 71: 145–155 (1972).

30  COGGIN, J. H., jr.; AMBROSE, K. R.; BELLOMY, B. B., and ANDERSON, N. G.: Tumor immunity in hamsters immunized with fetal tissues. J. Immun. 107: 526–533 (1971).

31  BALDWIN, R. W.; GLAVES, D., and VOSE, B. M.: Immunogenicity of embryonic antigens associated with chemically induced rat tumors. Int. J. Cancer 13: 135–142 (1974).

32  BALDWIN, R. W.; EMBELTON, M. J.; PRICE, M. R., and ROBINS, A.: Immunity in the tumor-bearing host and its modification by serum factors. Cancer 34: 1452–1460 (1974).

33  TING, C. C.; LAVRIN, D. H.; SHIU, G., and HERBERMAN, R. B.: Expression of fe-tal antigens in tumor cells. Proc. natn. Acad. Sci. USA 69: 1664–1668 (1972).

34  PORTER, R. R.: The hydrolysis of rabbit-$\gamma$-globulin and antibodies with crys-talline papain. Biochem. J. 73: 119–126 (1959).

35  KRAEHENBUHL, J. P.; GALARDY, R. E., and JAMIESON, J. D.: Preparation and characterization of an immunoelectron microscope tracer consisting of he-meoctapeptide coupled to Fab. J. exp. Med. 139: 208–223 (1974).

36  GONATAS, N. K.; STIEBER, A.; GONATAS, J.; GAMBETTI, P.; ANTOINE, J. C., and AVRAMEAS, S.: Ultrastructural autoradiographic detection of intracellular im-munoglobulins with iodinated Fab fragments of antibody. J. Histochem. Cyto-chem. 22: 999–1009 (1974).

37 Sternberger, L. A.; Hardy, P. H., jr.; Cuculis, J. J., and Meyer, H. G.: The unlabelled antibody enzyme method of immunohistochemistry. Preparation and properties of soluble antigen-antibody complex (horseradish peroxidase-antiperoxidase) and its use in the identification of spirochetes. J. Histochem. Cytochem. *18:* 315–333 (1970).

Dr. Geoffrey Rowden, McGill University Cancer Research Unit, McIntyre Medical Sciences Bldg., 3655 Drummond Street, *Montreal, PQ H3G 1Y6* (Canada)

Pigment Cell, vol. 2, pp. 235–238 (Karger, Basel 1976)

# Immunotherapeutic Approaches to Malignant Melanoma

## Clinical Experience

R. L. IKONOPISOV

Center of Oncology at The Medical Academy, Sofia

In recent years, immunological studies on malignant melanoma have provided the basis for a more rational approach to this most insiduous malignant disease. The results of previous studies have suggested that patients with localized disease possess circulating tumor-specific cytotoxic antibodies reacting against their own melanoma cells [4]. These could be lost once the disease becomes generalized with distant and massive metastases interfering with the function of the lymphoreticular tissues. Our previous studies [3] have shown that autoimmunization with irradiated melanoma cells render the host capable of forming cytotoxic antibodies when they disappear from the circulation. CURRIE et al. [2], studying the effects of autoimmunization with irradiated melanoma cells, demonstrated increases in the cytotoxic effects of the patients' peripheral blood lymphocytes when tested on autologous melanoma cells.

It is now widely accepted that the live attenuated BCG vaccine (*Mycobacterium bovis* strain) is a potent immunotherapeutic adjuvant with a capacity to modify the action of carcinogens, prevent growth of tumor transplants, eliminate established tumors in experimental animal models, and alter the course of neoplastic disease in man [1]. The combination of BCG vaccine and autografting of irradiated tumor cells have been effective in animal tumor disease [5].

## Material and Methods

Our studies cover the observations on 3 separate groups of patients with malignant melanoma concerning the therapeutic effects of immunization with irradiated autologous melanoma cells, the administration of live attenuated BCG vaccine and the combination of these two modalities of specific and nonspecific immunostimulation. Each modality of immunotherapy in the 3 groups under study was administered in addition to the surgical and chemotherapeutic procedures as required by the clinical stage of the disease.

The first group consisted of 27 patients of both sexes, aged between 15 and 67 years, treated with single irradiated melanoma cell autografts. The latter consisted of $300–500 \times 10^6$ irradiated autologous cells administered by subcutaneous injection at 6 sites of lymph node drainage.

The second group was composed of 50 melanoma patients, half of whom received live attenuated BCG vaccine in addition to the fundamental therapeutic modalities (surgery or chemotherapy) as required by the clinical stage of the disease, the remaining 25 patients with malignant melanoma being deprived of BCG. BCG vaccine was given by percutaneous multipuncture with a Heaf gun using a Bulgarian lyophilized strain which contained up to $17 \times 10^6$ viable mycobacterial bodies per ml.

The third group of patients consisted of 15 individuals with malignant melanoma who were given combined immunotherapy comprising multiple (at fortnightly intervals) irradiated melanoma cells in auto- or homografts of fresh or thawed and resurrected deep-frozen melanoma cell suspensions, plus immunostimulation with weekly shots of live attenuated BCG vaccine.

Combined auto- and/or homografting and BCG vaccination were performed as two separate but simultaneous procedures and not as mixed vaccines.

*Results*

In the first group (receiving irradiated autografts only in addition to surgery or chemotherapy), subjective and objective improvement was recorded in the immediate period following the administration of autografts. Subjectively, these patients, most of whom were in a clinical stage of generalized disease (only five patients had localized and regional disease in this group), experienced an immediate improvement with a sense of well-being, improved appetite, improved sleep, and less pain. Objectively, three phenomena indicated a host response: (1) cutaneous flares surrounding skin metastatic deposits ending with a halo of depigmentation; (2) diminishing or altogether subsiding of pulmonary metastases as depicted by X-ray pictures, and (3) partial or complete regression of subcutaneous metastatic deposits. Unfortunately, the duration of the subjectively experienced 'bright' period extended from 14 to 21 days only, followed by a marked worsening of the subjective symptoms and a clinically detectable rapid progression of the disease.

In the second group, patients treated with BCG and found in clinical stage I (subjected to surgical excision of the primary) exhibited a 3-year survival of 84.6%, as opposed to patients in the same clinical stage, subjected to primary surgery but not given BCG, whose 3-year survival amounted to only 42.8%. For clinical stage II, the corresponding figures were 45.5 and 11.1%. No patient found in clinical stage III, of complete dissemination of the neoplastic disease, survived the 3-year control period. In this group, those treated with BCG had nevertheless a slower course of the disease, as opposed to the precipitated one in patients not given BCG.

The immediate results are thus far better in the third group of combined immunotherapeutic approach, including both specific and nonspecific modalities. These are manifested by a longer period of well-being and the lack of an abrupt and rapid enhancement of the tumor growth after the 2–3 weeks of temporary effect, observed when autografting was done alone. Unfortunately, the period of observation and the number of patients in this group are too small to allow for any valid comparisons and conclusions. But it does seem that multiple fortnightly auto- and homografting of irradiated melanoma cells combined with a weekly regimen of vaccination with an immunogenic, highly viable and virulent BCG vaccine may produce better results in the treatment of malignant melanoma, especially when administered to patients in whom radical surgery has left behind only a negligible number of viable melanoma cells *in situ* of the surgically removed tumor or in the circulation.

## Discussion

Autografting with irradiated melanoma cells undertaken as a sole immunotherapeutic modality in addition to surgery or chemotherapy seems to affect least the course of the disease. Two factors may account for this failure: (1) the mass of the residual tumor surely exerts an immunosuppressive effect of a magnitude incomparable with the weak effect of the autograft, and (2) the high number of the dead cells in the autologous melanoma vaccine certainly stimulate the production of serum antibodies 'blocking' the cancericidic effect of the cell immune response. This situation may be improved when BCG vaccine is used. Mycobacterial antigens are known T cell activators, reenforcing the action of intensively dividing and differentiating immunocompetent lymphocytes. Perhaps the combination of irradiated autografts and the adjuvant action of the live attenuated BCG vaccine complement each other in the direction of an antitumor effect.

## Summary

Our clinical experience with the immunotherapeutic approach to malignant melanoma covers three modalities: active specific immunotherapy with irradiated autologous melanoma cells, active nonspecific immunotherapy with live attenuated BCG vaccine, and a combination of both. Specific immunotherapy with irradiated autologous melanoma cells has resulted in a temporary improvement, including the subsidence of lung metastases and subcutaneous melanoma deposits, as well as the occurrence of erythematous and depigmentation halos surrounding tumor nodules. The immediate improvement in the general condition of the patient is transitory and deterioration in the long run is not uncommon (enhancement in result to immunostimulation?). Nonspecific immunotherapy with live attenuated BCG vaccine (Bulgarian strain, Sofia) has been clearly beneficial to patients receiving surgery and chemotherapy according to the requirements of their clinical stage. Despite BCG immunotherapy, a certain percentage of patients found in stage I and stage II of their disease have advanced into a further stage. Deterioration is delayed and survival improved when a combination of autologous irradiated melanoma cells and BCG is administered simultaneously.

## References

1   BAST, R. C., jr.; ZBAR, B.; BORSOS, T., and RAPP, H. J.: BCG and cancer (personal commun.).
2   CURRIE, G. A., LEJEUNE, F., and HAMILTON FAIRLEY, G.: Immunization with irradiated tumour cells and specific lymphocyte cytotoxicity in malignant melanoma. Br. med. J. *ii:* 305–312 (1971).
3   IKONOPISOV, R. L.; LEWIS, M. G.; HUNTER CRAIG, I. D.; BODENHAM, D. C.; PHILLIPS, T. M.; COOLING, C. I.; PROCTOR, J.; HAMILTON FAIRLEY, G., and ALEXANDER, P.: Autoimmunization with irradiated tumour cells in human malignant melanoma. Br. med. J. *ii:* 752–754 (1970).
4   LEWIS, M. G.; IKONOPISOV, R. L.; NAIRN, R. C.; PHILLIPS, T. M.; HAMILTON FAIRLEY, G.; BODENHAM, D. C., and ALEXANDER, P.: Tumour-specific antibodies in human malignant melanoma and their relationship to the extent of the disease. Br. med. J. *iii:* 547–552 (1969).
5   PARR, I.: Response of syngeneic murine lymphomata to immunotherapy in relation to the antigenicity of the tumour. Br. J. Cancer *26:* 174–182 (1972).

Dr. R. L. IKONOPISOV, Department of Dermato-oncology and Clinical Immunotherapy of Tumours, Center of Oncology, Medical Academy, *Sofia-Darvenitsa 56* (Bulgaria)

Pigment Cell, vol. 2, pp. 239–245 (Karger, Basel 1976)

# The Place of Cytodiagnosis in Black Tumors of the Skin: its Value and Limits

B. Fontanière, P. Noël, M. Mayer[1], J. Colon, C. Bailly and M. Faucon

Laboratoire de Cytologie, Laboratoire d'Anatomie Pathologique, Service de Chirurgie, Centre Léon Berard, Lyon

## Introduction

Cytological examinations of skin neoplasms have many advantages as an aid to diagnosis. Excisional biopsy followed by histological study is the most widely accepted procedure when a malignant melanoma is clinically suspected. Few reports deal with cytological studies of malignant melanoma [1, 2, 4, 8, 9, 11]. Cytodiagnosis on scraped material or on imprints of ulcerated tumors does not seem to be widely practiced, except by some authors [3, 6, 7, 10, 12, 13].

This study is a review of cytological specimens obtained from skin lesions, either primary or metastatic. An initial preliminary report by Faucon et al. [5] was presented at the *Journées Nationales de Dermatologie* – 'French National Dermatology Congress on Malignant Melanoma' – held in Besançon in June 1966. The aim of this report is to show that morphological identification of melanoma by cytological methods is possible and useful for diagnosis. This type of cytological study merely requires a few precautions when applied to patients.

## Material and Methods

Although the smear technique is well-established, it calls for comment. The collection of material for cytological examination is permissible only in certain cases. First, in ulcerated lesions: Using a metal instrument and with a definite lightness of touch to avoid bleeding, five or more smears are taken. It is not recom-

1    Director of the Léon Berard Center, Lyon.

*Table I*

| Number of patients | Number of specimens | | | Total number of specimens |
|---|---|---|---|---|
| | ulcerated lesions | subcutaneous masses | scars or wounds after surgery | |
| 121 | 114 | 16 | 52 | 182 |
| | 130 | | | |

mended to prick the surface of non-ulcerated superficial tumors with a sharp instrument. Second, in subcutaneous masses or lymph nodes: If *no* melanoma history is known, these formations may be investigated by fine needle aspiration. The content of the needle is sprayed onto slides. After fixation in ether-alcohol (a-a), the slides are automatically stained with Papanicolaou staining.

This study is based on 182 specimens from 121 patients with skin melanoma (table I). 114 smears were obtained from primary or metastatic ulcerated nodules of melanoma; 16 were obtained by fine needle aspiration of lymph nodes or subcutaneous masses. 52 smears were obtained from scars after surgical excision of primary lesion or regional lymph nodes removal. Cases without a histological study, or where the primary site was extracutaneous, were excluded.

## Results

The cellularity of skin melanoma smears is often considerable. Cells are arranged in a typical pattern; most often they are distributed singly. The cells rarely form epithelial-like clumps, and this tendency is never predominant. The cells are either round, oval, polygonal or elongated. Their size varies within a large range, as in the case of pleomorphic cells (fig. 1, 2).

The cytoplasm is generally abundant but sometimes narrow, particularly in small and round or fibrous cells. Brown-black granules are seen in some cells, fine or coarse, scanty or very abundant. It is important to note these granules, although melanin cannot be differentiated with certainty from other pigments by this staining (fig. 3, 4).

It is also important to study the nuclear morphology. Though usually in a central position, the nucleus may be eccentric. The first striking feature is a somewhat clear appearance. Nuclei are well defined, round or oval, with a fine granular network of chromatin and often a visible but thin nuclear membrane. Nucleoli are present, single or multiple and, not unfrequently, very large. In addition, some special formations are found,

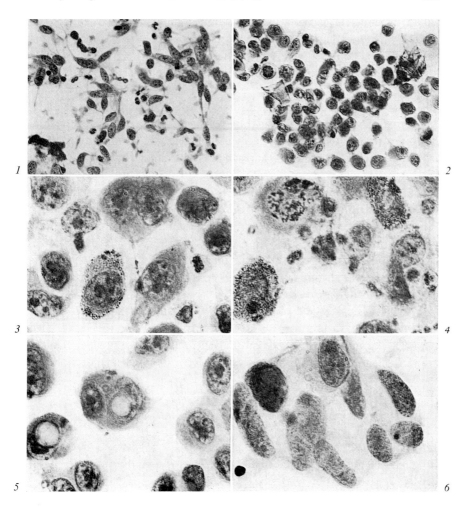

*Fig. 1.* Smear with elongated cells. × 280.

*Fig. 2.* Smear with small and round cells. A mitotic figure is visible. × 280.

*Fig. 3.* Pleomorphic cells. One cell is binucleated. Another cell shows small pigment granules in the cytoplasm. × 710.

*Fig. 4.* Large and round cells. Two of them contain a relatively great amount of pigment either in the form of small granules or aggregated in a large mass as in the lower left corner. × 710.

*Fig. 5.* Pleomorphic cells. Intranuclear vacuolations. × 710.

*Fig. 6.* Smear of Hutchinson's melanotic freckle. Apparently normal melanotic cells (right hand part) and large or hyperchromatic nuclei probably of neoplastic melanotic cells (left hand part). × 710.

called intranuclear vacuolations, sometimes simulating a true nucleolus (fig. 5). Single nuclei are most often seen, except in cases where cells are large and pleomorphic with frequent multinucleation. Mitoses are frequently seen in melanoma smears: this is important for cytological diagnosis.

In spite of these seemingly distinct morphological features, cytological examination can offer considerable difficulties. Smears of sparse cellularity are frequently found in cases of benign nevi. In this study, a true malignant melanoma gave a poorly cellular specimen, but its histological structure, showing a prominent fibrosis, explained the scanty smear. When pigment granules are absent in neoplastic cells or macrophages, the melanotic origin is rather difficult to recognize. A cytological diagnosis of reticulum cell sarcoma, undifferentiated carcinoma or sarcoma may be proposed in these cases. Melanin granules seem to be more easily detected in cytological preparations than in histological sections. Cytological specimens obtained from surgical scars or wounds may confirm a local recurrence of malignancy.

A cytological study of smears of Hutchinson's melanotic freckle provided an opportunity to observe both apparently 'normal' and 'neoplastic' types of melanotic cells on the same slide. These normal elements are difficult to distinguish from histiocytes (fig. 6). Nuclear morphology is the best criterion for the evaluation of their neoplastic transformation.


*Discussion*


Cytodiagnosis of tumors of the skin is an old method. However, this procedure, carried out with strict precautions, may provide useful information. Cellular configurations in cytological preparations were found to be divided into three main types: round, pleomorphic and fibrous, as YAMADA *et al.* have stated [13]. Differential diagnosis is facilitated by the particular cytological morphology: a special pattern of the smear; the morphology and size of nuclei and nucleoli, and the presence of pigment granules.

Table II gives some details about cytologically difficult smears: Smears of basal cell carcinoma show typical clumps of cells with oval-shaped and hyperchromatic nuclei. But melanin granules can be seen outside the cells, or in macrophages, and in 3 cases a melanoma was called 'pigmented basal cell carcinoma'.

*Table II*

| Histological classification | Number of specimens | Cytological classification |
|---|---|---|
| Malignant melanoma | 3 | pigmented basal cell carcinoma |
| | 4 | sarcoma |
| | 5 | poorly differentiated squamous cell carcinoma |
| | 2 | benign nevus |
| | 2 | neoplastic cells |
| | 1 | malignant dyskeratosis |
| Basal cell carcinoma | 1 | |
| Undifferentiated carcinoma | 2 | malignant melanoma |
| Reticulum cell sarcoma | 1 | |
| Malignant melanoma *or* undifferentiated squamous cell carcinoma *or* sarcoma | 4 | malignant melanoma *or* undifferentiated squamous cell carcinoma *or* sarcoma |

In 4 melanoma cases, melanin granules were lacking and the cells organized in large sheets. These were called 'sarcoma'.

If in addition the cells form clumps they can be classed as 'poorly differentiated squamous cell carcinoma'. Intranuclear vacuolation [13] if typical, i.e. an eosinophilic mass in the nucleus, is of considerable help, but this was not always found in our amelanotic melanomas. Two preparations from the same tumor led to a cytological diagnosis of benign nevus, whereas the clinical course was malignant and agreed with the histological classification. In 4 cases, histology, as well as cytology, could not classify the neoplastic cells.

However, out of 130 specimens from primary or metastatic, ulcerated or subcutaneous lesions, cytodiagnosis could not be properly established in only 25 cases (table III).

When dealing with surgical wounds the important thing is to find malignant cells. Clinically 3 situations exist: (1) incomplete repair of the excision zone; (2) a small nodule in the scar, or (3) a normal scar. In the latter case, the smears are mostly acellular. In the first two cases, difficulties may crop up when a majority of histiocytic cells are seen and pigment granules are found in scanty smears.

*Table III*

| Cytodiagnosis | Cutaneous smears | Fine needle aspiration | Postsurgical surveillance |
|---|---|---|---|
| Malignant melanoma | 84 | 7 | 20 |
| Absence of malignant cells With histological concordance | 7 (5 benign nevi) | 4 | 32 |
| False negatives, unsatisfactory smears | 2 | 1 | |
| | 105 | | |
| Smears difficult to interpret | 21 | 4 | |
| | 25 | | |

(Postsurgical surveillance 20 and 32 braced together = 52)

## Conclusions

The major advantage of cytological methods in establishing a preliminary diagnosis in black tumors of the skin is probably the elimination of other lesions such as pigmented basal cell carcinomas or even inflammatory processes, the behavior of which is very different from that of a melanoma. When compared with histological methods, this technique can provide additional information supporting the clinical impression and leading to a correct therapeutic attitude. Moreover, cytological examination after surgery may be a useful adjunct for detection of local recurrence. Valuable morphological information can be obtained by studying prints or smears of excised tumors.

## Summary

The diagnostic approach of malignant melanoma is clinical and its confirmation is histopathological. As cytodiagnosis is easy to practice on skin lesions, we have applied it for many years in the case of melanoma and 182 specimens have been examined. However, these tumors are rather unpredictable and very strict conditions must be respected when procuring material for smears.

The main interest of cytodiagnosis with respect to primary lesions is the distinction between melanoma and other pigmented tumors such as basal cell carcinoma, seborrheic keratosis, or pyogenic granuloma. In this situation, cytology and histology have been in agreement in 81% of the cases. Thus, cytodiagnosis appears to be a good preliminary method. Surveillance of repair after surgical excision is a further point of interest as is the etiology of some lymph nodes.

## References

1   ATKINSON, L. and HALLEY, J. B. W.: The place of cytology in the diagnosis of skin tumors; in McCARTHY Proc. Int. Cancer Conf., Sydney 1972, pp. 193–201.
2   BRODERICK, P. A.; ALLEGRA, S. R., and CORVESE, N.: Primary malignant melanoma of the esophagus. A case report. Acta cytol. 16: 159–164 (1972).
3   BONNEAU, H.; ROBERT-VAGUE, D.; CESARINI, J. P. et BONNEAU, H. P.: Les données cyto-biologiques actuelles des mélanomes malins. Revue Cytol. Clin. 2: 28–32 (1971).
4   EHRMANN, R. L.; YOUNGE, P. A., and LERCH, V. L.: The exfoliative cytology and histogenesis of an early primary malignant melanoma of the vagina. Acta cytol. 6: 245–254 (1962).
5   FAUCON, M.; GUILLAUD-BOURGEOIS, M. et DARGENT, M.: Confrontation cyto-histologique dans le diagnostic des tumeurs mélaniques. A propos de 60 observations. Bull. Soc. fr. Derm. Syph. 73: 732–739 (1966).
6   FAUCON, M.; NOËL, P. et DARGENT, M.: A propos de la cytologie des mélanomes malins. Revue Inst. Pasteur, Lyon 4: 383–392 (1971).
7   GARELY, E.: Cyto-diagnostic des tumeurs cutanées. Revue Cytol. Clin. 2: 28–32 (1969).
8   HADJU, S. I. and SAVINO, A. C. T.: Cytologic diagnosis of malignant melanoma. Acta cytol. 17: 320–327 (1973).
9   LINTHICUM, C. M.: Primary malignant melanoma of the vagina. A case report. Acta cytol. 15: 179–181 (1971).
10  LONGHIN, S.; DIMITRESCO, A. L., and TRIFU, P.: Value of cytodiagnosis in malignant melanoma. Inf. Med. Roumaine 12: 49–56 (1968).
11  PIVA, A. E. and KOSS, L. G.: Cytologic diagnosis of metastatic malignant melanoma in urinary sediments. Acta cytol. 8: 398–402 (1964).
12  TALAMAZZI, F.: Citologia del melanoblastoma. Tumori 50: 71–73 (1964).
13  YAMADA, T.; ITOU, U.; WATANABE, U., and CHASHI, S.: Cytologic diagnosis of malignant melanoma. Acta cytol. 16: 70–76 (1972).

Dr. B. FONTANIÈRE, Laboratoire de Cytologie, Centre Léon Berard, 28, rue Laénnec, F–69373 Lyon Cedex 2 (France)

Pigment Cell, vol. 2, pp. 246–253 (Karger, Basel 1976)

# Histopathological Classification of Primary Cutaneous Malignant Melanoma According to Clark's Biological Concepts

C. Bailly, J. Colon, P. Noël, M. Mayer, J. J. Bourgoin and B. Fontanière

Laboratoire d'Anatomie Pathologique, Centre Léon Berard
(Director: Prof. M. Mayer), Lyon

An electron microscopic study of malignant melanoma, based on a series of 27 cases, is reported. The specimens were taken from patients treated in Centre Léon Berard and from private patients.

*Material and Methods*

This material comprises: 20 primary cutaneous lesions, and 7 metastases or recurrences. In each case, the primary lesions were classed in one of the 3 histogenetical types and staged in one of the 5 levels of depth of invasion, using the photonic microscope and Sydney protocol [3–6].

Since 1972, we have used Clark's technics [1–4] to select in primary malignant melanoma with an 'adjacent intra-epidermal component' the cells which Clark calls 'surround cells' and the 'nodule' cells, for an ultrastructural study. We have compared our results concerning primary lesions with Clark's findings. We have also studied the metastases to try to show correlations with the histogenetical type of the primary lesion, when histological sections of the latter were available.

The series of primary cutaneous malignant melanomas studied included: 3 cases of Hutchinson melanotic freckle type; 12 cases of superficial spreading type, and 5 cases of nodular type.

The four main types of malignant melanoma cells are described in detail in Clark's papers. They are as follows:

Type I: The cell is close to the normal melanocyte but with an increased number of pigment granules and many melanosomes. The type I cell may sometimes contain numerous large autophagosomes (fig. 1).

Type II: In this type, the nucleolus is ramified (fig. 4), and nuclear inclusions are frequent (fig. 3). The cytoplasm contains spherical organelles which are an abortive form of normal melanosomes (fig. 2). Pigment synthesis may or may not be detected.

Type III: The nuclear membrane may be very infolded. In addition to organelles of type II, granular organelles, with (fig. 5) or without pigment synthesis, or lamellar organelles are found (fig. 6).

Type IV: Relatively undifferentiated cells, in which melanosomes are rare. A very large number of mitochondria and free ribosomes are to be found in the cytoplasm (fig. 8).

In each case we used the same protocol: the histological section of the primary lesion was classified in one of the 3 histogenetical types of malignant melanoma. We also studied 15 or 20 grids or more of the same tumor by electron microscope.

## Results and Discussion

### 1. Primary Lesions

The first thing noted was the great variability of cells in the same histogenetical type *and* in the same tumor. This calls for the examination of a large number of cells in different areas, to ensure a good approach to the main cell type.

a) In 3 cases of invasive malignant melanoma of Hutchinson melanotic freckle type: 'Surround' cells are generally of type I; 'nodule' cells are also of this type; many autophagosomes were also found. There findings are the same as CLARK's. A group of malignant melanocytes may also

---

*Fig. 1–5 (pp. 248/249).*

*Fig. 1.* Type I: Melanoma cell; nodule cell; malignant melanoma; Hutchinson's melanotic Freckle type; level IV. The nucleolus (Nu) is compact, the cytoplasm contains numerous completely melanized melanosomes (Me) and a large phagosome (Ph). × 4,800.

*Fig. 2.* Type II: Melanoma cells; surround cells; superficial spreading melanoma; level IV. The basement membrane (BM) of the epidermis is clearly seen; the keratinocytes (K) are darker than melanocytes (M) which form clumps; the nuclei (N) are large with dispersed nucleoli (Nu). × 3,600.

*Fig. 3.* Type II: Melanoma cell, surround cell; superficial spreading melanoma; level III. The nucleolus (Nu) is dispersed and nuclear inclusions (NI) are common. × 4,800.

*Fig. 4.* Type II: Melanoma cell; surround cell; superficial spreading melanoma; level IV. The nucleus is large; the nucleolus (Nu) is ramified; the cytoplasm contains spherical granular organelles. × 13,200.

*Fig. 5.* Type III: Melanoma cell; nodule cell; nodular melanoma; level IV. Granular organelles with pigment synthesis. × 24,000.

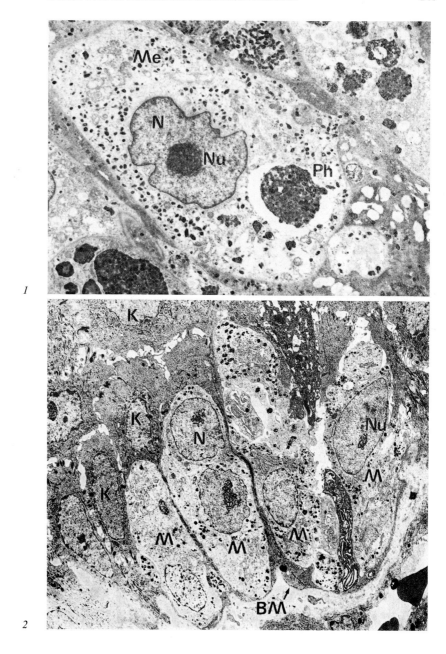

Fig. 1–5 *(for legends see p. 247).*

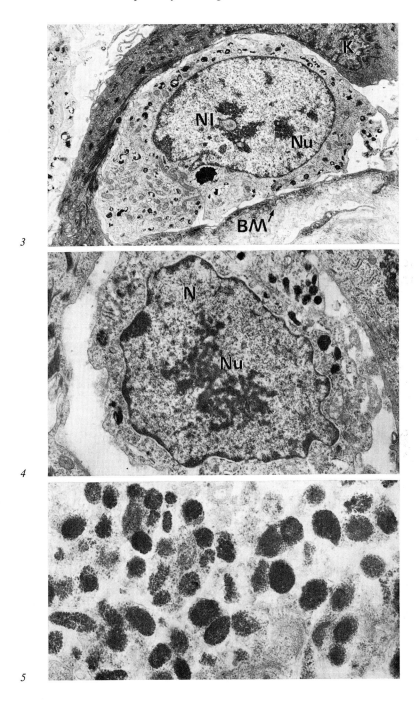

look like type IV with a very infolded nucleus, but contain melanosomes close to normal. They must not be classed as true type IV (fig. 7).

b) In malignant melanoma of superficial spreading type: The cell type appears more pleomorphic. The 'surround' component seems generally to be of type II. The 'nodule' contains a majority of type III cells and, occasionally, type IV.

c) In the nodular type: The cells are often poorly differentiated type IV cells, but generally type III.

The 'nodule cells' did not help us to form a precise diagnosis of the histogenetical type, but their morphology seems to have a prognostic signification. The risk of recurrence is high because the presence of this type of cell is a criterion of a great depth of invasion of the primary tumor. The level of invasion is deeper than grade III when a nodule arises on the surface of a malignant melanoma. There seems to be no *direct* correlation between cell type and level of invasion. Generally, a majority of type III cells were found in the 'nodule' of malignant melanoma of superficial spreading or nodular type, of levels III, IV or V. These results are summarized in table I.

2. Metastases

Only 7 cases were available: 5 cases with lymph node involvement, and 2 cases of local recurrence. The primary lesion was: nodular type in 2 cases, and superficial spreading type in 5 cases.

The metastatic cell type is more uniform than in the primary lesion. The cell is generally of type III or II, with or without pigment synthesis. Thus, we think that it is not possible to go back to the histogenetical type of the primary lesion (nodular or superficial spreading type). The metastatic cells have the same appearance as the 'nodule cells' of these two histogenetical types of malignant melanoma.

---

*Fig. 6.* Type III: Cell; nodule cell; nodular melanoma; level IV. Lamellar organelles. × 24,000.

*Fig. 7.* Nucleus of type IV melanoma cell. The nuclear membrane is very infolded. The cytoplasm is relatively uniform, but it contains mature melanosomes. This cell comes from the nodule component of a HMF – M. × 6,000.

*Fig. 8.* Type IV cell: Nodule cell; nodular melanoma; level IV; 'undifferentiated' cell. Melanosomes are rare (◄); mitochondria and free ribosomes are numerous. × 12,000.

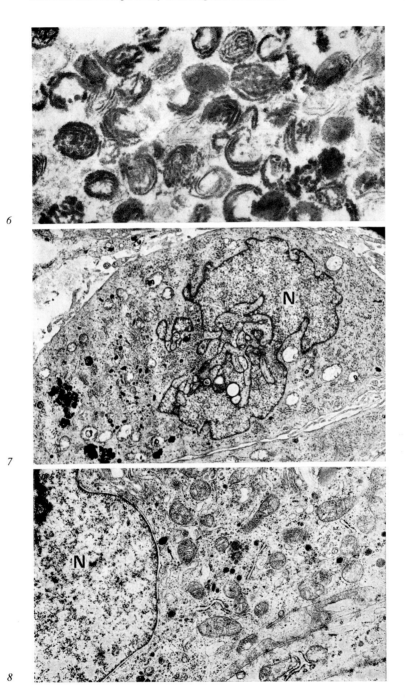

*Table I.* Correlations between light and electron microscope study in primary cutaneous malignant melanoma

| Light microscope: histogenetical type of primary tumors | Number of cases | Electron microscope: predominant cell type | |
| --- | --- | --- | --- |
| | | surround cell | nodule cell |
| HMF-M | 3 | I | I phagosomes + |
| SSM | 12 | II | III (II)  (IV) |
| NM | 5 | – | III (IV) |

## Therapeutic Applications

Ultrastructural study of the primary lesion does not alter the conclusions drawn from photonic examination. As far as our Institute is concerned, histological findings affect the management of a primary cutaneous malignant melanoma [1–5] of stage I of the extremities. Our protocol is the following: (1) a large surgical excision of the tumor, and (2) when the depth of invasion is over level III, a lymph node dissection must be decided and carried out 4 or 6 weeks later. If the lymph nodes are not involved, immunotherapy is given in accordance with EORTC protocol. If lymph nodes are concerned, chemotherapy or immunotherapy or both are done.

The prognostic evaluation given by an electron microscope study is less precise than that given by conventional histology and does not constitute a routine examination.

## Conclusions

These preliminary results do not bring anything new to the ultrastructural study of malignant melanoma, but merely constitute a modest contribution to a statistical report. Work including a wider series studied by light and electron microscope will be the subject of a later study.

## Summary

At the 'Centre Léon Berard' of Lyon (France) a series of primary cutaneous malignant melanomas have been studied with Clark's technics and correlations have been made in the three histogenetical types of tumors between light and electron microscopy.

In another study, lymph nodes from patients with metastatic disease or local recurrences have been analyzed by electron microscopy in an attempt to determine the histogenetical type of the primary lesions.

The limits of prognostic and therapeutic applications are discussed. The main purpose of this study has been to compare our cases of malignant melanomas with those in other countries, and to contribute to a statistical report.

## References

1    BAILLY, C.: L'histopronostic du mélanome malin cutané; thesis, Lyon (1972).

2    CESARINI, J. P. and CLARK, W. H.: Four variations of cytoplasmic fine structure associated with amelanotic melanoma. 8th Int. Pigment Cell Conf., Sydney 1972.

3    CLARK, W. H.; FROM, L.; BERNARDINO, E. A., and MIHM, M. C.: The histogenesis and biologic behavior of primary human malignant melanoma of the skin. Cancer Res. 29: 705–726 (1969).

4    CLARK, W. H.; TEN HEGGELER, B., and BRETTON, R.: Electron microscope observations of human cutaneous melanomas correlated with their biologic behavior; in MACCARTHY Melanoma and skin cancer. Proc. Int. Cancer Conf., Sydney 1972, pp. 121–2141.

5    COLON, J.; BAILLY, C.; BOURGOIN, J. J., and DARGENT, M.: Prognosis of malignant melanoma in function of its clinical and microscopic aspects – clinical study of proposed classifications. 8th Int. Pigment Cell Conf., Sydney 1972.

6    MCGOVERN, V. J.; MIHM, M. C.; BAILLY, C.; BOOTH, J. C.; CLARK, W. H.; COCHRAN, A. J.; HARDY, E. G.; HICKS, J. D.; LEVENE, A.; LEWIS, M. G.; LITTLE, J. H., and MILTON, G. W.: The classification of malignant melanoma and its histologic reporting. Cancer 32: 1446–1457 (1973).

Dr. CHRISTIANE BAILLY, Laboratoire d'Anatomie Pathologique, Centre Léon Berard, 28, rue Laénnec, F–69373 Lyon Cedex 2 (France)

Pigment Cell, vol. 2, pp. 254–263 (Karger, Basel 1976)

# An Automatic Analyzer for the Detection of Urinary Melanogens[1]

PHILLIP W. BANDA, ARLETTA E. SHERRY and MARSDEN S. BLOIS

Department of Dermatology, School of Medicine, University of California, San Francisco, Calif.

## Introduction

We have recently described the development of a new ion-exchange chromatographic system for detecting dihydroxyphenylalanine (dopa), its metabolites, and a number of other reducing constituents in urine [1]. The system is similar in general design to an amino acid analyzer, but it employs a unique colorimetric reagent for detection, diphenylpicrylhydrazyl (DPPH), and has its own set of operating parameters. The system provides a comprehensive chromatographic-peak profile of the melanogens in urine, and has been used to screen urines from melanoma patients representing a variety of clinical stages. We wish to report briefly on the correlations that have appeared.

## Materials and Methods

### a) Equipment

The operation of the analyzer is as previously described [1], with the following modifications. The detector is now a more recent Spectronic 20 (B&L No. 33-31-72) with a self-contained regulator and recorder jack. The external voltage regulator and resistor of the original system are no longer required. The volume of sample injected onto the column is now 0.5 ml, instead of the 1.0 ml previously used.

### b) Urines

The 24-hour urine specimens are collected and processed as previously described. For hydrolysis, a thawed aliquot of urine is passed through a 0.22-$\mu$m fil-

1  This investigation was supported by Public Health Service Research Grants No. CA-12043 and CA-13671 from the National Cancer Institute.

ter, brought to 0.1 N in HCl, and then heated for 1 h at 100 °C. In the discussions below, a hydrolyzed urine is always so designated.

Collections were obtained from patients seen at the Melanoma Clinic, University of California, San Francisco.

## Results

a) Chromatographic-Peak Profiles

The general appearance of a normal urine is shown in figure 1 (top). The characteristic feature here is the general absence of major peaks in the 1.5- to 3-hour elution range. The chromatograms for patients with disseminated melanoma, by contrast, show a number of major peaks in this range (fig. 2, bottom).

It is our general experience that the DPPH-chromatograms for patients with only a small primary tumor or a few recurrent cutaneous lesions resemble those of a normal urine, showing few peaks in the late elution range. A few urine samples from patients with primary or locally recurrent melanoma have shown major peaks in the 1.5- to 3-hour range, but these patterns fail to match those of the disseminated cases, and the late peaks can frequently be traced to the ingestion of medications, such as Aldomet. The most complex chromatographic patterns have always been found among the disseminated cases.

b) Hydrolysis of Normals

Figure 1 compares the DPPH-chromatogram of a normal urine (top) with the same urine after mild acid hydrolysis (bottom). After hydrolysis, the chromatogram shows a complex pattern of peaks that are absent from the non-hydrolyzed urine. The absence of these new peaks in the untreated urine is consistent with normal hepatic function in blocking reactive chemical groups, including the aromatic hydroxyls that reduce DPPH [1, 2, 5]. The mild acid hydrolysis removes the blocking groups, presumably glucuronides and sulfates, allowing the DPPH reaction to proceed. The conversion of a relatively simple chromatographic pattern in the 1.5- to 3-hour elution range into a more complex array of peaks upon hydrolysis is a consistent finding in all normal urines.

c) Disseminated Melanoma Urines

Figure 2 compares the DPPH-chromatogram of the urine from a patient with disseminated melanoma (bottom) with the same urine after mild

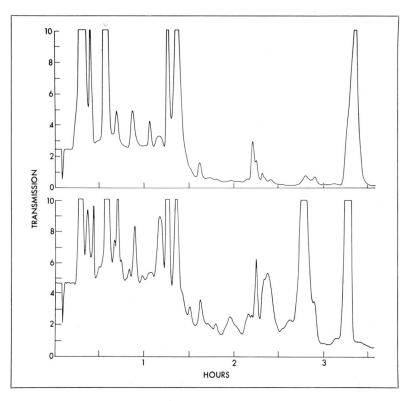

*Fig. 1.* Top = DPPH-chromatogram of a normal urine. Bottom = chromatogram of the same urine after mild acid hydrolysis. Urine volume, 2.50 ml each.

acid hydrolysis (top). The non-hydrolyzed urine displays a complex array of major peaks in the 1.5- to 3-hour elution range that is not observed in a normal urine (fig. 1, top). In addition, the hydrolyzed disseminated urine differs only slightly from the non-hydrolyzed urine, a finding consistent with the impairment of hepatic function in conjugating reactive groups. A close similarity between the chromatograms of hydrolyzed and non-hydrolyzed urines is commonly observed for patients with advanced hepatic metastases.

### d) Identity of Peaks

The prominent features most frequently observed in the chromatograms of urines from patients with disseminated melanoma are two peaks

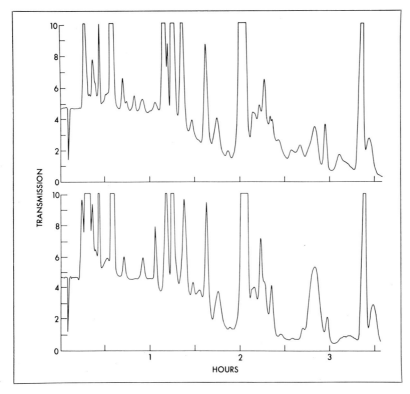

*Fig. 2.* Top = DPPH-chromatogram of a disseminated melanoma urine, after mild acid hydrolysis. Bottom = same urine before hydrolysis. Urine volume, 1.25 ml each.

found at approximately 120 and 170 min elution time. Several other distinguishing peaks are also observable in these samples, but the above two stand out as the most visually obvious in the DPPH-chromatograms. The two peaks have been observed in many different combinations: both equally, both with one or the other predominating, and one or the other but not both.

The identity of the peaks has not yet been firmly established, but a determination is actively in progress. The 120-min peak corresponds in elution position to methoxydopa (3-methoxy-4-hydroxy-phenylalanine, MOPA), but coincidence of chromatographic position is not sufficient to establish identity. Coincidence of position is valuable, however, for ruling out possible alternatives. Figure 3 compares the chromatogram of the ur-

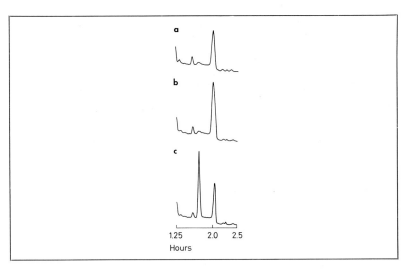

*Fig. 3. a* Disseminated melanoma urine, diluted; *b* same urine with MOPA added; *c* same urine with dopa added.

ine from a patient with disseminated melanoma (a) with the same urine to which MOPA has been added (b), and to which dopa has been added (c). Since dopa elutes at approximately 105 min, the 120-min peak cannot be dopa. In only one of the ten chromatographically disseminated cases (table I) has a major peak appeared at the dopa position, although a minor peak is not infrequent.

The 170-min peak fails to correspond in elution position to any presently known DPPH reactant. However, this peak elutes in a position corresponding closely to a constituent of hydolyzed normal urine (fig. 1, bottom).

e) Summary of Cases

Table I shows a summary of results for the clinically disseminated patients seen at the Melanoma Clinic during 1974. The results for primary and recurrent melanoma patients are not included. The cases summarized have presented with metastases to various internal organs, or with extensive nodal involvement, or both. Normal and disseminated chromatograms have been defined above. In the intermediate category, a chromatogram will show major peaks in the late elution range that fail to match those appearing in the majority of the disseminated cases. The 3

*Table I.* Classification of disseminated melanoma patients by DPPH-chromatographic profile

| Chromatogram | Cases | Status | |
|---|---|---|---|
| Normal | 3 | lung nodules only | (3) |
| Intermediate | 3 | +liver scan only | (1)[1] |
| | | −scans and tests | (2) |
| Disseminated | 10 | lung nodules only | (1) |
| | | +scans and tests | (9) |
| | | (liver scans: +3 | |
| | | ?3 | |
| | | −4) | |

1 Urine 10/74, scan 12/74.

intermediate chromatograms all show a major peak at approximately 140 min elution time.

The majority of the clinically disseminated cases (10 of 16) fall into the chromatographically disseminated category, as well; 9 of the 10 cases in this class have combinations of positive results for visceral metastases including chest X-rays, liver and bone scans, and blood chemistries, while one case with pulmonary metastases was normal with respect to other scans and tests. In the intermediate chromatographic category, 2 cases (one with brain metastases) appear to be clinically stable, while one case has recently shown a positive liver scan. The unusual chromatogram in this latter case dates from an earlier urine; a current specimen has not yet become available for analysis. In the patients with known metastases and normal chromatograms, all 3 cases have demonstrated only pulmonary metastases with all other scans and laboratory tests being normal. The chromatograms of the latter cases with pulmonary metastases show minor peaks distinguishable from both normal and disseminated urines. The chromatograms have been classed as normal until the significance of these minor peaks is resolved.

## Discussion

Past attempts at analyzing melanoma urines for dopa metabolites have taken several different approaches, involving various detecting reagents on either whole or fractionated urine. The diverse approaches have also resulted in a diversity of correlations between urinary melanogens and clinical state. In examining the urine concentrations of several melanogens, VOORHESS [7] found that only dopa appeared to be frequently elevated in patients with disseminated disease, and then in only half the cases. HINTERBERGER et al. [4], on the other hand, has reported urinary levels of 'free catechols' increasing with increased tumor burden.

We have developed an alternative approach to detecting urinary melanogens, using an automatic ion-exchange chromatographic system and a different reagent. We believe this analytical system offers many advantages over other techniques, not the least of which is avoiding the tedious manual steps previously required for isolating and detecting melanogens. The principal advantage of the DPPH-analytical system, however, lies in presenting a fairly comprehensive chromatographic picture of the melanogens and other reducing compounds in urine. The preselection of metabolites to be isolated, a procedure not without pitfalls, is now no longer necessary.

The results of our analyses have areas of agreement with both previous views, namely that dopa appears not to be a prominently excreted metabolite, but that other melanogens are commonly excreted at elevated levels in the urine of patients with disseminated melanoma. The major point of difference is that the peaks we find most prominent and characteristic in disseminated melanoma fail to correspond to the melanogens that have been previously mentioned in the literature [3].

Dopa and its metabolites, including phenols and indoles, have been assayed in melanoma urines by a number of different groups. The results of these studies have been summarized by DUCHON and MATOUS [3], showing that on the average dopa occurs at elevated levels in 65% of disseminated melanoma urines. We have also observed a peak at the dopa position in a number of disseminated melanoma cases, and its presence very likely represents an elevated level of dopa compared to normals. It is our conclusion, however, that even if dopa is present in elevated amounts, it is not the principal melanogen in the urine of patients with disseminated disease. The 120-min peak has predominated over dopa in 9 out of 10 of the chromatographically disseminated cases (table I).

It should be noted that the stoichiometry of the DPPH reaction with dopa is the highest of any melanogen thus far tested [2]. For another melanogen, including MOPA, to show a peak even equal in area to dopa, it would have to be present at concentrations greater than dopa. The only instances in which a major peak has been observed at the dopa position occurs when a patient (in the non-disseminated category) is taking Aldomet. Alphamethyldopa cannot be separated from dopa on our columns. RILEY et al. [6] have also noted elevated levels of unknown metabolites in mouse melanoma urines. Using amino acid analysis, these unknowns failed to correspond in elution position to dopa.

The presence of other melanogens in disseminated urines, such as phenolic acids, homovanillic acid, vanillactic acid, and dihydroxyphenylacetic acid, cannot be confirmed or excluded by the DPPH-chromatograms. Peaks close to the standard elution position of these metabolites have been observed in both normal and disseminated urines. Whether these peaks in normal urines represent the phenolic melanogens or other constituents has not yet been determined. The lack of a clear-cut difference at these positions between normal and disseminated urine chromatograms prevents any conclusions from being drawn at this time regarding the nitrogen-free melanogens.

The presence of dopamine in the urines received at the Melanoma Clinic has not been investigated. An automatic analyzer using DPPH has recently been developed in our laboratory for detecting the catecholamines, but the screening of melanoma urines for this class of highly basic metabolites has not yet commenced.

The classification of disseminated melanoma cases according to their DPPH-chromatographic profiles suggests that elevated urinary melanogens are closely associated with visceral metastases, particularly in the liver. The appearance of melanogens may not, however, be confined to liver involvement since abnormal liver function and enzyme tests were not demonstrable in all of the 10 cases with disseminated chromatograms. Table I also shows that urinary melanogens common to the widely disseminated cases are absent in 3 of 4 patients with (presumably) only pulmonary metastases. However, this latter finding may be attributable as much to the small size of detectable lung nodules as to their location.

It is important to point out the kind of information that is not contained in the summary table, particularly the chromatographic transitions from normal to disseminated profiles that have been observed as a patient progresses from a primary (or recurrent) to a clinically disseminated state. There also appears to be more than one trajectory by which the normal-to-disseminated chromatographic transition may be accomplished. Sufficient data have not yet been accumulated to determine how early a chromatographic transition may be detected, but preliminary evidence indicates that this can occur before other clinical or laboratory findings become positive. We thus believe that the proper role for testing urinary melanogens is on a regular basis, at least every three months for higher risk patients, and as often as monthly in special cases.

The unique complexity of each disseminated chromatographic profile is also difficult to convey in a summary table. Although many cases may appear clinically similar, no two patients with disseminated melanoma have identical chromatograms. The chromatographic profiles may thus contain further clinical information about melanoma patients and the course of their disease than has been recognized at the present time.

## Summary

We have described a new automatic ion-exchange chromatographic system for separating and detecting dihydroxyphenylalanine metabolites in the urine of patients with malignant melanoma. The system is similar to an amino acid analyzer, but uses the stable free radical diphenylpicrylhydrazyl (DPPH) as the colorimetric reagent, and has its own unique set of operating parameters. DPPH reacts with a wide range of reducing compounds of biological origin, particularly the hydroxy-methoxy-substituted indoles and phenols associated with the growth of pigmented tumors as melanin precursors, and is useful as a colorimetric indicator of elevated levels of melanogens in the urine of melanoma patients. An automatic DPPH-chromatography system was constructed in order to analyze urine for individual melanogens. The system has been used to obtain chromatographic scans of a urine series from normal controls and melanoma patients. 20–30 peaks are typically observed, showing a generally similar pattern for normal controls and for patients with local primary melanoma. Chromatograms of urine from patients with disseminated melanoma are quite different, however, showing a number of major peaks in the catechol-indole elution range that are not found in urine of normal controls or patients with primary melanoma. The distinguishing peaks in urine from patients with disseminated melanoma correspond to compounds of low molecular weight ($<$1,000), and remain to be identified.

## References

1    BANDA, P. W.; SHERRY, A. E., and BLOIS, M. S.: An automatic analyzer for the detection of dihydroxyphenylalanine metabolites and other reducing compounds in urine. Analyt. Chem. 46: 1772–1777 (1974).
2    BANDA, P. W.; SHERRY, A. E., and BLOIS, M. S.: The reaction of diphenylpicrylhydrazyl with physiological compounds. Anal. Lett. 7: 41–51 (1974).

3    Duchon, J. and Matous, B.: Dopa and its metabolites in melanoma urine. Pigment Cell, vol. 1, pp. 317–322 (Karger, Basel 1973).
4    Hinterberger, H.; Freedman, A., and Bartholomew, R. J.: Precursors of melanin in the blood and urine in malignant melanoma. Clin. chim. Acta 39: 395–400 (1972).
5    Papariello, G. J. and Janish, M. A. M.: Diphenylpicrylhydrazyl as an organic analytical reagent in the spectrophotometric analysis of phenols. Analyt. Chem. 38: 211–214 (1966).
6    Riley, V.; Spackman, D., and Fitzmaurice, M. A.: Plasma and urine amino acid changes associated with melanoma. Pigment Cell, vol. 1, pp. 331–345 (Karger, Basel 1973).
7    Voorhess, M. L.: Urinary excretion of dopa and metabolites by patients with melanoma. Cancer 26: 146–149 (1970).

Dr. Phillip W. Banda, Department of Dermatology, School of Medicine, University of California, San Francisco, CA 94143 (USA)

Pigment Cell, vol. 2, pp. 264–272 (Karger, Basel 1976)

# Demonstration of Cytotoxic Lymphocytes in Patients with Sutton's Disease against Melanoma Cells *in vitro*

M. MICKSCHE, C. CERNI, E. KOKOSCHKA and W. GEBHART

Institute for Cancer Research, and II. Department of Dermatology, University of Vienna, Vienna

*Introduction*

Extensive immunologic studies have revealed that malignant melanoma is highly immunogenic. It is therefore assumed that immunological mechanisms could be responsible for the spontaneous regression of primary and secondary manifestations associated with this tumor [12, 17]. Immunological parameters have been used to define the extent and prognosis of malignant disease [5]. A correlation between the presence of cytotoxic lymphocytes and the clinical stage of the disease has been found in some tumor systems [9, 14]. A pigment cell tumor which is also known to show spontaneous resolution is the so-called halo nevus – a nevus cell nevus which is predominantly located on the trunk and surrounded by a typical area of hypopigmentation. This dermatological phenomenon was first time described as leukoderma acquisitum centrifugum by SUTTON [18]. The natural history of this nevus is a gradual disappearance of the nevus cells accompanied by a centrifugal extension of the depigmented region in the overlying epidermis, due to a reduction or complete disappearence of melanocytes in this area [4]. There has been much speculation about the mechanisms involved in this spontaneous tumor involution [10, 13, 21]. Recently, COPEMAN *et al.* [3] have demonstrated circulating antibodies directed against cytoplasmic antigen of human malignant melanoma cells in patients with halo nevus.

The purpose of the present study was to investigate whether tumor-regression is mediated by cellular immune mechanisms and whether a common antigen on malignant melanoma cells and on nevus cells might exist.

## Material and Methods

### 1. Patient Selection

16 patients with different stages of leukoderma acquisitum centrifugum were included in this study. From 12 of these, a total number of 18 halo nevi was removed by surgery under general or local anesthesia. The specimens were immediately divided into small pieces and processed in different ways for various histopathological investigations. From all of these patients, peripheral blood was taken and lymphocyte reactivity was studied *in vitro* against cultured human malignant melanoma cells.

### 2. Histopathological Investigations

a) Light Microscopy

One part of the excised specimen was fixed in 10% formalin and embedded in paraffin for routine histology. Hematoxillin and eosin, Masson's silver and iron stains were performed on all biopsies.

b) Electron Microscopy

Small pieces of 5 excised tumors were prefixed with 3% glutaraldehyde. After several rinsing steps in buffer, postfixation was performed in 1% osmium tetroxide. The material was then dehydrated with ethanol and embedded in Epon 812. Ultrathin sections were then cut with a ultramicrotome (Reichert OMU 3) and after staining with uranylacetate and lead citrate examined with an electron microscope (Zeiss EM 9 S 2).

### 3. Immunological Investigations

a) Lymphocyte Preparation

50 ml heparinized peripheral blood was diluted and layered on a Ficoll-Ronpacon® gradient [1]. Purified lymphocytes were recovered from the gradient after low speed centrifugation After some washing steps with serum-free Hanks the lymphocyte suspension was passed through a nylon wool column (FT-242-Fenwal Laboratories, Ill.) to remove adherent cells and platelets. The final concentration was adjusted to $2.5 \times 10^6$ lymphocytes per ml.

b) Tumor Cell Preparation

As target cells for the cytotoxicity test, human malignant melanoma cells were grown as a continuous cell line *in vitro*. These were kindly supplied by Dr. G. HEPPNER (Brown University, Providence, R.I.). Waymouth medium with 30% newborn fetal calf serum (Gibco, Bio-Cult., Wash.) was used for culturing the cells.

c) Assay for Cell-Mediated Immunity

The microcytotoxicity test according to TAKASUGI and KLEIN [20] was used in HELLSTRÖM's modification [8].

Tumor cells were plated on Falcon Microtestplates II (3040) in an appropriate cell concentration depending on the plating efficiency of the cell line. The cultures were then incubated overnight at 37 °C. 24 h later, 0.2 ml of lymphocyte suspension from the test or control persons was added to each test well at dilutions of 1:5, 1:10

and 1:20 of the starting concentration. After 45 min incubation on a rocker, 0.05 ml Hanks solution containing inactivated fetal calf serum (50%) was added and the cultures incubated for 48 h in a humidified $CO_2$ incubator at 37 °C.

After this period, the microplates were carefully rinsed with phosphate-buffered saline. The remaining cells in the wells were fixed and stained with 1% crystal violet and counted by observing the plate under an inverted microscope.

Specific cell-mediated immunity of the patients was then calculated by the formula:

% cell-mediated immunity =

$$100 - \frac{\text{mean number of tumor cells left after incubation with test lymphocytes}}{\text{mean number of tumor cells left after incubation with lymphocytes of two control persons}} \times 100.$$

Statistical analyses were performed according to Student's t-test.

## Results

The clinical data of the patients are given in table I. They are in agreement with the accepted findings, that leukoderma acquisitum centrifugum occurs most frequently in young adults, and the predominant location of this lesion is the trunk (fig. 1a).

### Light Microscopic Findings

Histopathologically, the following, not strictly defined, stages of tumor involution could be found (fig. 1b).

a) Intact nevus cell nests in the upper corium or in the dermo-epidermal junction with only mild cellular infiltration in the surrounding connective tissue or slight invasion of the peripheral tumor islands.

b) Dense infiltration by lymphocytes, histiocytes and macrophages throughout the whole tumor, including the intraepidermal nevus cell nests. Progressive destruction of the tumor cell islands.

c) Exclusively cellular infiltrate consisting of the same cell types as above; nevus cells no longer identifiable; the pigment was found only within melanophages.

### Electron Microscopic Findings
a) Nevus Cells

The morphology of intact nevus cells varied in the investigated material, depending on the type of the primary nevus, the degree of melaniza-

*Table I*

| Patient | | Sex | Age | Halo nevus | | | | CMI[3], % |
|---|---|---|---|---|---|---|---|---|
| | | | | localization | num-ber[1] | duration | treatment[2] | |
| 1 | L. S. | F | 12 | trunk, chest, neck, l. arm | 5 | 2 years | – | 12** |
| 2 | P. C. | F | 28 | r. shoulder | 1 | 2 years | – | 35* |
| 3 | H. I. | F | 12 | l. thigh | 1 | 12 years | op. 1969 | –14 |
| 4 | G. A. | F | 9 | neck, r. knee | 2 | 6 months | – | 47* |
| 5 | B. G. | F | 13 | back | 3 | 3 years | op. 1972 | –40 |
| 6 | H. H. | F | 11 | back | 1 | 3 years | op. 1970 | 24** |
| 7 | A. A. | F | 62 | r. upper arm | 1 | 55 years | op. 1967 | 4 |
| 8 | N. A. | F | 12 | back | 2 | 2 years | – | 32* |
| 9 | N. S. | F | 24 | back | 1 | 1 year | op. 1972 | 20** |
| 10 | W. E. | M | 15 | trunk | >5 | – | – | 20* |
| 11 | H. G. | M | 18 | trunk | 1 | 3 years | op. 1971 | 0 |
| 12 | P. G. | M | 29 | trunk | >5 | 2 years | op. 1972 | 40* |
| 13 | D. K. | M | 16 | chest, trunk | 3 | 3 months | op. (2)72 | 18* |
| 14 | B. M. | M | 14 | back, neck | 3 | 11 years | op. (2)68 | 1 |
| 15 | S. F. | M | 22 | trunk | 1 | 6 years | – | 33* |
| 16 | S. S. | F | 19 | back | 1 | 1 year | – | 65* |

1 Number of halo nevi detected on the day of diagnosis.
2 When not indicated in parentheses, one nevus was excised.
3 The percent cell-mediated immunity was calculated by comparison between the mean number of target cells left after incubation with test lymphocytes and the mean number of target cells left after incubation with lymphocytes of two control persons.
* $p < 0.001$; ** $p < 0.01$.

tion, and the stage of the lesion. Most of the intact nevus cells showed a round or dentated nucleus, one or more nucleoli and a relatively high number of mitochondria. In the cytoplasm, a well-differentiated endoplasmatic reticulum, Golgi area, and a variable number of melanosomes could be identified.

Concomitant with the cellular infiltration, severe changes in the ultrastructure of the nevus cells were found (fig. 2a–d). The shape of the nuclei changed from round to polygonal. The nucleoplasm was more electron-dense and homogeneous and nucleoli were not as prominent as before. In the cytoplasm, many large vacuoles were present (fig. 2b) and mitochondria as well as endoplasmatic reticulum were swollen or ruptured. The nuclear membrane was widened and often detached from the nuclear

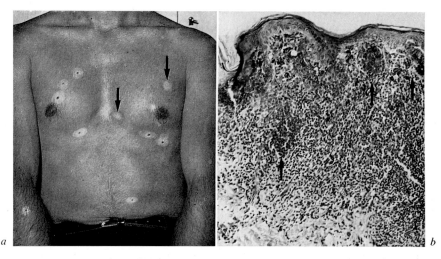

*a*  *b*

*Fig. 1. a* A 29-year-old patient with multiple halo nevi at different stages of tumor regression. Arrows indicate lesions with complete regression of the nevus. *b* Biopsy of a halo nevus showing dense cellular infiltrate underneath the nevus. Tumor cell nests (arrows) are hardly recognized. HE. × 105.

surface. Finally, the morphological organization of the cell was disrupted and, as a result of cytolysis, isolated parts of nuclei and round or amorphous masses of cytoplasmic compartments were found, sometimes floating freely in the extracellular space (fig. 2c).

b) Cellular Infiltrate (fig. 2a, d)

The cellular infiltrate consisted of: (1) lymphocytes without any special differentiation of their ultrastructure (fig. 2a); (2) many cells with dentated or lobulated nuclei, with a clear cytoplasm which contained a big number of free ribosomes or polyribosomes and only few cytoplasmic

*Fig. 2. a* Lymphocyte (L) in direct contact with the cell membrane of a nevus cell (N). ×13,500. *b* Nevus cell with vacuolization (V) of their cytoplasm as early signs of cell injury. × 20,000. *c* Cytolysis of the nevus cell in later stage of tumor cell damage. Cytolytic fragments are found between the collagen bundles (C) in the extracellular space. × 13,500. *d* Melanosomes from destroyed nevus cells are phagocytised by macrophages and collected in the melanophagolysosomes (M). × 16,000.

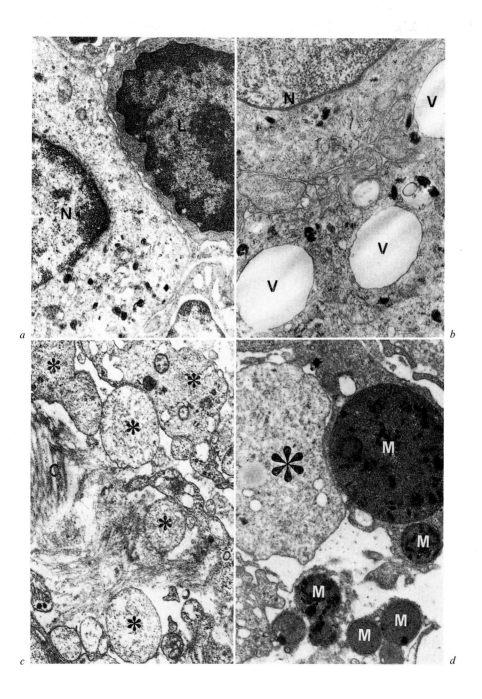

organelles (activated lymphocytes); (3) mast cells; (4) macrophages (fig. 2d). Some of them contained only few phagocytized particles, but more primary lysosomes. The majority contained a number of phagolysosomes. The predominant compartment in these lysosomes was melanin in different stages of degradation.

### Immunological Investigations

With the microcytotoxicity test, it was found that of 16 patients with halo nevus, 11 had lymphocytes which were specifically cytotoxic for the plated human malignant melanoma cells. In all cases, a comparison between the lymphocyte reactivity of the patients and of two healthy blood donors was performed. Values were expressed in percent cell-mediated immunity by the above-mentioned formula.

In 5 patients whose tumors had been surgically removed more than two years previously, no specific cytotoxic reaction of their lymphocytes against the melanoma cells could be detected.

### Discussion

The etiology of the dermatological phenomenon leukoderma acquisitum is only partially elucidated. Different authors have raised different hypotheses on the mechanism by which the tumor regression and the area of depigmentation might develop [6, 11, 22].

The generally accepted theory to date is that the phenomenon is the result of an immunological reaction by which the nevus cells and the melanocytes are destroyed.

This hypothesis was first proposed by RHODENBERG [15] in 1927. KOPF et al. [10] suggested that an immune reaction as in autoimmune disease or graft rejection might be responsible, but they were unable to substantiate this. STEGMAIER et al. [19] developed the working hypothesis that dermal nevus cells express an antigen which is recognized as 'non-self' and causes a delayed hypersensitivity reaction by which a cytotoxic substance is produced. A progressive destruction of the nevus cells and the melanocytes is the result.

COPEMAN et al. [3] have given evidence that the halo nevus cells have some antigenic identity with melanoma cells, by demonstrating circulating antibodies in patients with Sutton's disease, which were directed against cytoplasmic antigens of melanoma cells.

Our findings of a specific cytotoxic lymphocyte reaction in patients with halo nevus against the melanoma cells support the possibility that the tumor regression is mediated by cellular immune mechanisms. The reaction against the human melanoma cells might give evidence for a common antigen which is shared by the melanoma cells, the nevus cells and the melanocytes, as these three cell types are closely related embryonically. The re-expression of embryonic antigens due to malignant transformation has been demonstrated for animal [2] and human tumor systems [7] and these antigens can also be found in very low concentrations in normal tissue [16]. A quantitative difference in antigen expression and recognition could also be responsible in the halo nevus system and as a consequence, in the destruction of the target cells by immunocytes.

However, the phenomenon of a spontaneous tumor regression as found in the halo nevus provides an appropriate human model for *in vivo* and *in vitro* studies on tumor cell-immunocyte interactions.

## Summary

Histopathological findings and the demonstration of circulating antibodies directed against cytoplasmic melanoma antigen suggest that immunological mechanisms might be responsible for the regression of the halo nevus. We investigated lymphocyte reactivity of 16 patients, with clinically and histologically confirmed halo nevus, against cultivated human malignant melanoma cells in the microcytotoxicity test. Eleven of these patients had cytotoxic lymphocytes. Five patients, whose tumors had been removed by surgery more than two years ago, did not show a specific lymphocyte reaction against the melanoma cells. Our light and electron microscopic findings and the demonstration of cytotoxic lymphocytes give further confirmation that cellular immune mechanisms might be responsible for the spontaneous tumor regression.

## References

1   Bøyum, A.: Separation of blood leucocytes, granulocytes and lymphocytes. Tissue Antigens 4: 269–274 (1974).

2   Chou-Chik Ting; Lavrin, D. H.; Shiu, G., and Herberman, R. B.: Expression of fetal antigens in tumor cells. Proc. natn. Acad. Sci. USA 69: 1664–1668 (1972).

3   Copeman, P. W. M.; Lewis, M. G.; Phillips, T. M., and Elliott, P. G.: Immunological associations of the halo nevus with cutaneous malignant melanoma. Br. J. Derm. 88: 127–137 (1973).

4   EBNER, H. und NIEBAUER, G.: Elektronenoptische Befunde zum Pigmentver-
    lust beim Naevus Sutton. Dermatologica *137:* 345–357 (1968).
5   EIBLER, F. R. and MORTON, D. L.: Impaired immunologic reactivity and re-
    currence following cancer surgery. Cancer, Philad. *25:* 362–367 (1970).
6   FINDLAY, G. H.: Histology of Sutton's nevus. Br. J. Derm. *69:* 389–394 (1957).
7   GOLD, P. and FREEDMAN, S. O.: Specific carcinoembryonic antigens of the hu-
    man digestive system. J. exp. Med. *122:* 467–481 (1965).
8   HELLSTRÖM, I. and HELLSTRÖM, K. E.: Colony inhibition and cytotoxic assays;
    in BLOOM and GLADE *in vitro* methods in cell-mediated immunity, pp. 409–514
    (Academic Press, New York 1971).
9   HELLSTRÖM, I.; SJÖGREN, H. O.; WARNER, G., and HELLSTRÖM, K.: Blocking of
    cell-mediated immunity by sera from patients with growing neoplasms. Int. J.
    Cancer *7:* 226–237 (1971).
10  KOPF, A. W.; MORRILL, S. D., and SILBERBERG, I.: Broad spectrum of leukoder-
    ma acquisitum centrifugum. Archs Derm. *92:* 14–33 (1965).
11  LEIDER, M. and FISCHER, A. A.: Fate of central nevus in leukoderma acquisi-
    tum centrifugum. Archs Derm. *60:* 1160–1166 (1949).
12  LEWIS, M. G.: Possible immunological factors in human malignant melanoma
    in Uganda. Lancet *ii:* 91 (1967).
13  LEWIS, M. G. and COPEMAN, P. W. M.: Halo naevus – a frustrated malignant
    melanoma. Br. med. J. *ii:* 47–48 (1972).
14  O'TOOLE, C.; PERLMAN, P.; UNSGAARD, B.; MOBERGER, G., and ENDSMYR, F.:
    Cellular immunity to human primary bladder carcinoma. I. Correlation to clini-
    cal stage and radiotherapy. Int. J. Cancer *10:* 77–91 (1972).
15  RHODENBERG, G. L.: Spontaneous regression of multiple pigmented moles.
    Arch. Path. Lab. Med. *4:* 528–529 (1927).
16  ROSAI, J.; TILLACK, T. W., and MARCHESI, V. T.: Membrane antigens of human
    colonic carcinoma and non-tumoral colonic mucosa: results obtained with a
    new isolation method. Int. J. Cancer *10:* 357–367 (1972).
17  SMITH, J. L., jr. and STEHLIN, J. S., jr.: Spontaneous regression of primary ma-
    lignant melanoma with regional metastases. Cancer, Philad. *18:* 1399–1415
    (1965).
18  SUTTON, R. L.: An unusual variety of vitiligo leukoderma acquisitum centri-
    fugum. J. Cutan. Dis. *34:* 797–800 (1916).
19  STEGMAIER, O. C.; BECKER, S. W., jr., and MEDENICA, M.: Multiple halo nevi.
    Archs Derm. *99:* 180–189 (1969).
20  TAKASUGI, M. and KLEIN, E.: A microassay for cell-mediated immunity. Trans-
    plantation *9:* 219–227 (1970).
21  TANAKA, H.: Studies on pigmentation in nevoid, neoplastic and other diseases
    of the skin. Jap. J. Derm. *68:* 1–59 (1958).
22  WAYTE, D. M. and HELWIG, E. B.: Halo nevi. Cancer *22:* 69–90 (1968).

Dr. M. MICKSCHE, Institute for Cancer Research, University of Vienna, *A–1090
Vienna* (Austria)

Pigment Cell, vol. 2, pp. 273–283 (Karger, Basel 1976)

# 'Naevus caeruleus tardus' in Association with Progressive Systemic Scleroderma

Yoshiaki Hori, Shichiro Miyazawa and Shigeo Nishiyama

Department of Dermatology, Kitasato University Medical School, Sagamihara

Dermal melanocytoses (Mongolian spots) may occur on any portion of the body, but are seen most commonly in the sacral region. They usually are noted at birth and disappear within a few years [5]. Occasionally, dermal melanocytosis will persist beyond infancy [6].

Dermal melanocytosis (Mongolian spot), blue nevus (common type), oculocutaneous melanosis (nevus of Ota) and nevus of Ito are closely related. The nevus of Ota is located on the side of the face and involves the eye and/or oral mucous membrane. The nevus of Ito is unilaterally located on the shoulder girdle. The nevi of Ota and Ito are macular lesions, usually revealing a mixture of brown small patches and blue macules; they tend to persist and even to extend their area of patchy pigmentation.

The cells in a dermal melanocytosis are identical with blue-nevus cells and give a dopa-positive reaction. Unlike blue nevi, however, in which the cells occur in clumps and wavy groups, the cells in dermal melanocytosis are scattered widely in the dermis and do not disturb the normal architecture of the skin.

In the histopathology of the nevi of Ota and Ito, dermal melanocytes are observed to be widely spaced in the dermis and partial hyperpigmentation of basal layer of the epidermis is also recognized.

In progressive systemic sclerosis (scleroderma), brownish hyperpigmentation – histologically, basal hyperpigmentation of the epidermis – and depigmentation of the involved area of the skin have usually been observed.

No report has been presented of 'blue macules' in the patients with progressive systemic sclerosis until now. This paper deals with clinical and histopathological studies of 4 cases with progressive systemic sclerosis who developed blue macules on the back and/or upper arms in course of cutaneous sclerosis.

## Materials and Methods

Case 1: A 30-year-old woman who has been suffering from systemic sclerosis since the age of 26 and has developed blue macules on the left upper arm.

Case 2: A 32-year-old woman who has been suffering from subcutaneous calcinosis, Raynaud's phenomenon, teleangiectasia and cutaneous sclerosis since the age of 28 and has developed blue patches on the back and upper arms which are reticular and macular, and have gradually been increasing in their range and intensity of the blue tone.

Case 3: A 25-year-old woman, who has developed cutaneous sclerosis and blue macule on the back since the age of 23.

Case 4: A 44-year-old man who has been suffering from systemic sclerosis since the age of 38, who shows depigmentation and hyperpigmentation with blue macule on the back.

Biopsy specimens obtained from blue macules of the patients were fixed in 1% $OsO_4$ solution buffered with 0.2 M Na cacodylate for 2 h at 4° C and dehydrated in ethanol series, embedded in Epon 812. Ultra-thin sections were obtained with Porter-Blum MT-2B ultramicrotome, stained with uranyl acetate and lead citrate and observed with a Hitachi HU-12A electron microscope for ultrastructural study.

Light microscope and histochemical studies (dopa reaction) of the skin were also performed. X-ray microanalysis [3] was performed to analyze melanosomes in a dermal melanocyte as well as those in the epidermis of case 2. Thin sections (about 1,000 Å in thickness) were obtained, placed on platinum grids without any stain and observed with a JEM-100C transmission electron microscope with a scanning attachment combined with an EDAX energy dispersive type spectrometer for the X-ray microanalytic study.

## Results

Blue macules were recognized on the back and/or the upper arms on one side or on both sides. The blue macule consists mostly of linear blue lines and partially of small blue patches.

In the lower two thirds of the cutis, spindle-shaped and brown-pigment granule-bearing cells were recognized. These cells were widely spaced in the dermis and were observed between the connective and elastic tissue fibers, parallel to the epidermis, and did not disturb normal architecture (fig. 1, 2). Most of those cells were not clumped together, although some of them were recognized as a group. Dopa reaction of the spindle-shaped cells in the blue macules was positive (fig. 3).

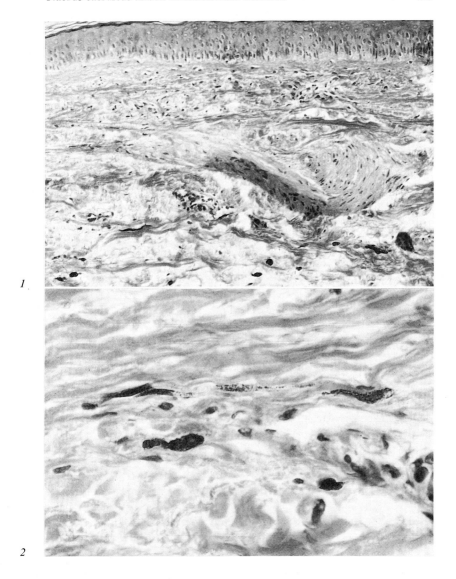

*Fig. 1.* Histology of blue macule of the upper arm of case 2. Spindle-shaped dermal melanocytes are recognized in the dermis. HE.

*Fig. 2.* The higher magnification of dermal melanocytes, case 2. HE.

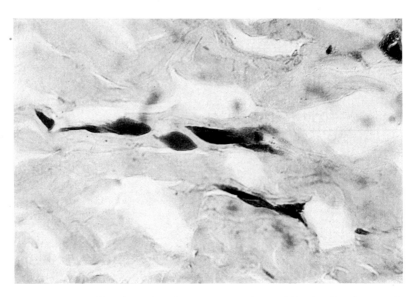

*Fig. 3.* Dopa-positive dermal melanocytes are observed in the dermis, case 3. Dopa reaction.

Electronmicroscopically, many full-melanized melanosomes (stage IV melanosomes) [4, 10] were contained in those spindle-shaped cells – dermal melanocytes. The melanosomes were rounded or elipsoid (fig. 4, 10, 11). Electron-lucent small granules [8] were recognized in the melanosomes (fig. 5, 6). A very few immature melanosomes (stages II or III melanosomes) were also observed (fig. 7, 8, 9). Almost all melanosomes, whatever the stage was, were solitarily distributed in the dermal melanocytes. The size of full-melanized melanosomes was 0.7 μm in the largest diameter.

By X-ray microanalysis combined with a transmission electronmicroscope with scanning attachment (fig. 12) the melanosomes of dermal melanocytes in blue macule, chlorine and sulfur were detected in melanosomes (fig. 13), and phosphorus was also detected, but it was recognized to be mixed with osmium and platinum. These data were almost the same as those of the melanosomes in the epidermal keratinocyte of the same subject (fig. 14), although at the peak of sulfur was lower than that of the melanosomes in the dermal melanocyte.

Basal lamina was recognized in most, but not all, dermal melanocytes.

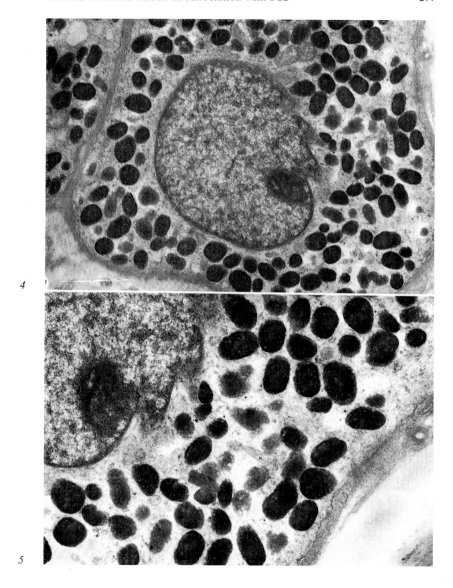

Fig. 4. Electron micrograph of a mature dermal melanocyte. Fully melanized melanosomes (stage IV melanosomes) are solitarily distributed in cytoplasm, case 2. Uranyl acetate and lead citrate stain. × 7,700.

Fig. 5. Higher magnification of figure 4. Electron lucent structure is recognized. Uranyl acetate and lead citrate stain. × 14,400.

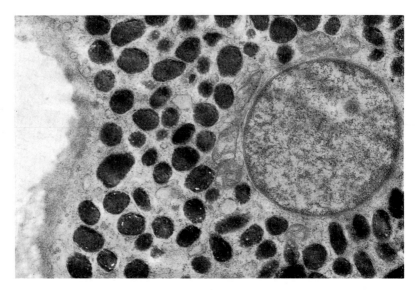

*Fig. 6.* Electron micrograph of a dermal melanocyte obtained from the upper arm of case 2. Electron lucent structure and microfibrils are observed. Uranyl acetate and lead citrate stain. × 14,400.

*Discussion*

The present study of blue macules in the patients with progressive systemic sclerosis revealed the existence of dermal melanocytes which were still producing melanosomes.

Histologically, the blue macules resemble the dermal melanocytosis (Mongolian spot); however, the blue macule is clinically different from dermal melanocytosis or the nevi of Ota or Ito. The blue macule consists of linear blue lines and blue patches.

Mongolian spot may occur on any portion of the body, although seen most commonly in the sacral region. They usually are noted at birth and disappear within a few years, but ocasionally will persist beyond infancy. Nevertheless, dermal melanocytes (Mongolian cells) were found in the bodies of all examined Japanese from the age of 18 to 82, although the dermal melanocytes were less frequently encountered in older persons [7].

Dermal melanocytes were also histologically found in the sacral region of Caucasians from the age of 5 months to 12 months [2]. ADACHI

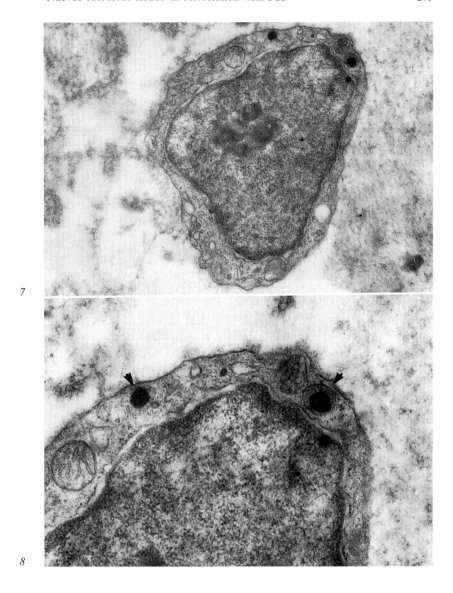

Fig. 7. Electron micrograph of an immature dermal melanocyte obtained from the upper arm of case 2. Uranyl acetate and lead citrate stain. × 14,400.

Fig. 8. Higher magnification of figure 7. Note stage III melanosome (arrows). Uranyl acetate and lead citrate stain. × 29,000.

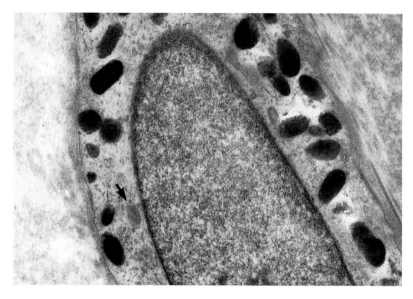

*Fig. 9.* Electron micrograph of a dermal melanocyte obtained from the upper arm of case 2. Stage II melanosomes (arrow) and many stage IV melanosomes are recognized. Uranyl acetate and lead citrate stain. × 14,400.

[1] stated that in apes, while there is some variation, the pigment cell is found almost uniformly in the deep part of the corium.

As the etiology of blue macules, manifestation of aberrant latent dermal melanocytosis, or reappearance of aberrant dermal melanocytosis which had disappeared grossly in early childhood, by the degeneration of dermal connective tissue, or reactivation or activation of dermal melanocytes by some irritation in the dermis, are considered. Also, migration of epidermal or follicular or hair bulb melanocytes to the dermis by inflammation or degeneration of the dermis due to scleroderma must be considered. Or, dermal melanocytes might have originated from nerve sheaths in adults [9] although transitional forms between the cells of the sheath of Schwann and the dermal melanocytes in the blue macule were not found. According to DORSEY and MONTGOMERY [6], not all blue nevi are present at birth or start in infancy and, in 17 out of 61 cases, the lesion first appeared between the ages of 30 to 50 years.

Therefore, the hypothesis of 'naevus caeruleus tardus', which is different from ordinal blue nevi, may be assumed.

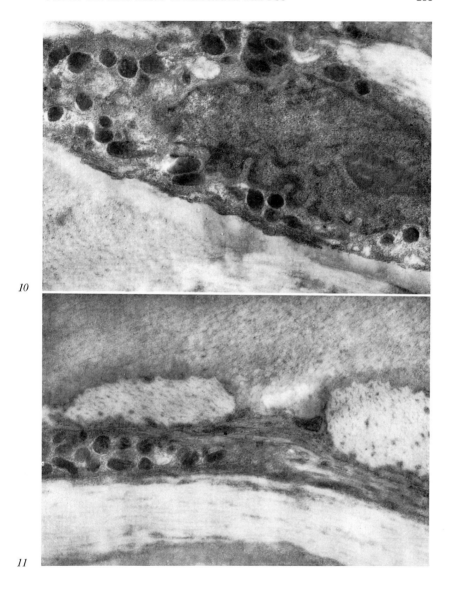

Fig. 10. Electron micrograph of a dermal melanocyte obtained from the back of case 3. Uranyl acetate and lead citrate stain. × 14,400.

Fig. 11. Electron micrograph of a peripheral portion of the same melanocyte of figure 10. Many stage IV melanosomes are recognized. Uranyl acetate and lead citrate stain. × 14,400.

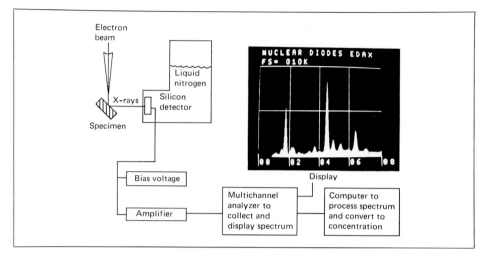

*Fig. 12.* Diagram of electron microscopic X-ray microanalysis system.

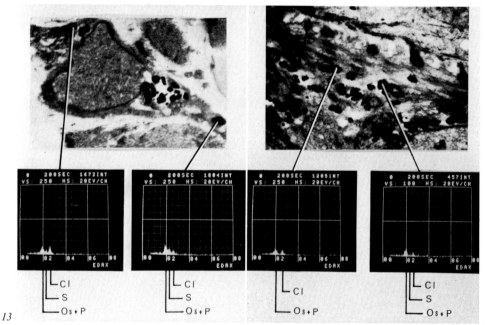

*Fig. 13.* Electron microscopic X-ray microanalysis of a melanosome in a dermal melanocyte of blue macule, case 2. Sulfur and chlorine were detected.

*Fig. 14.* Electron microscopic X-ray microanalysis of a phagocytized melanosome in a basal cell of case 2. Sulfur and chlorine were also detected.

## Summary

Lately appeared blue macules were recognized in 4 cases with progressive systemic sclerosis (scleroderma). Dermal melanocytes, which were producing melanosomes and dopa-positive, were observed in the lower two thirds of the dermis of blue macules.

The melanosomes in the dermal melanocytes of the blue macule were analyzed by electron microscopic X-ray microanalysis. Chlorine and sulfur were detected in these melanosomes.

As the etiology of blue macules, manifestation of latent aberrant dermal melanocytosis, reappearance of aberrant dermal melanocytosis, 'naevus caeruleus tardus' and other theories are considered.

## References

1  ADACHI, B.: Hautpigment beim Menschen und beim Affen. Z. Morph. Anthrop. 6: 1 (1903).

2  ADACHI, B.: Mongolen Kinderfleck bei Europäern. Z. Morph. Anthrop. 6: 132 (1903).

3  BEAMAN, D. R. and ISASI, J. A.: Electron beam microanalysis. Materials Res. Standards 11: 8–35 (1971).

4  CLARK, W. H., jr. and BRETTON, R.: A comparative fine structural study of melanogenesis in normal human epidermal melanocytes and in certain human malignant melanoma cells; in The skin, pp. 197–214 (Williams & Wilkins, Baltimore 1971).

5  COLE, H. N., jr.; HUBLER, W. R., and LUND, H. Z.: Persistent, aberrant Mongolian spots. Archs Derm. Syph. 61: 244–260 (1950).

6  DORSEY, C. S. and MONTGOMERY, H.: Blue nevus and its distinction from Mongolian spot and the nevus of Ota. J. invest. Derm. 22: 225–236 (1954).

7  ISHIKAWA, N.: Über den sogenannten Mongolenfleck bei japanischen Föten. Folia anat. jap. 2: 1–4 (1924).

8  JIMBOW, K. and KUKITA, A.: Fine structure of pigment granules in the human hair bulb. Ultrastructure of pigment granules; in Biology of normal and abnormal melanocytes, pp. 171–193 (University of Tokyo Press, Tokyo 1971).

9  MASSON, P.: Névromme myélisé dermique associé à un naevus bleu. Schweiz. med. Wschr. 77: 1154–1155 (1947).

10  TODA, K.; HORI, Y., and FITZPATRICK, T. B.: Isolation of the intermediate 'vesicles' during ontogeny of melanosomes in embryonic chick retinal pigment epithelium. Fed. Proc. Fed. Am. Socs exp. Biol. 27: 722 (1968).

Dr. Y. HORI, Kitasato University Medical School, Sagamihara, Kanagawa (Japan)

Pigment Cell, vol. 2, pp. 284–289 (Karger, Basel 1976)

# Exposure to Sunlight and Urinary Excretion of 5-S-Cysteinyldopa[1]

H. RORSMAN, G. AGRUP, B. FALCK, A.-M. ROSENGREN and E. ROSENGREN

Departments of Dermatology, Histology, Biochemistry, and Pharmacology, University of Lund, Lund

The recent detection of a new amino acid, 5-S-cysteinyldopa, in malignant melanomas has led to the finding of this compound also in the urine of melanoma patients [1–3, 6, 7, 12]. 5-S-Cysteinyldopa is also present in normal skin [11], and is excreted in small amounts in the urine of healthy subjects [4,5]. Individuals with white hair show the lowest concentrations, and the quantity of 5-S-cysteinyldopa in the urine seems to reflect certain conditions of the melanin metabolism [5].

Analysis of 5-S-cysteinyldopa in the urine is apparently the most reliable and sensitive method for the chemical diagnosis of metastasizing melanomas [2]. At our department, 5-S-cysteinyldopa determinations have been used in the follow-up of melanoma patients over the past two years. During the summer of 1973, we recorded several unexpectedly high concentrations in normal subjects and in melanoma patients with no clinical evidence of metastases. We assumed that the raised excretion of 5-S-cysteinyldopa was due to stimulation of or damage to the melanocytes owing to exposure to sunlight. It was decided to make a systematic study of the seasonal variations in this amino acid.

1 This investigation has been supported by grants from the Swedish Cancer Society, the John and Augusta Persson Foundation for Scientific Medical Research, and the Walter, Ellen and Lennart Hesselman Foundation for Scientific Research.

## Material and Method

The investigation was performed at Lund, Sweden. 18 healthy subjects were studied with regard to their urinary excretion of 5-S-cysteinyldopa. One woman became pregnant, one failed to produce the sample of urine at the right time, one was excluded after taking acetylsalicylic acid and one because he had spent a winter holiday in the Mediterranean area. The series thus came to comprise 14 subjects, 6 men and 8 women, aged 26–57 years. Details of age, sex and hair colour and the presence or absence of freckles are given in table I.

24-hour specimens of urine were collected in plastic bottles containing 1 g sodium metabisulphite. 20 ml of the collected urine was adsorbed onto $Al_2O_3$ and eluted with 0.1 N HCl. 5-S-Cysteinyldopa was determined fluorimetrically by a method described previously [10]. Urine sampling was performed in autumn 1973 (September, October), winter 1974 (January), spring 1974 (April), and after the summer vacation 1974 (July and August).

The town of Lund is situated on latitude 55° 43′N and longitude 13° 12′E. The weather conditions during the investigation are evident from table II.

An unusually sunny summer with 913 h of sunshine during the months June to August preceded our investigation. At least 4 weeks had passed after the 1973 summer holiday before the autumn urine specimens were collected. The summer of 1974 was rather poor, and our subjects had had less exposure to sunlight than usual. All the subjects had regular jobs and exposure to sunlight was therefore limited mainly to the weekends and summer vacations.

No particular increase in pigmentation was noted in any subject when examined in the spring. All but one of the subjects considered themselves to have a sun tan at the end of the summer.

*Table I.* Age, sex, hair color and freckles in the investigated subjects

| Subject No. | Age | Sex | Hair color | Freckles |
|---|---|---|---|---|
| 1 | 57 | F | grey | |
| 2 | 54 | M | grey, blonde | |
| 3 | 48 | F | grey, brown | |
| 4 | 44 | F | dark brown | |
| 5 | 43 | M | red | + |
| 6 | 43 | F | warm blonde | |
| 7 | 40 | M | ash blonde | |
| 8 | 37 | M | red | + |
| 9 | 37 | F | brown | |
| 10 | 29 | M | blonde | |
| 11 | 28 | F | warm blonde | |
| 12 | 28 | M | brown | |
| 13 | 27 | F | blonde | |
| 14 | 26 | F | blonde | + |

*Table II.* Average temperature and hours of sunshine in Lund September 1973 to August 1974

|            | Temperature °C | Sunshine h |
|------------|----------------|------------|
| September  | +12.7          | 143        |
| October    | + 6.7          | 139        |
| November   | + 2.7          | 70         |
| December   | + 0.5          | 43         |
| January    | + 2.1          | 14         |
| February   | + 2.5          | 48         |
| March      | + 3.2          | 168        |
| April      | + 7.5          | 288        |
| May        | +10.4          | 258        |
| June       | +14.5          | 255        |
| July       | +15.0          | 224        |
| August     | +16.4          | 225        |

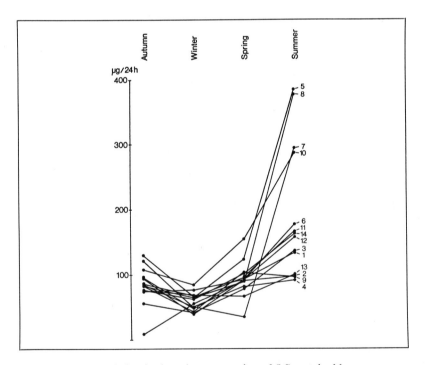

*Fig. 1.* Seasonal variation in the urinary excretion of 5-S-cysteinyldopa.

*Results*

The variations in urinary 5-S-cysteinyldopa are evident from figure 1. The mean excretion in autumn was 84 $\mu$g, in winter 60 $\mu$g, in spring 94 $\mu$g, and in summer 191 $\mu$g/24 h. It is evident that the scatter of values was lowest in winter, intermediate in autumn and spring, and clearly highest in the summer. The highest values (378 and 384 $\mu$g/24 h) were noted in the two red-haired, freckled subjects (Nos. 5 and 8) in the summer. The woman who considered herself not suntanned at the summer examination (No. 4) had a 24-hour excretion of 93 $\mu$g; she had the darkest hair and skin of all subjects investigated.

*Discussion*

The determination of 5-S-cysteinyldopa under standardized conditions is clinically useful in the diagnosis of melanoma metastases [2]. However, the findings we now present demonstrate that 5-S-cysteinyldopa concentrations must be interpreted with caution. The normal range in winter is most easily defined. In autumn and spring, exposure to sunlight affects the normal findings and the range increases. In summer, the normal range is so great that 5-S-cysteinyldopa becomes of small diagnostic value in the follow-up of melanoma patients.

These findings are relative and do not necessarily apply at other latitudes or to individuals of other complexion.

If the urinary 5-S-cysteinyldopa is to be of general use in the follow-up of melanoma patients, it will be necessary to make detailed analysis of the normal variations of 5-S-cysteinyldopa excretion at other latitudes, in other climates and in other populations.

5-S-Cysteinyldopa is a precursor of the phaeomelanin present in red hair [8, 9]. A previous study disclosed no correlation between red hair and the excretion of 5-S-cysteinyldopa when there had been no exposure to sunlight [5]. However, the highest summer concentrations of 5-S-cysteinyldopa were seen in the two red-haired subjects, who showed less suntan than some of the other persons investigated. It is possible that the formation of 5-S-cysteinyldopa is more pronounced in the readily sunburned skin of the red-haired and that it is related to the damage induced by the irradiation.

The variations in 5-S-cysteinyldopa that we now present seem to be the first report of a seasonal variation of an amino acid. This variation is related to exposure to sunlight, and the findings illustrate how sensitively the excretion of 5-S-cysteinyldopa reflects what is going on in the melanocytes.

## Summary

The urinary excretion of 5-S-cysteinyldopa was studied in 14 subjects in autumn, winter, spring, and summer. The summer values were considerably higher than those recorded at other seasons. The range was greatest in summer, intermediate in the autumn and spring, and smallest in winter. The raised excretion of 5-S-cysteinyldopa in summer was recorded after the summer vacations, when exposure to sunlight had been increased. Previous exposure to sunlight must be borne in mind in the assessment of urinary 5-S-cysteinyldopa when following up patients treated for melanoma.

## References

1 AGRUP, G.; AGRUP, P.; ANDERSSON, T.; FALCK, B.; HANSSON, J.-A.; JACOBSSON, S.; RORSMAN, H.; ROSENGREN, A.-M., and ROSENGREN, E.: Urinary excretion of 5-S-cysteinyldopa in patients with primary melanoma or melanoma metastasis. Acta derm.-vener., Stockh. 55: 337–341 (1975).

2 AGRUP, G.; AGRUP, P.; ANDERSSON, T.; FALCK, B.; HANSSON, J.-A.; JACOBSSON, S.; RORSMAN, H.; ROSENGREN, A.-M., and ROSENGREN, E.: 5-S-Cysteinyldopa in the urine of melanoma patients. Acta derm.-vener., Stockh. (to be published, 1976).

3 AGRUP, G.; FALCK, B.; JACOBSSON, S.; RORSMAN, H.; ROSENGREN, A.-M., and ROSENGREN, E.: 5-S-Cysteinyldopa in melanomas of Caucasians. Acta derm.-vener., Stockh. 54: 21–22 (1974).

4 AGRUP, G.; FALCK, B.; KENNEDY, B.-M.; RORSMAN, H.; ROSENGREN, A.-M., and ROSENGREN, E.: Dopa and 5-S-cysteinyldopa in the urine in healthy humans. Acta derm.-vener., Stockh. 53: 453–454 (1973).

5 AGRUP, G.; FALCK, B.; FYGE, K.; RORSMAN, H.; ROSENGREN, A.-M., and ROSENGREN, E.: Excretion of 5-S-cysteinyldopa in the urine of healthy subjects. Acta derm.-vener., Stockh. 55: 7–9 (1975).

6 BJÖRKLUND, A.; FALCK, B.; JACOBSSON, S.; RORSMAN, H.; ROSENGREN, A.-M., and ROSENGREN, E.: Cysteinyldopa in human malignant melanoma. Acta derm.-vener., Stockh. 52: 357–360 (1972).

7 DAHLQVIST, I.; FALCK, B.; JACOBSON, S.; RORSMAN, H.; ROSENGREN, A.-M., and ROSENGREN, E.: 5-S-Cysteinyldopa in the urine of melanoma patients. Commun. No. 7, Department of Anatomy, University of Lund, Lund (1972).

8 PROTA, G.: Structure and biogenesis of phaeomelanins; in RILEY Pigmenta-

tion: its genesis and biologic control, pp. 615–630 (Appleton Century Crofts, New York 1972).

9  PROTA, G. and NICOLAUS, R. A.: On the biogenesis of phaeomelanins; in MONTAGNA and HU Advances in biology of skin: the pigmentary system, vol. 8, p. 323 (Pergamon Press, Oxford 1967).

19  RORSMAN, H.; ROSENGREN, A.-M., and ROSENGREN, E.: A sensitive method for determination of 5-S-cysteinyldopa. Acta derm.-vener., Stockh. *53:* 248–250 (1973).

11  RORSMAN, H.; ROSENGREN, A.-M., and ROSENGREN, E.: Determination of 5-S-cysteinyldopa in melanomas with a fluorimetric method. Yale J. Biol. Med. *46:* 516–522 (1973).

12  VOGEL, C. L.; DHRU, D.; RORSMAN, H.; ROSENGREN, A.-M., and ROSENGREN, E.: Dopa and 5-S-cysteinyldopa in melanoma in Ugandan Africans. Acta derm.-vener., Stockh. *54:* 19–20 (1974).

H. RORSMAN, MD, Department of Dermatology, Lasarettet, *S-221 85 Lund* (Sweden)

Pigment Cell, vol. 2, pp. 290–296 (Karger, Basel 1976)

# Quantitative Histochemical Analysis of Metabolic Enzymes in Human Melanomas and in Premalignant Lesions

D. Cerimele, M. Gerna Torsellini and F. Serri

Department of Dermatology, Skin Aging and Cancer Research Center, University of Pavia, Pavia

Malignant tumors are usually characterized by numerous metabolic alterations; acceleration of the glycolytic pathway and inhibition of the specific tissue functions are common features [12]. Melanoma can be considered one of the most malignant human tumors because of its capacity to produce metastases and because of its high rate of growth.

Quantitative histochemical methods are very useful in the study of the activity of the enzymes in fast-growing tumors, such as melanoma. These methods allow the researcher to discard normal tissues and necrotic parts of tumors and therefore to isolate tumorous tissues and to perform estimations on these selected specimens.

Murine and hamster melanomas have been investigated with these methods [1, 2], however, only scanty data on human melanomas have been obtained. Consequently, we sought to investigate some possible alterations of fundamental functions, like those connected with the utilization of glucose and the production of energy in human melanoma. Preliminary results suggested increased activity of many enzymes in human melanoma [4]. Therefore, we decided to extend our studies in this direction.

## Material and Methods

Ten human melanomas obtained immediately after surgical excision were studied. In three cases, the melanoma developed from a pre-existing lentigo maligna; in seven cases the melanoma developed from a pre-existing nevus.

In all cases, the surgeon excised in a whole piece the melanoma, the pre-existing lentigo or nevus, and a large extension of normal skin; the entire surgical block was immediately frozen in liquid nitrogen. In each case, three samples were taken:

the first from the normal skin, at the periphery of the block, at least 2 cm away from the pigmented lesions; the second from the lentigo maligna or from the pigmented nevus; the third from the melanomatous growth. All the specimens were cut 20 $\mu$m in thickness in a cryostat at $-20$ °C. The frozen sections thus obtained were dried in a vacuum in order to preserve the activity of the enzymes, and to avoid diffusion and loss. The sections were dissected free-hand with a knife under a stereomicroscope. Samples of normal epidermis, of precancerous tissue and of melanoma were thus obtained. The samples (0.5–1 $\mu$g) were weighed on a quartz fishpole balance and then transferred into small (3×50 mm) test tubes for fluorometric enzyme estimations. From each specimen, five samples were taken and analyzed; every single datum, therefore, is the average of five estimations.

Quantitative histochemical techniques for the assay of enzymatic activity in very reduced samples were first described by LOWRY [8]; these methods have been applied to the study of the skin [6] and to the study of pigmented tumors in animals [1] and other skin conditions [5]. A detailed description of these techniques and of their results have been published [9].

In order to obtain a complete picture of the alterations of the energy metabolism, we decided to assay some key enzymes of the glycolytic pathway, the tricarboxylic cycle, the pentose phosphate pathway, two transaminases and $\beta$-hydroxyl-acyl-dehydrogenase; the detailed list of enzymes assayed is described separately (table I).

*Table I.* Enzymes studied

*I. Glycolysis*

Hexokinase
Phosphofructokinase
$\alpha$-Glycero-phosphate-dehydrogenase
Glyceraldehyde-3-phosphate dehydrogenase (G-3-PDH)
Enolase
Lactic dehydrogenase

*II. Tricarboxylic acid cycle*

Isocitric dehydrogenase (ICDH)
Malic dehydrogenase (MDH)
Malic enzyme (ME)

*III. Pentose phosphate cycle*

Glucose-6-phosphate dehydrogenase (G-6-PDH)
6-Phosphogluconic dehydrogenase (6-PGDH)

*IV. Amino acid metabolism*

Alanine transaminase
Aspartate transaminase

*V. Fatty acid metabolism*

$\beta$-Hydroxylacyl-dehydrogenase ($\beta$-OH-DH)

## Results

In the premelanoma and in melanoma, most of the enzymes studied showed a significantly increased activity, in comparison with normal epidermis; the only exceptions were malic enzyme and alanine transaminase, which showed a significantly decreased activity in melanoma (table II). The enzymes of the glycolytic pathway showed an increased activity in premelanoma and in melanoma: the increase of hexokinase was statistically significant, the increase of all other enzymes was highly significant (table III). The activity of the enzymes of the tricarboxylic acid cycle (isocitric dehydrogenase and malic dehydrogenase) was highly increased both in premelanoma and in melanoma, while the activity of the malic enzyme was decreased (table IV). The two enzymes of the pentose phosphate pathway (glucose-6-phosphate dehydrogenase and 6-phosphogluconic dehydrogenase) were increased in premelanoma and in melanoma in a highly significant way (table V).

Among the other enzymes assayed, the activity of alanine transaminase was decreased in premelanoma and melanoma in a statistically sig-

*Table II.* Enzyme activities in normal skin, premelanoma and melanoma

| Enzymes | Normal | Premelanoma | Melanoma |
|---|---|---|---|
| Hexokinase | 0.488 | 0.608 | 0.918 |
| Phosphofructokinase | 0.695 | 1.042 | 2.382 |
| α-Glycerophosphate dehydrogenase | 0.175 | 0.276 | 0.528 |
| Glyceraldehyde-3-phosphate dehydrogenase | 3.568 | 6.986 | 13.073 |
| Enolase | 8.628 | 12.677 | 22.440 |
| Lactic dehydrogenase | 19.897 | 37.767 | 58.453 |
| Isocitric dehydrogenase | 1.255 | 1.380 | 2.212 |
| Malic dehydrogenase | 15.330 | 22.656 | 53.237 |
| Malic enzyme | 0.276 | 0.202 | 0.168 |
| Glucose-6-phosphate dehydrogenase | 0.792 | 0.912 | 1.930 |
| 6-Phosphogluconic dehydrogenase | 0.402 | 0.691 | 1.107 |
| Alanine transaminase | 0.763 | 0.483 | 0.440 |
| Aspartate transaminase | 1.724 | 2.884 | 5.042 |
| β-Hydroxylacyl-dehydrogenase | 1.153 | 1.690 | 2.760 |

Each activity is expressed as mol/kg dry weight/h.
All the data are the mean of ten different samples; each one being the mean of five determinations.

*Table III.* Enzyme activities of the glycolytic pathway in normal skin, premelanoma and melanoma

| Enzymes | Normal, mean ± SD | Premelanoma, mean ± SD | Melanoma, mean ± SD | p[1] |
|---|---|---|---|---|
| Hexokinase | 0.488 ± 0.176 | 0.608 ± 0.210 | 0.918 ± 0.339 | <0.05 |
| Phosphofructokinase | 0.695 ± 0.251 | 1.042 ± 0.361 | 2.382 ± 0.860 | <0.01 |
| a-Glycerophosphate dehydrogenase | 0.175 ± 0.073 | 0.276 ± 0.106 | 0.528 ± 0.225 | <0.01 |
| Glyceraldehyde-3-phosphate dehydrogenase | 3.568 ± 1.237 | 6.986 ± 2.034 | 13.073 ± 4.569 | <0.01 |
| Enolase | 8.628 ± 3.021 | 12.677 ± 4.288 | 22.440 ± 7.625 | <0.01 |
| Lactic dehydrogenase | 19.897 ± 6.698 | 37.767 ± 12.809 | 58.453 ± 20.264 | <0.01 |

1 Variance analysis.

*Table IV.* Enzyme activities of the tricarboxylic acid cycle (Krebs' cycle) in normal skin, premelanoma and melanoma

| Enzymes | Normal, mean ± SD | Premelanoma, mean ± SD | Melanoma, mean ± SD | p[1] |
|---|---|---|---|---|
| Isocitric dehydrogenase | 1.255 ± 0.531 | 1.380 ± 0.472 | 2.212 ± 0.742 | <0.01 |
| Malic dehydrogenase | 15.330 ± 5.360 | 22.656 ± 11.254 | 53.237 ± 15.134 | <0.01 |
| Malic enzyme | 0.276 ± 0.095 | 0.202 ± 0.070 | 0.168 ± 0.059 | <0.01 |

1 Variance analysis.

*Table V.* Enzyme activities of the pentose-phosphate pathway in normal skin, premelanoma and melanoma

| Enzymes | Normal, mean ± SD | Premelanoma, mean ± SD | Melanoma, mean ± SD | p[1] |
|---|---|---|---|---|
| Glucose-6-phosphate dehydrogenase | 0.792 ± 0.274 | 0.912 ± 0.309 | 1.930 ± 0.675 | <0.01 |
| 6-Phosphogluconic dehydrogenase | 0.402 ± 0.147 | 0.691 ± 0.238 | 1.107 ± 0.389 | <0.01 |

1 Variance analysis.

*Table VI.* Other enzyme activities in normal skin, premelanoma and melanoma

| Enzymes | Normal, mean ± SD | Premelanoma, mean ± SD | Melanoma, mean ± SD | p[1] |
|---|---|---|---|---|
| Alanine transaminase | 0.763 ± 0.268 | 0.483 ± 0.163 | 0.440 ± 0.152 | <0.05 |
| Aspartate transaminase | 1.724 ± 0.602 | 2.884 ± 0.962 | 5.042 ± 1.771 | <0.01 |
| β-Hydroxylacyl-dehydrogenase | 1.153 ± 0.410 | 1.690 ± 0.576 | 2.760 ± 0.937 | <0.01 |

1 Variance analysis.

nificant manner, while the activity of aspartate transaminase and of β-hydroxylacyl-dehydrogenase was increased in a highly significant manner (table VI).

## Discussion

Quantitative histochemistry of many enzymes has been done in many tissues during last 20 years. It has been demonstrated to be a useful research tool, even if it has not solved the problems to which it has been applied. The best way to obtain information about the quantitative enzymatic organization of metabolism would be to measure metabolite fluxes. The measurement of the activity of the enzymes under optimum conditions could be less significant from the physiological point of view. If more than one enzyme is studied, and particularly if the enzymes of the central part of the main metabolic pathways are studied, it is possible to gain sufficiently significant information [7]. The results we have obtained are in agreement to a large extent with the data obtained by other authors in mouse melanoma using quantitative histochemical methods [1] and in human melanoma with histochemical methods [3]. Human melanoma, like mouse melanoma, has high activities of most of the enzymes related to the main metabolic pathways, particularly of the enzymes of the glycolytic pathway; the activity of alanine transaminase is decreased, but does not disappear as it does in mouse melanoma [1]. The finding that the enzymes of the glycolytic pathway in human melanoma show a highly increased activity could be in agreement with, but it is not sufficient to affirm, the hypothesis that a cancer cell can originate because of impairment of respiratory metabolism leading to markedly enhanced glycolysis

[10]. The demonstration that no evidence of respiratory derangement is found in the mouse melanoma mitochondria, and that the rate of ATP synthesis in melanoma mitochondria appears to be comparable to that in the mitochondria of normal tissues [2], is at variance with Warburg's hypothesis [11].

In conclusion, we can say that human melanoma has a typical pattern of enzymatic activity, characterized by the increased activity of most enzymes, and mainly of the enzymes of the glycolytic pathway and by a lessened activity of alanine transaminase. We have no reason to affirm that the pattern of the metabolic enzymes in human melanoma is a primary alteration; as far as we know, the theory that the enzymatic alterations are secondary to the basic malignant defect [3] is equally acceptable.

## Summary

Quantitative histochemical analysis of 14 enzymes of the main metabolic pathways has been performed on ten human melanomas and on the lesions (nevi and lentigo maligna) from which the melanomas developed. Most of the enzymes assayed, particularly those representative of the glycolytic pathway, showed highly increased activities in melanoma and, to a lesser degree, in lentigo maligna and nevi. However, in melanoma the activities of alanine transaminase and of malic enzyme were reduced by about 50%.

## References

1  ADACHI, K.: Enzyme activities in mammalian pigment cells. Advances in biology of skin, vol. 8, pp. 223–240 (Pergamon Press, Oxford 1967).
2  ADACHI, K.; KONDO, S.; HIRAGA, M.; HU, F., and BELL, M.: Energy metabolism of mouse melanoma; in RILEY Pigmentation: its genesis and biological control, pp. 551–569 (Appleton-Century Croft, New York 1972).
3  BRAUN-FALCO, O. und BURG, G.: Zur Enzym-Histochemie des malignen Melanoms. Untersuchungen an Primärtumoren und Metastasen. Arch. Derm. Forsch. 246: 303–316 (1973).
4  CERIMELE, D.; TORSELLINI, M., and SERRI, F.: Pattern of some enzyme activities during carcinogenesis in human melanoma. Dermatology, pp. 577–578 (Excerpta Medica, Amsterdam 1974).
5  CERIMELE, D.; YAMASAWA, S., and SERRI, F.: The effect of chronic sun damage on the activity of metabolic enzymes of the epidermis of human skin. Br. J. Derm. 87: 149–153 (1972).
6  HERSHEY, F. B.; LEWIS, C., jr.; MURPHY, J.; SCHIFF, T.: Quantitative histochemistry of human skin. J. Histochem. Cytochem. 8: 41–50 (1960).

7   HÖHMANN, B. and ZWIEBEL, R.: Selection of enzymes for active measurements in energy metabolism. A new parameter of reference for active measurements in tissue structures. Recent advances in quantitative histo and cytochemistry, pp. 348–350 (Huber, Bern 1971).
8   LOWRY, O. H.: The quantitative histochemistry of the brain. Histological sampling. J. Histochem. Cytochem. *1:* 420–431 (1953).
9   LOWRY, O. H. and PASSONNEAU, J. V.: A flexible system of enzymatic analysis (Academic Press, New York 1972).
10  WARBURG, O.: On the origin of cancer cells. Science *123:* 309–314 (1956).
11  WEINHOUSE, S.: On respiratory impairment in cancer cells. Science *124:* 267–269 (1956).
12  WENNER, C.: Progress in tumor enzymology. Adv. Enzymol., vol. 29, pp. 321–390 (Wiley & Sons, Chichester 1967).

Dr. F. SERRI, Clinica Dermatologica dell'Università, *I–27100 Pavia* (Italy)

Pigment Cell, vol. 2, pp. 297–309 (Karger, Basel 1976)

# Comparison of Various Methods for Determination of Melanogens as a Diagnostic Test for Melanoma

H. F. HABERMAN, E. V. GAN and I. A. MENON

Clinical Science Division, Dermatology Division, University of Toronto, Toronto, Ont.

Since melanomas synthesize varying quantities of melanin, it is logical that intermediates and/or their derivatives in the synthesis of melanin would be present in blood and urine from melanoma patients. Various authors have attempted to determine the levels of these compounds in urine from melanoma patients. These compounds (melanogens) are of two types, namely phenol melanogens and indole melanogens.

The melanogens have been determined by using colorimetric methods and paper chromatography. Two kinds of colorimetric methods have been mainly used for the determination of melanogens: (1) oxidation reactions in which the development of melanin or other reaction products are followed, and (2) the Thormahlen test in which nitroferricyanide is added to urine [1].

The Thormahlen test was first reported by THORMAHLEN [2] in 1887 and subsequently applied by DUCHON and PECHAN [1] as well as by several other investigators [3–5]. This test is rather specific for indole melanogens. The indole melanogens have been found to be mainly derivatives of 5,6-dihydroxyindole (Thormahlen-positive indole melanogens) and of 5,6-dihydroxyindole-2-carboxylic acid (Thormahlen-negative indole melanogens). It has been said that the principle behind the Thormahlen test is that sodium nitroprusside is reduced to ferrocyanide by the reducing action of melanogen. However, this cannot be the full explanation, because it does not explain the rather high specificity of this test for indole melanogens. The other widely used method is the ferric chloride test which measures phenol melanogens. This test was first reported by JAKSCH [6] in 1889 and applied by LEONARDI and other investigators to melanoma patients [7–9]. The rationale behind this test is that ferric ions and phenols form complexes and not just salts. It should be noted that not all phenols give color with $FeCl_3$. Moreover, the colors can last for hours or only seconds. With some phenols a slight excess of reagent may destroy the color. With other phenols an excess of reagent is essential [10].

Individual catecholic compounds have been measured by a few investigators in the urine of patients with malignant melanoma. SCOTT [11] separated 3,4-dihydroxyphenylalanine (dopa) and similar compounds from urine of melanoma patients and observed that a band corresponding to dopa was present in 20 out of 28 patients studied. Corresponding bands were not observed in samples from 22 patients with other diseases. VOORHESS [12] determined the levels of dopa, dopamine, norepinephrine and epinephrine in urine samples from 16 patients with advanced melanoma. Abnormally high levels were found only in half of the cases; the pattern varied among the patients. Dopa was the single compound which was most frequently excreted in large amounts. HINTERBERGER et al. [13, 14] separately determined the levels of dopa, 3,4-dihydroxy-phenylethanolamine, and 3,4-dihydroxyphenylacetic acid in urine from patients with melanoma. Varying levels of these catecholic compounds were observed in their samples. It was concluded that a definite correlation appears to exist between these three catechols in urine and increasing weight of tumor tissue. TAKAHASHI and FITZPATRICK [15] determined the levels of dopa in a small number of patients with melanoma as well as healthy individuals and observed elevated levels of dopa in several of the patients with melanoma.

This paper includes a method for the quantitative determination of catechols in urine and discusses the usefulness of this test for malignant melanoma. This method utilizes a ferrocitrate reagent which was originally described by DOTY [16] as a method for determination of adrenaline in fluids. ROUTH and BANNOW [17] applied this test to patients with Parkinson's disease on L-dopa for monitoring L-dopa therapy. They used a semiquantitative paper strip method. This paper reports modifications of this test so that it is quantitative and can be used in solution. The chemical specificity of this test has been studied and it has been employed for the determination of catechols in urine from patients with melanoma, patients with other diseases and healthy individuals [18].

There are more than 40 phenol melanogens such as p-hydroxyphenyl-acetic acid, salicyluric acid, homovanillic acid, p-hydroxyphenyl-propionic acid, salicylic acid, etc. [19–24, 42]. The results of these investigators as well as the results obtained in our laboratory have shown that different phenolic compounds are present in higher levels in various melanoma patients; however, no specific phenol(s) were always present in high concentrations in melanoma patients. It therefore appears that the time-consuming procedures for determining individual compounds are not suitable as a screening test.

We have also developed a method for measuring phenolic compounds in urine by means of a diazo test and have determined the levels of phenolic compounds in urine from melanoma patients [25–27]. This method involves the reaction of an aromatic diazonium salt with phenolic compounds to yield colored diazo compounds [28]. WEIS [29] has reported a qualitative method for the determination of urinary melanogens using the diazo reaction. In our studies, the diazo compound formed was quantitatively assayed spectrophotometrically. The reaction has been confirmed with several phenolic compounds as described below. We have determined the tyrosinase and dopa oxidase activities in serum from patients with melanoma. These activities seem to be present only in patients with advanced malignant melanoma.

We have not employed other biochemical tests for melanoma such as the fluorometric method for the measurement of cysteinyl dopa [30–33], determination of individual compounds such as dopa and other phenolic compounds [11, 12, 15, 19–24, 34, 35], amino acids in urine [36], or other colorimetric methods for melanogens [37].

## Materials and Methods

*Tyrosinase activity.* Tyrosinase activity was determined as described previously [38, 39] .

*Dopa oxidase activity.* Dopa oxidase activity was determined by measuring the oxygen uptake of the reaction system which consisted of: 3.75 mM L-dopa, 0.5 ml serum, 0.05 M $PO_4$ buffer pH 6.8 in a total volume of 2.0 ml. The oxygen utilization was measured by using a Gilson Medical Electronics Oxygraph, model KM.

*Thormahlen test.* 0.4 ml 1.25% sodium nitro-prusside and 0.5 ml 40% NaOH were added to 2.5 ml urine and the contents were thoroughly mixed. 0.6 ml glacial acetic acid was then added and the absorbance at 625 nm was read after exactly 1.0 min. A standard curve was prepared using various concentrations of indole. The results are expressed in terms of mg equivalents of indole per 24-hour urine sample.

*Ferric chloride test.* 1.0 ml of 10% $FeCl_3$ in 10% HCl was added to 5.0 ml of the urine sample. Absorbance at 419 nm was determined immediately. A standard curve was prepared using various concentrations of L-dopa, the results being expressed in terms of mg equivalent of dopa per 24-hour urine sample.

*Ferrocitrate test.* 0.5% $FeSO_4$ $7H_2O$ was dissolved in 0.005 N HCl containing 0.5% $NaHSO_3$ and 5% sodium citrate was added. Immediately before use this solution was diluted 10-fold with 3 M Tris-HCl buffer pH 8.5. 0.1 ml of this reagent was mixed with 1.0 ml of the test solution and absorbance at 540 nm was read within 30 min. A standard curve was prepared using L-dopa. The results are expressed as mg equivalents of dopa per 24-hour urine sample.

*Diazo test.* The diazo test was performed as previously described [27].

*Collection of urine samples.* 24-hour urine samples were collected in bottles containing 10 ml glacial acetic acid, 1 g sodium sulfite and 1 g sodium oxalate as recommended by Hinterberger *et al.* [13]. None of the patients or healthy individuals were taking salicylates during the 24 h preceding and during the collection period.

*Clinical state of melanoma.* At the time of collecting the test specimens, the patients were classified by the referring physicians into the following three groups: (A) no evidence of residual disease, (B) local lymph node involvement and/or local skin recurrence, (C) widely metastatic disease.

## Results

The chemical specificity of the four tests employed in our studies is summarized in table I. Besides indole and 5-hydroxyindole which gave strongly positive reactions to the Thormahlen test, bilirubin also was faintly positive in this test. The $FeCl_3$ test was positive for the phenolic compounds, although the intensity of the reaction varied considerably. Moreover, a few non-phenolic compounds, e.g. indole, phenyllactic acid, pyruvic acid and tryptophane gave positive reaction to this test. The ferrocitrate test was intensely positive for the catecholic compounds, namely dopa, dopamine, epinephrine and norepinephrine, and faintly positive for bilirubin. The diazo test was intensely positive for all the phenolic compounds; there was less diversity in the intensity of the reaction given by the various phenolic compounds for the diazo test compared to the $FeCl_3$ test. The diazo test was also positive to a few compounds that are not phenols.

The results of the tests for melanogens for all the three groups, namely healthy individuals, patients with melanoma, and patients with other diseases, are shown in figures 1–4. An analysis of the percentage of positive results given by each of the 4 tests is given in table II. For this purpose, a test was considered to be positive if the value for the sample was higher than the mean +3 times standard deviation derived from a group of 23 normal individuals. Altogether, samples from 105 patients with malignant melanoma were tested. Among the total number of patients with me-

*Table I.* Specificity of various tests used for the determination of melanogens

| Compound | Thor-mahlen | Ferric chloride | Ferro-citrate | Diazo |
|---|---|---|---|---|
| L-Tyrosine | − | + | − | + + + + |
| Salicylic acid | − | + + + + | − | + + + + |
| Bilirubin | + | + | + | + + + + |
| Biliverdin | − | + + | − | + + + + |
| L-Dopa | − | + + + | + + + + | + + + + |
| Dopamine | − | + + + | + + + + | + + + + |
| Epinephrine | − | + + + | + + + + | + + + + |
| Norepinephrine | − | + + + | + + + + | + + + + |
| Indole-2-carboxylic acid | − | + + | − | + + + |
| 5-Hydroxyindole | + + + + | + | − | + + + + |
| Indole | + + + + | + | − | + + + |
| 5-Hydroxyindole-3-acetic acid | − | + + | − | + + + + |
| B-Phenyl-L-lactic acid | − | + | − | + |
| Pyruvic acid | − | + | − | − |
| Tryptophane | − | + | − | + + |
| Phenylalanine | − | − | − | + |

lanoma, approximately 13% gave positive results for the Thormahlen test; the ferrocitrate test was positive for 24% and diazo and FeCl$_3$ tests were positive for 40 and 45%, respectively. The clinical state of melanoma was known only in the case of 63 patients; they were classified under the 3 groups mentioned above. The group of patients with widely metastatic disease (group C) had the largest percentages of positive results for all the tests. Among all the groups, the FeCl$_3$ test and the diazo test had the largest percentage of positive results. The Thormahlen and ferrocitrate tests had very small percentages in the groups A and B. In group C, the ferrocitrate had a significantly larger percentage of positive results than the Thormahlen test.

Urine samples from 24 patients hospitalized with various diseases other than cancer were tested. In this group, the Thormahlen test had the largest percentage of positive results, followed by the FeCl$_3$ test; the ferrocitrate and diazo tests had the lowest percentage of positive results.

A statistical analysis of the above results is given in table III. The mean and standard deviation were calculated for the values of each group. The results for the patients with melanoma were compared to the results for healthy individuals and patients with other diseases. Similarly, the results for patients with other diseases were compared to those for the

*Table II*

| Test | Percent positive[1] test | | | | |
|------|-------|-------|-------|-------|-------|
| | other diseases (n = 24) | melanomas total (n = 105) | melanomas (subgroups)[2] | | |
| | | | group A (n = 25) | group B (n = 20) | group C (n = 18) |
| 1. Thormahlen | 20.8 | 13.3 | 7.7 | 0 | 27.8 |
| 2. Ferrocitrate | 8.3 | 23.8 | 3.8 | 15.0 | 44.4 |
| 3. Diazo | 8.3 | 40.6 | 26.9 | 40.0 | 42.1 |
| 4. FeCl$_3$ | 16.7 | 45.3 | 34.6 | 60.0 | 52.6 |

1 Positive test = value higher than mean + 3 times standard deviation derived from a normal group of 37 individuals.
2 Groups: A = disease-free; B = local skin recurrences and/or regional nodes; C = systemic matastases.

group of healthy individuals. Because the variances of the concerned two samples were different, Wallace's method was employed to calculate the degrees of freedom for the Student's test [40, 41]. It was found that the results for the Thormahlen test for patients with melanoma and patients with other diseases were higher than the results for the group of healthy individuals at 1 and 5% probability levels of significance. The results for the patients with melanoma were not higher than those for patients with other diseases at 5% probability level of significance. The results of the FeCl$_3$ test for the patients with melanoma were higher than the results for healthy individuals and those for patients with other diseases at 0.1 and 5% probability levels of significance, respectively; the results for the patients with other diseases were higher than those for the healthy individuals at 5% probability level. With the ferrocitrate test, the results for the patients with melanoma were higher than those for healthy individuals and those for patients with other diseases at 1 and 5% levels of significance; the results for patients with melanoma were not higher than those for the patients with other diseases at 5% probability level of significance. The results of diazo test for the patients with melanoma were higher than

*Fig. 1–4.* Results of the Thormahlen (1), ferric chloride (2), ferrocitrate (3) and diazo (4) tests upon urine samples from healthy individuals, patients with melanoma and patients with other diseases.

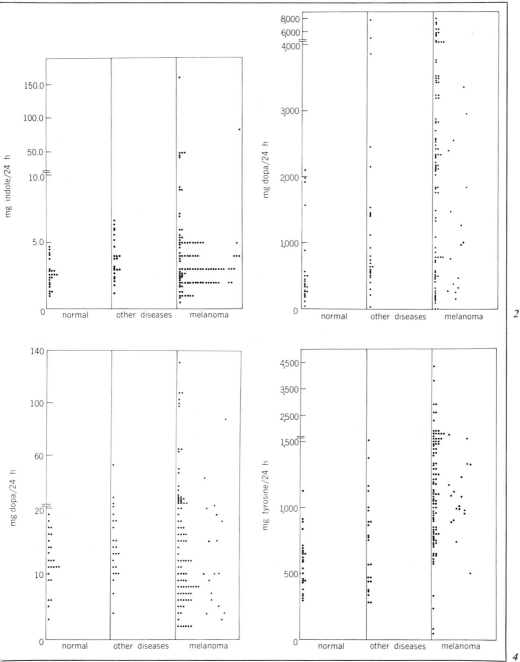

*Table III.* Comparison of the tests for melanogens

| | Thor-mahlen test | FeCl₃ test | Ferro-citrate test | Diazo test |
|---|---|---|---|---|
| Healthy individuals, mean | 2.62 | 559 | 11.87 | 583 |
| Healthy individuals, standard error | 0.22 | 124 | 0.90 | 45 |
| Patients with melanoma, mean | 6.74 | 2,154 | 19.63 | 1,184 |
| Patients with melanoma, standard error | 1.56 | 154 | 2.15 | 54 |
| Patients with other diseases, mean | 4.28 | 1,459 | 15.68 | 719 |
| Patients with other diseases, standard error | 0.46 | 391 | 2.12 | 78 |
| Z and significance (patients with melanoma versus healthy individuals) | 2.61** | 8.08*** | 3.32** | 8.54*** |
| Z and significance (patients with other diseases versus healthy individuals) | 3.24** | 2.20* | 1.65* | 1.51n.s. |
| Z and significance (patients with melanoma versus patients with other diseases) | 1.51n.s. | 1.65* | 1.31n.s. | 89*** |

Number of specimens tested: healthy individuals $= 23$; patients with melanoma $= 105$; patients with other diseases $= 22$.
Z = Standardized normal variant.
Significance: *, ** and *** = significant at 5, 1, and 0.1% probability, respectively; n.s. = not significant at 5% probability.

those for healthy individuals as well as those for patients with other diseases at 0.1% level; the results for the patients with other diseases were not higher than those for healthy individuals at 5% level of significance.

The serum samples from 10 patients with melanoma did not contain abnormally high levels of melanogens as determined by the above methods, although some of these tests were positive in the urine from these patients.

We have employed the tyrosinase and dopa oxidase activities in serum from patients for the detection of melanoma. None of the healthy individuals tested gave a positive result for this test. However, only 15% (13 out of 87 patients tested) and 13% (9 out of 69 patients) gave positive results for the tyrosinase and dopa oxidase tests.

*Discussion*

None of the tests employed in our studies was found to be absolutely specific for any one type of compounds. However, each test gave relatively more intense reactions with certain types of compounds. Thus, the Thormahlen test was intensely positive for indole compounds; the $FeCl_3$ and diazo tests gave intensely positive reactions for phenolic compounds; the ferrocitrate test was strongly positive for catechols. It may, therefore, be inferred that none of these tests would be strictly specific for melanoma. A number of disease states as well as drugs and drug metabolites are likely to interfere with these tests.

Our results show that the Thormahlen test gave the lowest percentage of positive tests for patients with melanoma and highest percentage of positive results for patients with other diseases. The $FeCl_3$ test gave a large percentage of positive results for patients with melanoma, but this test was also positive for a large number of patients with other diseases. The ferrocitrate test was positive only in a small percentage of patients with other diseases; but this test appears to be positive mainly for patients with melanoma in advanced states. The diazo test was positive in a large percentage of patients with melanoma and gave a very low percentage of positive results for patients with other diseases. The activities of tyrosinase and dopa oxidase in serum seem to be positive only when the tumor is in an advanced stage.

When considered individually, the diazo test seems to be the most suitable one for the detection of melanoma. However, different tests were positive for different patients. It may, therefore, be concluded that none of the above tests is sufficiently specific and sensitive for the diagnosis of melanoma. However, each of these tests appears to have some merit. These four tests are simple to perform and are relatively non time-consuming. We would like to suggest that these tests may be useful in detecting occult secondaries, as a warning of relapses and as a biochemical indication of response to therapy.

## Summary

Four methods for the determination of melanogens (intermediates in the synthesis of melanin and their derivatives) in urine were compared with respect to the usefulness of these tests for the diagnosis of melanoma. These tests included two widely employed tests, namely the Thormahlen test, which gives positive reaction mainly for indole derivatives, and the $FeCl_3$ test, which is positive for a number of phenolic compounds, and two tests recently developed in our laboratory, namely the ferrocitrate test, which is positive mainly for catechols, and the diazo test, which is positive for a number of phenolic compounds. None of these tests was strictly specific for any particular type of compound. 24-hour urine samples from 23 healthy individuals, 105 patients with melanoma and 37 patients hospitalized with various diseases other than cancer were examined. The $FeCl_3$ and diazo tests gave positive results for the highest percentage of patients with melanoma. However, the $FeCl_3$ test was also positive for a large number of patients with other diseases. The ferrocitrate test was positive for a relatively small percentage of patients with melanoma, but it also gave positive results for only a very low percentage of patients with other diseases. The Thormahlen test was positive for only a low percentage of patients with melanoma and gave positive results for the highest percentage of patients with other diseases. The patients with melanoma were classified into three groups: (A) no evidence of residual disease, (B) local lymph node involvement and/or local skin recurrence, and (C) widely metastatic disease. Group C had the highest and group A had the lowest percentages of positive results for all the four tests. Tyrosinase and dopa oxidase activities could be detected in serum from the patients only in a very low percentage of patients with melanoma. Among the tests for melanogens employed in our studies, different tests were positive for different patients. Therefore, each test appears to have some merit.

## Acknowledgments

We would like to acknowledge the excellent technical assistance of HELEN LI.

The authors wish to acknowledge the Medical Research Council of Canada for a grant (MA-5043) and a Fellowship to E. V. GAN, and Ontario Geriatric Society and Ontario Cancer Treatment and Research Foundation for grants. H . F. HABERMAN is an Associate of Ontario Cancer Treatment and Research Foundation.

## References

1  DUCHON, J. and PECHAN, Z.: The biochemical and clinical significance of melanogenuria. Ann. N.Y. Acad. Sci. *100:* 1048–1068 (1963).

2  THORMAHLEN, J.: Mitteilung über einen noch nicht bekannten Körper im pathologischen Menschenharn. Arch. Path. Anat. *108:* 317 (1887); cited by DUCHON and PECHAN [1].

3   ROTHMAN, J. M.: Studies on melanuria. J. Lab. clin. Med. *27:* 687–692 (1942).

4   DUCHON, J.: Tyrosine metabolism in melanoma. Nature, Lond. *194:* 976 (1962).

5   PECHAN, Z.: Studien über Melanine und Melanogenese. III. Auswertung der Thormahlenschen Reaktion für die Bestimmung des Indol-Melanogens. Neoplasma *6:* 397–403 (1959).

6   JAKSCH, R.: Beiträge zur Kenntnis des Verhaltens des Harnes bei der Melanurie. Hoppe-Seyler's Z. physiol. Chem. *13:* 385 (1889); cited by DUCHON and PECHAN [1].

7   BEELER, M. B. and HENRY, J. B.: Melanogenuria – evaluation of several commonly used laboratory procedures. J . Am. med. Ass. *176:* 52–54 (1961).

8   LEONARDI, G.: Zur Charakterisierung der Harnmelanogene. Naturwissenschaften *41:* 305–306 (1954).

9   LEONARDI, G.: Papierchromatographische Trennung von Harnmelanogenen. Naturwissenschaften *41:* 141 (1954).

10  SCHNEIDER, F. L.: Qualitative organic microanalysis, p. 202 (Springer, Berlin 1964).

11  SCOTT, J . A.: 3,4-Dihydroxyphenylalanine (dopa) excretion in patients with malignant melanoma. Lancet *ii:* 861–862 (1962).

12  VOORHESS, M. L.: Urinary excretion of dopa and metabolites by patients with melanoma. Cancer *26:* 146–149 (1970).

13  HINTERBERGER, H.; FREEDMAN, A., and BARTHOLOMEW, R. J.: Precursors of melanin in the urine in malignant melanoma. Clin. chim. Acta *18:* 377–382 (1967).

14  HINTERBERGER, H.; FREEDMAN, A., and BARTHOLOMEW, R. J.: Precursors of melanin in the blood and urine in malignant melanoma. Clin. chim. Acta *39:* 395–400 (1972).

15  TAKAHASHI, H. and FITZPATRICK, T. B.: Quantitative determination of dopa; its application to measurement of dopa in urine and in the assay of tyrosinase in serum. J. invest. Derm. *42:* 161–165 (1964).

16  DOTY, J. R.: Photometric determination of epinephrine in pharmaceutical products. Analyt. Chem. *20:* 1166–1168 (1948).

17  ROUTH, J. I. and BANNOW, R. E.: Development of a screening test for L-dopa and its metabolites in urine. Clin. Chem. *17:* 872–874 (1971).

18  HABERMAN, H. F. and MENON, I. A.: A modified method for the determination of catechols in urine and its application to melanoma. Clin. Res. *22:* 327A (1974).

19  ARMSTRONG, M. D.; SHAW, K. N. F., and WALL, P. E.: The phenolic acids of human urine paper chromatography of phenolic acids. Acta physiol. scand. *44:* 293–303 (1958).

20  BADINAND, A.; PASQUIER, J.; VALLON, J. J.; GUILLERY, R. et MILON, E.: Identification chromatographique en couche mince de deux melanogenes indoliques urinaires. Clin. chim. Acta *25:* 357–364 (1969).

21  DUCHON, J. and GREGORA, V.: Homovanillic acid and its relation to tyrosine metabolism in melanoma. Clin. chim Acta *7:* 443–446 (1962).

22  DUCHON, J.; MATOUS, B., and PROCHOZKOVA, B.: The vanillactic acid in the urine of melanoma patients. Clin. chim. Acta *18:* 318–319 (1967).

23  DUCHON, J.; MATOUS, B., and PROCHOZKOVA, B.: Vanillactic acid in the urine of melanoma patients. Clin. chim. Acta *18:* 487–488 (1967).

24  DUCHON, J. and MATOUS, B.: Dopa and its metabolites in melanoma urine; in RILEY Pigment Cell, vol. 1, pp. 317–322 (Karger, Basel 1973).

25  MENON, I. A.; GAN, E. V., and HABERMAN, H. F.: A new method for the determination of phenolic compounds in urine from melanoma patients. Clin. Res. *20:* 886 (1972).

26  GAN, E. V.; MENON, I. A., and HABERMAN, H. F.: Determination of phenolic compounds in urine from melanoma by diazo test. Clin. Res. *21:* 982 (1973).

27  GAN, E. V.; HABERMAN, H. F., and MENON, I. A.: A simple and sensitive test for the determination of phenolic compounds in urine and its application to melanoma. J. invest. Derm. *64:* 139–144 (1975).

28  ZOLLINGER, H.: Azo and diazo chemistry (Interscience, New York 1961).

29  WEISS, M.: Die Urochromogenprobe und andere Harnreaktionen. Klin. Wschr. *1:* 694–697 (1922).

30  FALCK, B.; JACOBSSON, S.; OLIVERCRONA, H.; OLSEN, G.; RORSMAN, H., and RO-SENGREN, E.: Determination of catecholamines, 5-hydroxytryptamine and 3,4-dihydroxyphenylalanine (dopa) in human malignant melanomas. Acta derm.-vener., Stockh. *46:* 65–67 (1966).

31  RORSMAN, H.; ROSENGREN, A. M., and ROSENGREN, E.: Fluorometry of a dopa peptide and its thioether. Acta derm.-vener., Stockh. *51:* 179–182 (1971).

32  RORSMAN, H.; ROSENGREN, G. M., and ROSENGREN, E.: Fluorometry of catechol thioethers. Acta derm.-vener., Stockh. *52:* 353–356 (1972).

33  RORSMAN, H.; ROSENGREN, A. M., and ROSENGREN, E.: Determination of 5-S-cysteinyldopa in melanomas with a fluorimetric method. Yale J. Biol. Med. *46:* 516–522 (1973).

34  GOODALL, McC.: Metabolism of L-dopa-3-[14]C(3,4-dihydroxyphenylalanine) in human subjects; in McGOVERN and RUSSELL Pigment Cell, vol. 1, pp. 308–311 (Karger, Basel 1973).

35  HINTERBERGER, H.; FREEDMAN, A., and BARTHOLOMEW, R. J.: Precursors of melanin in the urine and 3,4-dihydroxyphenylalanine in the blood of patients with malignant melanoma; in McGOVERN and RUSSELL Pigment Cell, vol. 1, pp. 312–316 (Karger, Basel 1973).

36  RILEY, V.; SPACKMAN, D., and FITZMAURICE, M. A.: Plasma and urine amino acid changes associated with melanoma; in McGOVERN and RUSSELL Pigment Cell, vol. 1, pp. 331–345 (Karger, Basel 1973).

37  TASKOVICH, L.; BANDA, P. W., and BLOIS, M. S.: Chemical studies on urinary melanogens; in McGOVERN and RUSSELL Pigment Cell, vol. 1, pp. 323–330 (Karger, Basel 1973).

38  MENON, I. A. and HABERMAN, H. F.: Tyrosinase activity in serum from normal and melanoma-bearing mice. Cancer Res. *28:* 1237–1241 (1968).

39  HABERMAN, H. F. and MENON, I. A.: Presence and properties of tyrosinase in sera of melanoma-bearing animals. Acta derm.-vener., Stockh. *51:* 407–412 (1971).

40 WELCH, B. L.: Specification of rules for rejecting too variable a product with particular reference to an electric lamp problem. J. R. Statist. Soc. Suppl. *3:* 29–48 (1936).

41 WELCH, B. L.: The generalization of 'students' problem when several different population variances are involved. Beometrika *34:* 28–35 (1974).

42 VALLON, J. J.; BADINAND, A. et BICHON, C.: Isolement chromatographique sur Sephadex G-10 des metanephrines et des melanogenes des urines. Clin. chim. Acta *36:* 397–404 (1972).

Dr. H. F. HABERMAN, Clinical Science Division, University of Toronto, Medical Sciences Building, *Toronto, Ont. M5S 1A8* (Canada)

Pigment Cell, vol. 2, pp. 310–315 (Karger, Basel 1976)

# Melanosis in Visceral Organs

B. Oberman, M. Belicza and B. Krstulović

Department of Pathology, Faculty of Medicine, University of Zagreb, Zagreb

Data about visceral melanosis is rare in pathological literature. Some authors believed that it appeared in cases of melanoma where the tumor had metastasized, as did Zeller [16] who first described melanuria in 1883. This idea was later supported by Lubarsch [8] and Masson [9]. Kettler [6] described melanosis in cases where melanomas were necrotic, especially when they had metastasized. Wells [15] reported that melanosis appeared in only 20% of the cases with melanoma. Rosenberg [14] and Goodall et al. [3] likewise believed it a rare occurrence. Jacobsen and Klinck [5] showed findings of melanin in kidneys of Negroes who did not have melanoma. Agress and Fishman [1] observed melanin in Kupffer cells of the liver in cases of lipomelanotic reticulosis. Rivière et al. [13] and Oberman and Rivière [10] described melanosis in golden hamsters with melanoma.

## Methods and Materials

We received melanoma from golden hamsters *(Mesocricetus auratus)* from the Institut de Recherches Scientifiques sur le Cancer, in Villejuif. In a series of subcutaneous transplants in hamsters over a period of four years, the tumor did not metastasize. It grew fast and was approximately 5 cm in the largest diameter after two or three months. At this point, ten animals, six months of age, were sacrificed. Most of the tumor was necrotic and contained a large quantity of melanin. Ultrastructurally, it had been studied earlier by Oberman and Ljubešić [11] and typical melanosomes were found.

For a comparative study, material from healthy hamsters of the same age was also examined.

Pieces of tumors and visceral organs were fixed in 10% neutral formalin. Besides the coloration with hematoxylin and eosin, we applied the following meth-

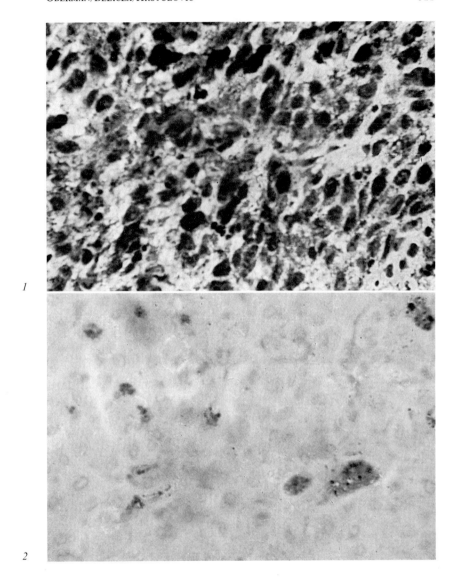

*Fig. 1.* Numerous melanin granules in a completely necrotic melanoma (ferrous ion uptake by Lillie's method). × 285.

*Fig. 2.* Liver of hamster with melanoma. Note enlarged Küpffer's cells containing abundant pigment granules (ferrous ion uptake by Lillie's method). × 285.

ods: the reduction of ferricyanide to ferrocyanide, the so-called Schmorl's reaction [12]; ferrous ion uptake method (fig. 1, 2) [7]; PAS reaction; bleaching with 10% hydrogen peroxide for 24–48 h; silver impregnation after Fontana; ferrocyanide reaction for iron (Prussian blue); and testing for bilirubin with Fouchet reagent [4].

Using the same methods, we analyzed one human metastatic melanoma.

For electron microscopy, specimens from different parts of liver of hamsters with and without melanoma were obtained and immediately fixed in 2% cold phosphate-buffered glutaraldehyde. They were then transferred into phosphate buffer at pH 7.3 with 1% osmium tetroxide for post-fixation and dehydrated by graded acetone and embedded in Durcupan ACM (Fluka). Ultrathin sections were cut by LKB Ultratome microtome, and stained with uranyl acetate followed by lead citrate. Electron photomicrographs were produced by electron microscope 'Opton EM 9A'.

## Results

In the examined organs of hamsters with melanomas, pigment in granular shape was observed mainly in the liver. In the other organs, only insignificant granules were discerned in the kidney and in the spleen. The pigment was located mostly in Küpffer's cells of the liver (fig. 3, 4), and a very small amount of granules with similar appearance was found in hepatocytes and histiocytes in the portal region. With hydrogen peroxide this pigment was bleached like the melanin in the tumor. Schmorl's and Lillie's reaction and impregnation with silver were all positive. Reaction for demonstrating the presence of iron and bilirubin were negative. In the liver of the control animals, a few granules which were similar to those found in animals with tumors were seen.

In the case of human melanoma, melanin in the tumor and the pigment in the visceral organs had the same reaction as the animal material. In Küpffer's cells, there was also a large amount of pigment.

Using the electron microscopy in the Küpffer's cells of hamsters with tumors, phagosomes with mostly double membranes and containing numerous granules, which were similar to melanosomes, were discovered. In some hepatocytes, the phagosomes with similar appearance were also recognized. Glycogen was not usually found in the hepatocytes; however, there were many vacuoles and vesicles, the endoplasmic reticulum was dilated, and the mitochondria were swollen. In the control animal group, similar phagosomes were found, but in an insignificant amount. Granules in the shape of lipofuscin, bilirubin or iron pigment were not observed.

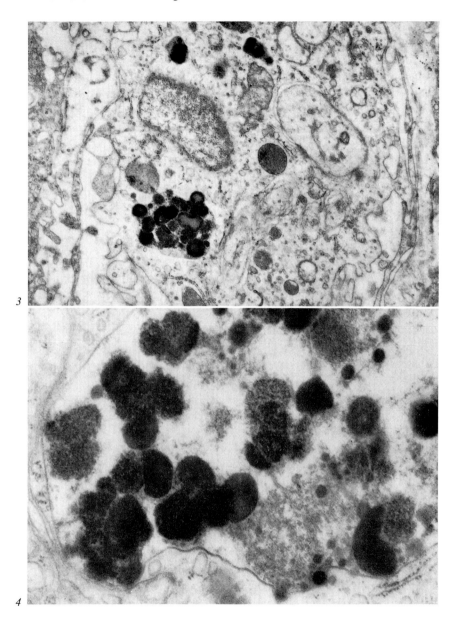

*Fig. 3.* A large phagosome in a Küpffer's cell of a hamster with melanoma. Pigment granules in phagosome. Orig. magnif. × 5,100.

*Fig. 4.* Increased magnification of the same phagosome. Orig. magnif. × 14,600.

## Comments

Earlier work with hamsters, mice and rats with various other non melanotic tumors did not show such pigment in the visceral organs as in hamsters with melanomas. This pigment in visceral organs was bleached with hydrogen peroxide like melanin in the melanoma. Many granules, especially in the phagosomes in the Küpffer's cells, were shaped like melanosomes in melanoma. In this work, we applied only a few methods which are usually used for melanin demonstration, and the results were positive. For this reason, we believe that this pigment found in the visceral organs of hamsters came from melanoma. The insignificant amount in the liver of hamsters without melanoma more than likely came from the skin and flank organ.

In our previous research on hamsters with melanoma which had metastasized [10, 13], we found pigment in the kidney, and in the liver and spleen. The melanoma with which we are now working did not metastasize, and the pigment was mostly distinguished in Küpffer's cells of the liver. Thus, in this group of hamsters, these cells played a dominant role in the process of melanosis. This work shows that in hamsters, this process in the visceral organs can appear without the development of metastasis. The tumors were mostly necrotic and perhaps this factor played some role in the increased mobilization of the melanin.

Necrosis of the tumor and even malnutrition of the animals more than likely caused secondary, regressive changes which we found ultrastructurally in the liver of the hamsters with melanoma.

Although one cannot always compare all elements of an experimental tumor with a human one, the pigment does have a similar localization in the human visceral organs, and it gives a similar histochemical reaction as in the experiments.

In our analysis, we were not able to determine the exact mode of pigment entering the cells during the process of melanosis, but we suppose that it enters through pinocytosis. The form in which it is transported from the tumor is under discussion: it can be transported in its defined form [9], or its intermediary products are transported, which then transform, through the oxidation process, into melanin [2]. In any case, we have seen that melanin transported by blood from the tumor in cells of the visceral organs can retain the same form and can give the same histochemical reaction as in melanoma.

The question of melanosis is very complex. Some of the methods presented here do have limited value, but there are some general results obtained which may serve as a basis for further research.

## Summary

Visceral melanosis was studied in golden hamsters with nonmetastisizing melanoma. Histologically, histochemically and ultrastructurally, granules with characteristics of melanin were especially found in Küpffer's cells of liver.

## References

1 AGRESS, C. M. and FISHMAN, H. C.: Lipomelanotic reticulosis. J. Am. med. Ass. *143:* 957 (1950).

2 FITZPATRICK, T. B.; MONTGOMERY, H., and LERNER, A. B.: Pathogenesis of generalized dermal pigmentation secondary to malignant melanoma and melanuria. J. invest. Derm. *22:* 163–172 (1954).

3 GOODALL, P.; SPRIGGS, I., and WELLS, F. R.: Malignant melanoma with melanosis and melanuria and with pigmented monocytes and tumor cells in the blood. Br. J. Surg. *48:* 549–555 (1961).

4 HALL, M. J. A.: A staining reaction for bilirubin in sections of tissue. Am. J. clin. Path. *34:* 313–316 (1960).

5 JACOBSEN, V. C. and KLINCK, G. H.: Melanin. I. Its mobilization and excretion in normal and in pathologic conditions. Archs Path. *7:* 141–151 (1934).

6 KETTLER, L. H.: in KAUFMANN Lehrbuch der Spez. Pathol. Anatomie 11/3 (Gruyter, Berlin 1958).

7 LILLIE, R. D.: Histopathologic technic and practical histochemistry (McGraw-Hill, New York 1965).

8 LUBARSCH, O.: in HENKE und LUBARSCH Handbuch der Spez. Pathol. Anatomie u. Histologie VI–1 (Springer, Berlin 1925).

9 MASSON, P.: Tumeurs humaines (Maloine, Paris 1956).

10 OBERMAN, B. et RIVIÈRE, M. R.: Etude de la mélanose apparaissant chez le hamster doré après implantation du mélanome M 622. Path. Biol., Paris *11:* 315–321 (1963).

11 OBERMAN, B. and LJUBEŠIĆ, N.: Electronic microscopic investigation of melanotic and amelanotic melanoma in hamster. Lij. Vjesnik. *91:* 947–953 (1969).

12 PEARSE, A. G. E.: Histochemistry, theoretical and applied (Churchill Livingstone, Edinburgh 1972).

13 RIVIÈRE, M. R.; OBERMAN, B.; CHOUROULINKOV, I. et GUERIN, M.: Etude anatomopathologique et comportement biologique d'un mélanome (M. 622) greffable et métastasant d'un hamster doré. Bull. Ass. fr. Etude Cancer *49:* 44–72 (1962).

14 ROSENBERG, J. C.: Melanuric nephrosis. Archs Path. *62:* 399–402 (1956).

15 WELLS, H. G.: Chemical pathology (Saunders, Philadelphia, 1926).

16 ZELLER, A.: Über Melanurie. Arch. klin. Chir. *29:* 245–253 (1883).

Dr. B. OBERMAN, Department of Pathology, Faculty of Medicine, University of Zagreb, *Zagreb* (Yugoslavia)

Pigment Cell, vol. 2, pp. 316–320 (Karger, Basel 1976)

# Melanin-Binding Drugs and Ultrasonics-Induced Cytotoxicity

JOHN E. MCGINNESS, PETER M. CORRY and E. ARMOUR

Physics Department, The University of Texas System Cancer Center, Texas Medical Center, Houston, Tex.

## Introduction

The importance of electron-phonon coupling (i.e. the coupling of electronic states to vibrational states of the material) in the amorphous semiconductor switching [5] and perhaps in the protective role of melanins *in vivo* [4] suggests the use of ultrasonics as an intracellular probe of the relationship of the melanosome to its environment. Another probe can be obtained by using a melanin-binding drug. The choice of drugs and ultrasonics is further guided by a considerable volume of literature which indicates a consistent preferential killing of melanin-containing tissue under apparently related conditions [1, 3, 6, 7]. The objective of our work *in vitro* is then to determine under laboratory conditions the requirements for the reproducible generation of drug-potentiated killing of melanized tissue by ultrasound.

## Methods and Results

Figure 1 contains cell survival data determined by traditional colony formation techniques after treatment with drugs and ultrasound. The amelanotic cells were assayed for pigment content and typically contain from 3 to 4 pg per cell. Data obtained on cells containing 40 pg per cell is presented elsewhere [2]. The amelanotic line is pertinent to the present discussion due to the existence of a shoulder on the survival curve in the absence of drugs. This shoulder, which is absent in cell lines with higher pigment content, allows some assessment of the creation of sublethal, and lethal damage within the cell and possible changes in the type of damage created by different treatments.

Data was obtained initially by exposing cells to chlorpromazine (say 10 μg/ml) for 1 h and then washing and resuspending in fresh medium to allow any loosely bound drug to escape. Experiments with amelanotic cells plated in tubes and allowed to uptake [35]S-chlorpromazine (CPZ) indicated that nonpigmented cells released almost all chlorpromazine within 1 h, and pigmented cells reach a point of equilibrium typically retaining 0.1 pg CPZ per picogram of melanin.

The amelanotic cells were then exposed to ultrasound at 10 kHz as indicated in figure 1. No significant killing of the cells occurred with chlorpromazine alone. However, the killing induced by the ultrasound is clearly potentiated by the drug and the survival shoulder out to 5 sec disappears.

Our work on isolated materials has indicated that melanins would polymerize in the presence of a number of charge transfer compounds and that these drugs dramatically alter the electrical characteristics of the

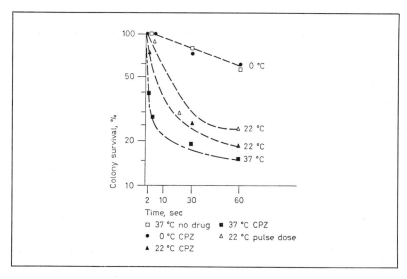

*Fig. 1.* The effects of 10 kHz ultrasonics on lightly pigmented cells is presented as a function of temperature at which the irradiation was carried out. Incubation of the cells with chlorpromazine (CPZ) in the growth medium at a concentration of 10 μg/ml for 1 h is compared with incubation at 1 μg/ml for periods longer than one generation time.

melanins [2]. This observation suggested the following experiment. When cells were grown in CPZ for periods much longer than a cell generation time ($\approx$14 h), it was observed that 1 $\mu$g/ml of drug was capable of potentiating approximately the same amount of killing by ultrasound previously induced by 10 $\mu$g/ml for 1 h pulse incubation.

The effects of temperature on the ultrasonic drug interaction were investigated to provide further insight into the nature of the interaction. Amelanotic cells were grown in the presence of the drug and then washed and resuspended in fresh medium. 1 ml of cells from 500 to $10^3$ cells/ml were pipeted into tubes and cooled to 0 °C in an ice water bath. The cells were heated to temperature for 5 min, sonicated and immediately cooled to 0 °C. The cells were incubated in dishes at 37 °C and colony counts were obtained at maturity.

Further results of the effect of the drug kanamycin are shown in figure 2. As seen in figures 1 and 2, drug effects at higher temperatures can be essentially reversed by maintaining the cells at 0 °C. As the shoulder to the survival curve is also restored, implying a change from lethal to sublethal damage, there are two possible explanations for these observations. These are that the ultrasonic energy is not being converted into

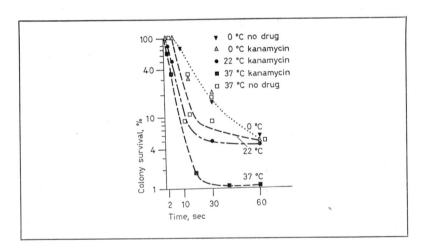

*Fig. 2.* The effects of 1 MHz ultrasonics on human amelanotic cells are examined by traditional colony survival experiments as a function of temperature with and without kanamycin. The cells were incubated in the presence of kanamycin (4 $\mu$g/ml) in the growth medium for periods longer than one generation time, usually 48 h. This drug is known to tightly bind to melanins *in vivo* and in some cases induces deafness in humans.

higher cytotoxic form or that the cytotoxic product is prevented from expressing damage. If increasing the temperature allows the cytotoxic products to diffuse farther before they decay, and lowering the temperature insures that they decay before reaching a target (i.e. if the products are free radicals), the curves might be explained.

Experiments to assay single and double-strand scission (if the cytotoxic products are metastable free radicals), as well as other survival studies, are in progress in an attempt to distinguish between these two possibilities.

*Discussion*

Historically, most physical systems were well understood in classical terms. The development of energy transfer devices which operated by manipulating objects of low mass (electrons or holes) through small distances required the application of the uncertainty principle, and thus could not be understood in terms of Newtonian physics. Melanin represents an electronic energy transfer device which derives its main characteristics from the manipulation of electrons and phonons by electric fields over small distances. It is not surprising, therefore, that a final elucidation of its biological roles requires a quantum mechanical description.

The ability of water and other molecules with high permanent dielectric constant to drastically modify conductivity without participating in conduction itself [2, 5] indicates that a large number of electrons near the Fermi level in melanin are in localized states which will polarize the nuclei of surrounding atoms. In turn, movement of these nuclei will greatly affect the energy of the electrons in the vicinity, hence producing an electron-phonon coupling and a sensitivity to vibrations of the molecule. A tendency for these localized states to be singly occupied could also account for the ESR signal in these materials. A further coupling can result from vibrations of any charged (e.g. amine or carboxyl) groups which may be present in the melanin. An interesting picture of the drug-ultrasonic interaction evolves from this discussion. The ultrasonic energy is apparently relaxed out uniformly in the nonpigmented tissue. The melanosome, however, relaxes out energy from the field within a small volume and couples it to the production of some cytotoxic species. The application of the melanin-binding drug apparently increases the production of cytotoxic products.

The observation of drug-induced potentiation of ultrasonic killing in pigment-containing cells suggests a similar mechanism for kanamycin-induced ototoxicity in humans [3].

## Summary

In vitro experiments with human melanoma cells indicate that ultrasonic induced killing of melanin-containing cells can be potentiated by the proper choice of temperature and drugs. These agents appear to be interacting through electron-phonon coupling in the melanins within the melanosome itself. As the mechanism of these interactions becomes clearer, it may be possible to relate these phenomena to some human syndromes and perhaps develop controlled methods to kill pigmented tumor cells.

## Acknowledgments

The authors wish to express their gratitude to Dr. Marvin Romsdahl for supplying the cultured melanoma cells. This research was supported in part by AEC Contract AT-(40-1)-2832 and Training Grant CA-05099 from the Public Health Service.

## References

1   Blois, M. S.: The binding properties of melanins: in vivo and in vitro. Adv. Biol. Skin 12: 65–79 (1972).
2   Corry, P. M.; McGinness, J. E., and Armour, E.: Semiconductor properties of melanins related to preferential killing of melanoma cells (this volume).
3   Lindquist, N. G.: Accumulation of drugs on melanins. Acta radiol., suppl. 325: 1–92 (1973).
4   McGinness, J. E. and Proctor, P. H.: The importance of the fact that melanin is black. J. theor. Biol. 39: 677–678 (1973).
5   McGinness, J. E.; Corry, P. M., and Proctor, P. H.: Amorphous semiconductor switching in melanins. Science 183: 853–855 (1974).
6   Proctor, P.: Electron-transfer factors in psychosis and dyskinesia. Physiol. Chem. Physics 4: 349–360 (1972).
7   Proctor, P.; McGinness, J. E., and Corry, P.: A hypothesis on the preferential destruction of melanized tissues. J. theor. Biol. 39: 677–678 (1973).

Dr. John E. McGinness, Physics Department, The University of Texas System Cancer Center, Texas Medical Center, Houston, TX 77025 (USA)

Pigment Cell, vol. 2, pp. 321–326 (Karger, Basel 1976)

# Semiconductor Properties of Melanins Related to Preferential Killing of Melanoma Cells

PETER M. CORRY, JOHN E. MCGINNESS and ELWOOD ARMOUR

Department of Physics, The University of Texas System Cancer Center, Texas Medical Center, Houston, Tex.

The relationship of the electronic properties of biological macromolecules to their function within the cell has been a matter of great controversy for many years. The suggestion that energy conversion and transduction may occur as a result of electronic conduction through biological macromolecules [11] has never been widely accepted due to a lack of evidence that such molecules have semiconductor properties. Recently, it was shown that the melanins are not only amorphous semiconductors, but also possess the more exotic property of amorphous semiconductor threshold switching at biologically attainable electric field strengths [6]. Hydration of the melanins was found to be essential to the demonstration of these characteristics; however, it was shown that the conduction was not ionic in nature. These properties were also found to persist in intact melanosomes isolated from a human melanoma.

The observation of these highly unique properties led to further experimental work to determine the extent to which they could be altered by other molecules of biological importance. The results of one such study are shown in figure 1, which demonstrates the effect of including diethyl amine at various concentrations in the reaction mixture during synthesis of the melanins. Figure 2 shows the effect of the addition of the drug chlorpromazine on the threshold switching potential subsequent to polymerization. The melanins were synthesized by auto-oxidation of L-3-4-dihydroxyphenylalanine (dopa).

These data clearly indicate that the melanins may be 'doped' both during and after their synthesis. This doping results in dramatic alteration of both the conductivity and the threshold switching characteristics of these molecules. These effects coupled with low temperature specific heat

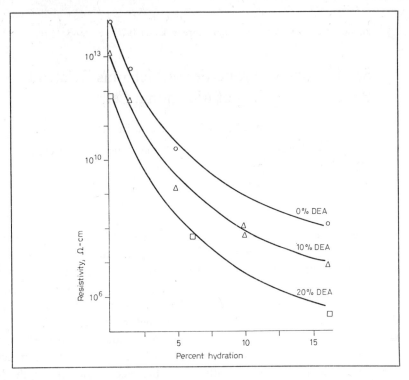

*Fig. 1.* The resistivity of dopa melanin samples as a function of percent hydration for 3 samples synthesized in the presence of 0, 10, and 20% diethyl amine (DEA) in the reaction mixture. The resistivity of each sample is seen to drop some 6 orders of magnitude. The parallel nature of these curves indicates independent roles for the diethyl amine and water of hydration.

measurements on these melanins [8] make consistent the interpretation that the doping molecules are contributing carriers to conduction states and the water of hydration acts by alteration of local dielectric constants. A curious parallel is seen between the data of figure 2 and the observation of COTZIAS *et al.* [3], which notes that in some normal patients the administration of small doses of chlorpromazine induces the symptoms of Parkinson's disease, but at much higher doses the symptoms disappear.

In light of the above observations and evidence in the literature that many human disorders involve the melanized tissues in energy transduction areas [5], a hypothesis was developed relating the electronic properties of the melanins to their function within the cell [9]. This hypothesis is

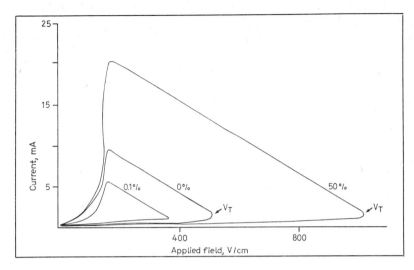

*Fig. 2.* The variation of threshold switching potentials ($V_T$) of dopa melanin, as a function of chlorpromazine added to the sample subsequent to polymerization. At low concentrations of 0.1%, $V_T$ is seen to decrease; however, when the concentration is increased to 50%, a large increase in $V_T$ over that for the undoped melanins is observed. Similar patterns in electrical conductivity properties are also observed. The methods of measurement and an explanation of threshold switching characteristics are detailed in [6]. The $V_T$ for undoped melanins is approximately 50 mV/$\mu$m, well within the range of those generated by biological systems.

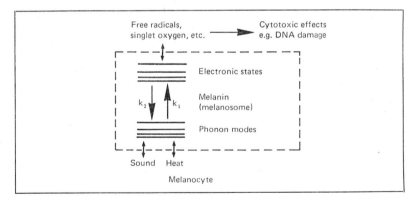

*Fig. 3.* Schematic representation of the hypothesized role of the electronic properties of the melanins within the cell. Energy absorbed in electronic states can be transferred to the phonon modes, and vice versa, by electron-phonon coupling. This mechanism may behave in either a cytoprotective or a cytotoxic manner, depending on the mode and rate of energy introduction.

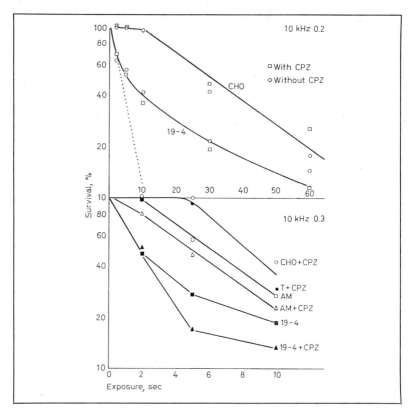

*Fig. 4.* Colony survival of pigmented tumor cells and non-pigmented cells in culture as a function of the exposure to 10 kHz sonic irradiation. CPZ = Chlorpromazine at 1 μg/ml for 24 h in growth medium; CHO = Chinese hamster ovary cells; T = human T cells; AM = human 'amelanotic' melanoma cells, 3 pg of melanin per cell; 19-4 = highly pigmented human melanoma cells, 40 pg of melanin per cell. The final stage input power to the irradiating cavity was 35 and 53 for the upper and lower panels, respectively.

shown diagramatically in figure 3. The main feature of this hypothesis is that the melanins behave as a non-linear energy transduction device operating by phonon-electron coupling. Another feature is that the melanins will behave as a 'phonon bottleneck' at high energy input, resulting in a switch from a cytoprotective state at low energy input rates, to a cytotoxic state at the high energy input rates. The rate constants for energy transduction and conversion from one state to another are obviously affected by the extent of electron-phonon coupling, which in turn is intimately related to the molecules electronic properties. Another interesting implication is that melanized cells should be more susceptible to energy introduced in the phonon modes than non-melanized tissues, and synergism between drugs which alter the electronic properties and a physical agent such as ultrasonics should be observed.

As a test of this hypothesis, colony survival studies were carried out to assay effects of ultrasonics on pigmented human melanoma cells and control unpigmented cells in culture. The results of some such experiments which clearly demonstrate the increased killing efficiency as a function of pigment content of the cells, are shown in figure 4. (Pigment content of the cells was assayed by the method of ROSENTHAL et al. [10].) This preferential killing of the melanized cells also appears to be a function of the presence of the drug chlorpromazine. Other drugs (e.g. kanamycin), temperature and ultrasonic frequency have also been shown to be factors [7].

Using established procedures [1, 2, 4], the production of single- and double-strand DNA scission within the pigmented cell was investigated as an indirect assay of free radical production. The results of these studies show a reduction in single-strand DNA molecular weights (initially $4.5 \times 10^8$ daltons) as a function of ultrasonic dose. The double-strand molecular weight decrease (initially $9 \times 10^8$ daltons) appeared to be a dose-squared function. These data are consistent with the idea that free radicals or some other excited state species are being produced and attack the DNA near the nuclear membrane of pigmented cells, resulting in single-strand breaks. Such molecular weight decreases were not evident for similar ultrasonic treatment of non-pigmented cells.

All of the above observations support the hypothesis presented. The question of whether or not all of the electronic properties of these macromolecules are relevant to their role in vivo can only be answered by future experimental studies. However, the information learned to date has provided some insight into the biological role of the melanins, their involvement in some human disorders and perhaps into some of the general mechanisms by which the cell produces and uses energy. Other questions, such as the response of normal pigmented cells and pigmented tumor cells in animals, have yet to be investigated. At present, there is no reason to expect that the response of these cells will differ radically from that observed for the tissue culture systems, and should they prove to behave similarly, it may be possible to develop new modalities for the treatment of human malignant melanoma.

## Summary

The effect of various drugs on the conductivity and amorphous semiconductor switching properties of the melanins has been studied. From the results of these investigations, it is postulated that the melanins behave as a non-linear energy transduction device within the melanized cell. Experimental studies using melanized cells in culture support this hypothesis and demonstrate that melanized tumor cells can be preferentially killed by sonic irradiation. Some evidence indicates that free radical production is involved in this process.

## Acknowledgements

The authors wish to express their gratitude to Dr. MARVIN ROMSDAHL for supplying the cultured melanoma cells. This research was supported in part by AEC Contract AT-(40-1)-2832 and Training Grant CA-05099 from the Public Health Service.

## References

1 CORRY, P. M. and COLE, A.: Radiation-induced double-strand scission of the DNA of mammalian metaphase chromosomes. Radiat. Res. 36: 528–543 (1968).

2 CORRY, P. M. and COLE, A.: Double strand rejoining in mammalian DNA. Nature new Biol. 245: 100 (1973).

3 COTZIAS, G. C.; PAPAVASILOV, P. S.; WOERT, M. H. VAN, and SAKAMOTO, A.: Melanogenesis and extrapyramidal diseases. Fed. Proc. Fed. Am. Socs exp. Biol. 23: 713 (1964).

4 LETT, J. T.; CALDWELL, I.; DEAN, C., and ALEXANDER, P.: Rejoining of X-ray induced breaks in the DNA of leukemia cells. Nature, Lond. 214: 790 (1967).

5 LINDQUIST, N. G.: Accumulation of drugs on melanin. Acta radiol. suppl. 325 (1973).

6 MCGINNESS, J. E.; CORRY, P. M., and PROCTOR, P. H.: Amorphous semiconductor switching in melanins. Science 183: 853 (1974).

7 MCGINNESS, J. E.; CORRY, P. M., and ARMOUR, E.: Melanin-binding drugs and ultrasonic induced cytotoxicity (this volume).

8 MIZUTANI, U.; MASSACSKY, T. B.; MCGINNESS, J. E. and CORRY, P. M.: Low temperature specific heat anomalies in Melanins and tumour melanosomes. Nature 259: 505 (1976).

9 PROCTOR, P. H.; MCGINNESS, J. E., and CORRY, P. M.: A hypothesis on the preferential killing of melanized tissues. J. theor. Biol. 48: 19 (1974).

10 ROSENTHAL, M.; KREIDER, J. W., and SHIMAN, R.: Quantitative assay of melanin in melanoma cells in culture and in tumors. Analyt. Biochem. 56: 91 (1973).

11 SZENT-GYORGYI, A.: II. Energy migration in organized biological systems. Disc. Faraday Soc. 27: 111 (1959).

Dr. PETER M. CORRY, Department of Physics, The University of Texas System Cancer Center, Texas Medical Center, Houston, TX 77025 (USA)

Pigment Cell, vol. 2, pp. 327–338 (Karger, Basel 1976)

# Effects of Dimethyltriazeno Imidazole Carboxamide (DTIC, NSC 45,388) on Melanoma Metabolites and Enzymes [1]

L. R. Morgan, jr., M. S. Samuels, R. D. Carter and E. T. Krementz

Clinical Cancer Research Center, Department of Surgery, Tulane University School of Medicine, and Department of Pharmacology, Louisiana State University Medical Center, New Orleans, La.

## Introduction

5-Amino-imidazole-4-carboxamide and its analogues have been shown to be incorporated into RNA and to block metabolic pathways of nucleotide synthesis of $\alpha$-n-formyl-glycinamide ribonucleotide formation [9]. 5-(3,3-Dimethyl-1-triazeno)-imidazole-4-carboxamide (DTIC) exhibits antitumor activity in patients with malignant melanoma [1, 3–6, 8–12, 18–20]. We participated in the Central Oncology Group's Phase Trial protocols for DTIC and support the observation that DTIC exhibits antitumor activity in patients with malignant melanoma [4].

As part of our interest in the melanin cell cycle of malignant melanoma [13, 15, 17], we have continued to measure the urinary excretion of homovanillic acid (HVA) and arylsulfatase B and tumor tissue tyrosinase-dopa oxidase and arylsulfatase in patients with melanoma who are receiving chemotherapy. We previously reported several patients with melanoma who did not respond to DTIC therapy, but did demonstrate a decrease in their urine HVA levels and an increase in urine arylsulfatase B activities while on therapy [16]. The lesions continued to grow on DTIC therapy and many of the satellite lesions became amelanotic and with decreased dopa oxidase levels [16]. This is in contrast to the trend for untreated melanoma, i.e. both urine HVA and arylsulfatase B values increase with advancing disease [14].

1 Supported by Grants CA-05108 and CA-08087, National Cancer Institute, Bethesda, Md.

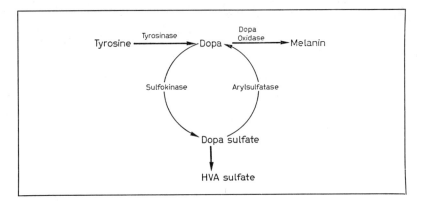

*Fig. 1.* Relationship between HVA, dopa and arylsulfatase in melanoma.

Arylsulfatase is a lysosomal enzyme present in all tissues, except for mature erythrocytes, and exists in isoenzymic forms A, B and C. Forms B and C are present in elevated quantities in many visceral and soft tissue neoplasms, including melanoma, in which elevated quantities of the B isoenzyme also appear in the urine [7, 14, 15]. Dopa and HVA are metabolites of melanin synthesis and are excreted in elevated quantities in the urine in malignant melanotic melanoma [14]. The quantitative relationship between urine arylsulfatase B and HVA in malignant melanoma have been described previously [14]. Figure 1 summarizes some possible relationships between dopa, HVA and arylsulfatase.

The appearance of elevated quantities of dopa and HVA is thought to be due to increased activity of the tyrosinase-dopa oxidase complex [17]. They are excreted in urine in part as sulfates. These sulfates are substrates for the enzyme arylsulfatase and could stabilize the enzyme within the lysosomal vacuoles. These sulfates could stabilize the arylsulfatase localized within the tumor (stabilization of lysosomal membrane). In the presence of reduced concentrations of dopa and HVA, i.e. amelanotic melanomas, the enzyme is released and appears in the urine. There is an increase in the ratio of urine arylsulfatase/HVA in amelanotic melanomas [14]. At present, we wish to report an interesting pattern in 33 patients with melanotic melanomas of decreased urine HVA and tumor dopa oxidase, accompanied by an increase in urine arylsulfatase B activities while on DTIC therapy. These observations are compared to the pattern seen in a group of melanotic melanoma patients that responded to DTIC therapy.

## Materials and Methods

All patients involved in this study had histologically proven disseminated melanoma and the presence of one or more measurable lesions to serve as an objective indicator of response to therapy. No patient was admitted to the study who had had immunotherapy, chemotherapy, irradiation, or extensive surgery within the preceding four weeks.

38 patients with disseminated malignant melanoma were involved in the present study. These patients were involved in both the Central Oncology Group's Phase I and II studies which consisted of DTIC 4.5–6.0 mg per kg body weight per day intravenously for 5 days, with a 9-day rest period between courses and DTIC 4.5 mg per kg body weight per day intravenously, for 10 days, with a 28-day rest period respectively [5]. DTIC was supplied by the Cancer Chemotherapy Division, National Service Center, National Cancer Institute.

The patients were comprised of Negro and Caucasian males and females, aged 17–76 years. All of the patients possessed normal renal and hematopoietic functions upon admission to the study.

Urine homovanillic acid (HVA): 24-hour urine samples were collected on ice (0–5 °C) without preservatives before each course and 5–8 days after each course was completed. HVA was assayed according to the modified electrophoretic procedure recently described [14]. The HVA is reported in reference to creatinine to account for any renal variation.

Urine arylsulfatase B: The procedure of BAUM et al. [2] was employed to determine arylsulfatase B activity on the 24-hour urine samples.

Tissue dopa oxidase: Melanoma biopsies were assayed for dopa oxidase according to the previously described procedure [13]. Dopa oxidase activity is reported as microliters of oxygen consumed per mg of protein per unit of time ($\mu$l $O_2$ per mg protein per 3 h).

DTIC metabolism by melanoma homogenates: DTIC was dissolved in 0.1 M phosphate buffer, pH 6.8, to give concentrations from 1 to 60 $\mu$mol per 3 ml of buffer. Melanoma dopa oxidase was prepared from melanotic human melanomas according to the procedure above. A typical assay mixture contained 1 ml of L-dopa (2 $\mu$mol per ml of 0.1 M phosphate buffer, pH 6.8, 1 ml of tumor homogenate, and 1 ml of DTIC in phosphate buffer). The reaction mixture was incubated at 37 °C for 3 h in a standard Warburg apparatus [13]. Appropriate controls and blanks were assayed in duplicate so that the inhibitory effect of DTIC on L-dopa oxidation could be calculated.

## Results

Clinical studies: In present study, five patients had partial responses (>50% but <100% regression of measurable lesions); ten had no change for one or more courses of therapy, and 23 had progressive disease.

*Table I.* Effect of DTIC phase I and II studies on urine HVA and arylsulfatase B in five patients with melanoma demonstrating partial remissions

| Case No. (age/sex) | Disease sites | Total dosage, g | Treatment period, weeks | Urine HVA 1.56 (0.15–1.82)[1] $\mu g/ml$ creatinine | | Urine arylsulfatase B 5.05 (2.63–8.27)[1] $\mu g/ml/h$ | |
|---|---|---|---|---|---|---|---|
| | | | | before | after | before | after |
| 1  43/M | soft tissue | 11.6 | 16 | 3.50 | 1.70 | 10.21 | 3.95 |
| 2  51/F | soft tissue | 11.6 | 16 | 2.77 | 0.98 | 8.96 | 11.09 |
| 3  35/F | lung | 10 | 6 | 1.04 | 1.14 | 13.30 | 3.64 |
| 4  55/M | soft tissue | 2.6 | 4 | 1.70 | 1.07 | 4.61 | 7.71 |
| 5  61/M | soft tissue, lung | 8.1 | 4 | 0.38 | 1.16 | 19.30 | 8.18 |

1 Mean average and range for 40 normal subjects of same age ranges.

In table I are the changes noted in urine HVA and arylsulfatase B that accompanied the partial responses to DTIC therapy. No attempt was made to record the concentration of arylsulfatase A which also appeared in the urine. Although the A isoenzyme is also excreted in the urine, it is not elevated in patients with malignant melanomas [14]. The changes noted in table I were seen during both phase I and II studies. No difference between phases I and II were noted. In these patients, the general tendency was for the HVA and arylsulfatase B to become or approach normal values. Patient No. 2 expired one month after the last urine assay reported here. At postmortem, a melanoma brain metastasis was found, and was felt to be the cause of death although pulmonary metastases were regressing at the time of death. The brain lesion supported the rising arylsulfatase B noted.

Figure 2 is a graph of the urine HVA and arylsulfatase B after each course of DTIC for those patients with progressive disease or with lesions that remained unchanged. The total courses ranged from 1 to 18. Only one patient received ten or more. In figure 2, we have included amelanotic as well as melanotic tumors, since even the low HVA values of the amelanotic tumors were reduced during therapy. Phase I and II studies are included together since the figures for the two protocols were not sig-

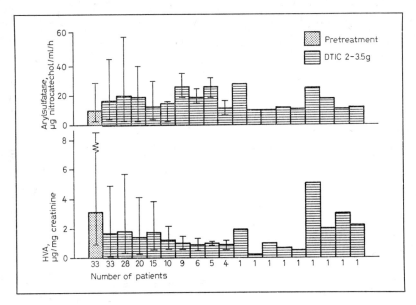

*Fig. 2.* The effect of DTIC on urine HVA and arylsulfatase B in patients with disseminated malignant melanoma that demonstrated no change in lesions or progressive disease. The first dotted column represents the values before drug therapy. The top of the columns is the average for each course and the high and low brackets the extreme values. Each shaded column represents the values 5–8 days after a course of therapy was completed. All 33 patients received at least one course of phase I or II therapy. The normal mean average and ranges for HVA = 1.56 (1.05–1.82) $\mu$g/ml creatinine, and for arylsulfatase B = 5.05 (2.63–8.87) $\mu$g/ml/h.

nificantly different. Of interest is that the patient with the lowest HVA value in each column was also the lowest throughout courses 1–9 and the highest was the same patient throughout all 18 courses. The latter patient's lesions remained unchanged and he seemed to be asymptomatic; however, during the 15th course a pulmonary lesion, as well as a lower extremity lesion, increased in size with melanotic satellite lesions appearing and, as noted, a rise in HVA occurred.

Many of the patients had cutaneous satellite lesions and lymph nodes that could be biopsied at intervals during DTIC therapy. In table II are listed the DTIC dosage, changes in tumor histology, dopa oxidase activities, and HVA levels before and after therapy in five patients that had progressive disease while on DTIC therapy. Figures 3–6 compare the his-

Table II. Changes in melanoma histology, dopa oxidase and urine HVA after DTIC therapy

| Patient | Disease site | Total dosage, g | Treatment period, weeks | Histology[a] | | Tumor dopa oxidase 0.01 (0–0.11)[b] $\mu l\ O_2$/mg protein/3 h | | Urine HVA 1.56 (0.15–1.82)[c] $\mu g$/ml creatinine | |
|---|---|---|---|---|---|---|---|---|---|
| | | | | before | after | before | after | before | after |
| 6 | soft tissue | 9.5 | 12 | Melanin: +2. Cell types: spindle. Grade: 2 | Melanin: +1. Cell types: epithelial, nevoid, spindle. Grade: 2 | 0.5 | 0 | 2.4 | 0.7 |
| 7 | soft tissue, lung | 8.8 | 16 | Melanin: +2. Cell types: nevoid cells. Grade: 2 | Melanin: +1. Cell types: epithelial, nevoid cells. Grade: 1 | 3.0 | 0.5 | 4.7 | 0.7 |
| 8 | soft tissue, pelvic | 1.0 | 6 | Melanin: +3. Cell types: epithelial, spindle, bizarre cells. Grade: 3 | Melanin: 0. Cell types: spindle, bizarre. Grade: 3 | 2.3 | 0 | 3.1 | 2.1 |
| 9 | soft tissue, lung | 2.4 | 3 | Melanin: +3. Cells: epithelial, dendritic. Grade: 3 | Melanin: +1. Cell types: spindle, bizarre, nevoid. Grade: 3 | 1.9 | 0.3 | 2.1 | 2.5 |
| 10 | soft tissue | 2.5 | 3 | Melanin: +4. Dendritic cells. Grade: 4 | Melanin: +2. Bizarre cells. Grade: 3 | 8.9 | 2.4 | 1.4 | 0.6 |

[a] Grades 1–4 refer to degree of differentiation – 1 being the most anaplastic, 4 the most well-differentiated.

[b] Mean average and range values for 20 normal Caucasians and Negroes. Dopa oxidase values were from skin-punch biopsies.

[c] Mean average and range values for 40 normal Caucasians and Negroes from the same age range and sex distribution as the patients.

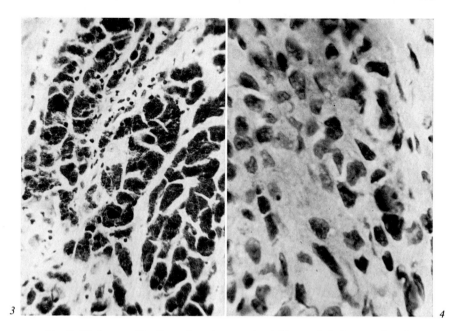

3                                                                                  4

*Fig. 3.* High magnification of a pigmented satellite nodule in case 7, prior to
DTIC therapy. Note the dense melanin granules present.

*Fig. 4.* High magnification of an amelanotic lesion that developed in case 7 adjacent to the site of the nodule described in figure 3 following DTIC therapy (total
dosage 8.8 g over a 4-month period). Note the pleomorphic amelanotic cells.

tology of two of these patients, cases 6 and 7. In general, the cell types
did not change as much as did the dopa oxidase activities. As can be seen,
the epithelial and dendritic cell types predominated in the melanotic lesions. The changes in urine HVA, which are an indirect product of the tyrosinase-dopa oxidase conversion of tyrosine and dopa to melanin, also
paralleled the decrease in the tissue dopa oxidase. One patient, case 9,
demonstrated decreased dopa oxidase, but little or no change in HVA,
probably due to the massive tumor volume present.

DTIC metabolism *in vitro:* The inhibitory effect of DTIC on L-dopa
oxidation by human melanoma dopa oxidase is presented in table III.
DTIC in varying concentrations (1–60 $\mu$mol) has an inhibitory effect on
L-dopa (2 $\mu$mol) oxidation as measured by a decrease in oxygen consumption over a 3-hour period. Appropriate blanks and controls were used to
account for auto-oxidation and dopa-DTIC interaction.

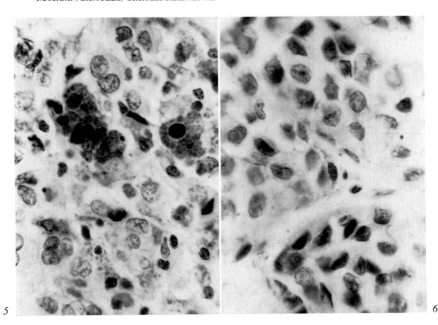

5
6

*Fig. 5.* High magnification of a pigmented nodule in case 6 before therapy.

*Fig. 6.* High magnification of an amelanotic nodule that developed in case 6 adjacent to the original melanotic lesion after DTIC therapy (total dosage 9.5 g over a 3-month period).

*Table III.* The effect of DTIC on the oxidation of dopa by melanoma dopa oxidase

| DTIC concentration, $\mu$mol | Dopa oxidase inhibition, % |
|---|---|
| 60.0 | 65 |
| 11.0 | 70 |
| 7.0 | 72 |
| 6.0 | 64 |
| 4.0 | 30 |
| 2.0 | 10 |
| 1.0 | 0 |

Reaction mixture contained L-dopa ($\mu$mol), DITC ($\mu$mol indicated in column 1) and human melanoma dopa oxidase (1 mg) in a total volume of 3.0 ml of 0.1 M phosphate buffer (pH 6.8) and incubated for 3 h at 37°C in a Warburg apparatus as described in Materials and Methods.

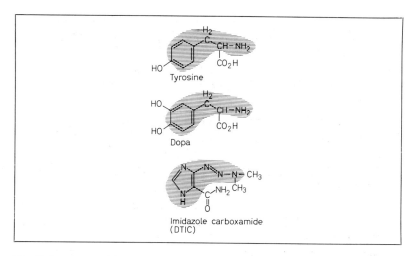

*Fig. 7.* Structures of tyrosine, dopa and DTIC. Shaded areas represent structurally isosteric moieties.

## Discussion

DTIC was originally prepared as an analog of 5-aminoimidazole-4-carboxamide. However, it does not primarily inhibit purine biosynthesis; it is not cross-resistant with the thiopurines and, in general, its mechanism remains obscure.

During our participation in the phase I study of DTIC, we noticed that a number of our patients developed amelanotic satellite lesions [16]. This suggested that a possible interaction of DTIC at the level of the melanin cell cycle might also be occurring. When the structures of DTIC, tyrosine and dopa were compared, at first they seem very different, and they are (fig. 7). DTIC is a structurally designed antimetabolite of a purine precursor necessary for nucleic acid synthesis. Tyrosine and L-dopa are amino acids and precursors of the catecholamines and substrates for tyrosinase-dopa oxidase. However, all three possess a center of unsaturation separated from a nitrogen by a two-atom chain (shaded area in fig. 7). These simple relationships make the three structures isosterically related and capable of similar biological properties.

Decreased urine HVA concentrations as well as decreased tumor dopa oxidase activities with increasing amelanotic satellite lesions while on DTIC therapy suggest that there were inhibitions of the melanin cell cycle in the present study. However, in the natural course of melanoma, new metastases tend to become amelanotic and less well-differentiated and, therefore, these changes might be nonspecific.

Arylsulfatase is a hydrolytic enzyme that exists as three isoenzymes, A, B, C. All three forms are present in most normal tissues. A and B isoenzymes are soluble in nature and excreted in the urine [7]. Isoenzyme C is particulate and not excreted in the urine. All three forms are found elevated in melanomas with the elevation of arylsulfatase B in urine most consistent [14]. DZIALOSZYNSKI et al. [7] and MORGAN et al. [15] have reported elevated concentrations of arylsulfatase B and C in both melanotic and amelanotic human melanoma. Amelanotic melanomas contain less arylsulfatase B and C than do the melanotic varieties. However, urine arylsulfatase B levels are higher in the former patients than in the latter patients. The rise in urine arylsulfatase B with reduction of HVA, noted in the patients in this study, supports previous observations that there is an inverse relationship between urine HVA and arylsulfatase B [14]. The fact that many of the tumors which did not respond to therapy changed patterns is of interest. An inverse relationship between urine HVA and arylsulfatase B is observed for most patients with melanotic and amelanotic malignant melanomas [14]. Urine HVA and arylsulfatase B increase in melanotic melanomas as organ involvement and volume of disease increase. However, one system is always higher than the other; in the melanotic variety, HVA >arylsulfatase B; and in the amelanotic variety, arylsulfatase B >HVA [14].

One explanation is that since dopa and HVA are excreted in part as sulfates and are substrates for arylsulfatase, they may stabilize the enzyme as substrates within the tumor lysosomal membrane. In the absence of dopa and HVA, e.g. amelanotic melanomas, the arylsulfatase is more labile and lost easier from the cell. In figure 2, as the urine HVA concentration decreased, the arylsulfatase B concentration increased. It should be mentioned that in neither the Negro (two in the present study) nor the Caucasian patients were any abnormal depigmentations of the outside of the lesions noticed while on DTIC therapy.

The chemical similarities of DTIC, dopa and tyrosine and the inhibition of L-dopa oxidation in vitro are good evidence that DTIC can interfere in vitro with the melanin cell cycle. This supports the data seen in table III. Thus, in addition to the possible inhibitory action of DTIC on cellular replication, it may also be interfering with melanin synthesis in melanomas. This property of DTIC is desirable, if interference with melanin metabolism interferes with cell growth. However, if it causes increased appearances of amelanotic melanoma metastases in the unresponsive patient, this is undesirable.

## Summary

Effects of DTIC on tumor and urine metabolites and enzymes was investigated in 38 patients with disseminated malignant melanoma. Urine assays for homovanillic acid (HVA) and arylsulfatase B and tumor assays for dopa oxidase were performed before and after therapy.

Those patients who had a partial remission following DTIC therapy (5/38) demonstrated decreased urine HVA and arylsulfatase B content as well as a reduction in melanoma dopa oxidase activities. In contrast, 33 nonresponders demonstrated a pattern of decreased urine HVA content and tumor dopa oxidase activities, while urine arylsulfatase B activities increased. Many of the nonresponders ($>50^0/_0$) developed amelanotic satellite lesions while on therapy.

## References

1  AHMANN, D. L.; HAHN, R. G., and BISEL, H. F.: A comparative study of 1-(2-chloroethyl)-3-cyclohexyl-1-nitrosourea (NSC 79037) and imidazole carboxamide (NSC 45, 388) with vincristine (NSC 67574) in the palliation of disseminated malignant melanoma. Cancer Res. 32: 2432–2434 (1972).

2  BAUM, H.; DODGSON, K. A., and SPENCER, B.: The assay of arylsulphatases A and B in human urine. Clin. chim. Acta 4: 453–455 (1958).

3  BURKE, P. J. MCCARTHY, W. H., and MILTON, G. W.: Imidazole carboxamide therapy in advanced malignant melanoma. Cancer 27: 744–752 (1971).

4  CARTER, R. D. and KREMENTZ, E. T.: Combination treatment of metastatic malignant melanoma with 1-(2-chloroethyl)-3-cyclohexyl-1-nitroso (CCNU), vincristine (VCR) and dimethyltriazeno imidazole carboxamide (DIC). Proc. Am. Ass. Cancer Res. 12: 88 (1971).

5  CARTER, S. K. and FRIEDMAN, M. A.: 5-(3,3-dimethyl-1-triazeno)-imidazole-4-carboxamide (DTIC, DIC, NSC-45388). A new antitumor agent with activity against malignant melanoma. Eur. J. Cancer 8: 85–92 (1972).

6  COHEN, S. M.; GREENSPAN, E. J.; WEINER, M. J., and KABAKOW, B.: Triple combination chemotherapy of disseminated melanoma. Cancer 29: 1489–1495 (1972).

7  DZIALOSZYNSKI, L. M.; KROLL, J. L., and FROHLICH, A.: Arylsulphatase in human tumors. Clin. chim. Acta 14: 450–456 (1966).

8  GARDERE, S.; HUSSAIN, S., and COWAN, D. H.: Treatment of metastatic malignant melanoma with a combination of 5-(3,3-dimethyl-1-triazeno)-imidazole-4-

carboxamide (NSC-45388), cyclophosphamide (NSC-26271), and vincristine (NSC-67574). Cancer Chemother. Rep. *56:* 357 361 (1972).

9   HANO, K.; AKASHI, A.; YAMAMOTO, I.; NAVURNI, S.; HORII, S., and NINOMIYA, I.: Antitumor activity of 4 (or 5)-aminoimidazole-5-(or 4)-carboxamide derivatives. Gann *56:* 417–420 (1965).

10  LOO, T. L.; LUCE, J. K.; JARDINE, J. H., and FREI, E., III: Pharmacologic studies of the antitumor agent 5-(dimethyltriazeno) imidazole-4-carboxamide. Cancer Res. *28:* 2448–2453 (1968).

11  LUCE, J. K.; TORIN, L. B., and FREI, E. III: Combination dimethyl triazeno imidazole carboxamide (NSC-45388: DTC), vincristine (NSC-67574: VCR, and 1,3 bis (2-chloroethyl)-1-nitrosourea (NSC 409962: BCNU) chemotherapy for disseminated malignant melanoma. 10th Int. Cancer Congr., Houston 1970 (abstr. 762). Houston, Tex. (Medical Arts Publishing, 1970).

12  MACDONALD, C.; WOLLNER, N.; CHAVINII, F., and ZWEIG, F.: Phase I study of imidazole carboxamide dimethyltriazeno (ICD). Proc. Am. Ass. Cancer Res. *8:* 43 (1967).

13  MORGAN, L. R.; LOLLEY, F.; MADDUX, B.; SAMUELS, M. S., and KREMENTZ, E. T.: Urine homovanillic acid and tissue dopa oxidase in patients with melanoma. Cancer *33:* 1601–1606 (1974).

14  MORGAN, L. R. and KREMENTZ, E. T.: The clinical correlation of melanin metabolites and arylsulphatase in malignant melanoma. Revue Institut Pasteur, Lyon *4:* 427–434 (1972).

15  MORGAN, L. R.; REEHLMANN, N. J.; MADDUX, B.; SAMUELS, M. S., and KREMENTZ, E. T.: Arylsulphatase and the melanin pigment cell cycle. Int. J. Biochem. *1:* 257–262 (1970).

16  MORGAN, L. R.; SAMUELS, M. S., and KREMENTZ, E. T.: Effects of dimethyltriazeno imidazole carboxamide on melanoma metabolites and enzymes. Abs. of Am. Ass. Cancer Res., S.W. Section, New Orleans 1970.

17  MORGAN, L. R.; SYLVEST, V., and WEIMORTS, D.: Oxidation of *o*-aminophenols by mouse and human melanoma dihydroxyphenylalanine oxidase and dihydroxyphenyl-alanine. Cancer Res. *27:* 2395–2407 (1967).

18  NATHANSON, L.; HORTON, J.; TAYLOR, S., and KRAUT, M.: Effectiveness of 5 (or 4)- (3-dimethyl-1-triazeno)-imidazole 4 (or 5)-carboxamide (DTIC: NSC 45, 388) in malignant melanoma. J. invest. Derm. *54:* 94–100 (1970).

19  SAVLOV, E. D.; HALL, T. C., and OBERFIELD, R. A.: Intra-arterial therapy of melanoma with dimethyl triazeno imidazole carboxamide (NSC-45388). Cancer *28:* 1161–1164 (1971).

20  WAGNER, D. G.; RAMIREZ, G.; WEISS, A. S., and HILL, G. J.: Combination I-II study of imidazole carboxamide (NSC 45, 388). Am. Soc. clin. Oncol. *51* (1971).

L. R. MORGAN, jr., MD, PhD, Department of Pharmacology, Louisiana State University Medical Center, School of Medicine, *New Orleans, LA 70112* (USA)

Pigment Cell, vol. 2, pp. 339–346 (Karger, Basel 1976)

# Influence of Tyrosine Phenol-Lyase and Phenylalanine Ammonia-Lyase on Growth of B-16 Melanoma

Gary W. Elmer, Gary G. Meadows, Christopher Linden, John DiGiovanni and John S. Holcenberg

Department of Pharmaceutical Sciences, School of Pharmacy and Division of Clinical Pharmacology, School of Medicine, University of Washington, Seattle, Wash.

## Introduction

A useful strategy in cancer chemotherapy is to exploit metabolic differences between normal and neoplastic cells. One unique feature of most malignant melanocytes is the presence of an active melanin synthesizing system in these cells. It is reasonable to expect that the tyrosine requirements for pigmented malignant melanomas may be higher than for normal cells since tyrosine is needed for both protein and melanin synthesis. A promising therapeutic approach, therefore, would be to limit the amount of tyrosine or phenylalanine (which can be converted to tyrosine in the liver) available to these neoplastic cells. Since tyrosine is an essential amino acid, this can be accomplished by dietary restrictions. Some provisional success has been achieved in animal and human malignant melanomas by feeding diets depleted in tyrosine and/or phenylalanine [4, 5, 7, 10]. A serious limitation to this therapy, however, has been the long period of time necessary to decrease serum tyrosine levels and to achieve objective remissions. Also, the unpalatable nature of the diets has made human compliance difficult [5]. An alternative therapeutic approach for depleting these amino acids that would avoid some of these difficulties is to administer an enzyme that will rapidly degrade tyrosine or phenylalanine. To be therapeutically useful, this enzyme should ideally: (1) degrade the amino acid rapidly and irreversibly under physiological conditions; (2) be easily obtained in reasonable yields and purity, and (3) have a sufficiently low Km value that it could compete with tumor enzymes for the low substrate concentrations found in serum. With these considerations in mind, two microbial enzymes, tyrosine phenol-lyase and phenylalanine ammonia-lyase, were selected for study.

Tyrosine phenol-lyase catalyzes the conversion of L-tyrosine to phenol, pyruvate, and ammonia. The enzyme has been described from *Erwinia herbicola* [8] and *Escherichia intermedia* [9]. KUMAGAI *et al.* [8] have reported that the crystalline enzyme from *Erwinia herbicola* has a specific activity of 0.94 IU/mg and a Km of 0.28 mM. Phenylalanine ammonia-lyase has been purified from *Rhodotorula glutinis* by HODGINS [6]. The purified enzyme from this source had a specific activity of 1.07 and a Km of 0.25 mM. The enzyme catalyzes the conversion of L-phenylalanine to L-cinnamate and ammonia. ABELL *et al.* [2] have reported that administration of phenylalanine ammonia-lyase rapidly depletes serum tyrosine and phenylalanine in normal mice. They achieved inhibition of growth of both murine and human leukemic lymphocytes *in vitro* [2] and inhibition of growth of murine L-5178Y lymphoblastic leukemia *in vivo* [1].

It has been reported that the benign murine lactate dehydrogenase (LDH) elevating virus has a profound effect in prolonging clearance of EC-2 asparaginase [15] and glutaminase asparaginase GA:1.2 in mice [16]. Therefore, the effect of this LDH virus on the plasma half-life of phenylalanine ammonia-lyase and tyrosine phenol-lyase was determined.

## Materials and Methods

Enzymes: Purification of phenylalanine ammonia-lyase and tyrosine phenol-lyase will be described elsewhere. Phenylalanine ammonia-lyase from *Rhodotorula glutinis* was purchased from PL Biochemicals, Inc., Milwaukee, Wisc., and partially purified to a specific activity of 1.0 IU/mg. Tyrosine phenol-lyase was purified from *Erwinia herbicola* to a specific activity of 1.25 IU/mg. A unit of enzyme activity is defined as the amount of enzyme catalyzing the formation of 1 $\mu$mol of pyruvate (tyrosine phenol-lyase) or L-cinnamate (phenylalanine ammonia-lyase) per minute. The plasma levels of lactate dehydrogenase, for normal and LDH virus-infected mice, were determined by the method of BERGMEYER *et al.* [3] and the activity reported as Wroblewski units [17].

Mice employed: $BDF_1$ female mice weighing from 18 to 21 g were obtained from Charles River Laboratories, Willmington, Mass. Mice were given Purina Chow and water *ad libitum* and were acclimatized at least 7 days prior to experimentation. Some mice were purposefully infected with the LDH virus by injecting i.p. a 0.1 ml dose of a 1:10 dilution of serum from LDH virus-infected mice.

Influence of tyrosine phenol-lyase on tyrosine and phenylalanine plasma levels: The mice in this experiment were purposefully infected with the LDH virus 7 days prior to enzyme administration. Blood samples were collected from the tail vein prior to and at 7 and 26 h after injection of enzyme. The samples were prepared for amino acid analysis by the following procedure developed by SPACKMAN [personal communication]. The plasma from groups of three mice was pooled and transferred into tared vials containing 15% sulfosalicylic acid and the weight of plasma was determined. The samples were centrifuged and the resulting pellet washed three times with cold 5% sulfosalicylic acid. The supernate and washings were pooled, adjusted to pH 2.6 with NaOH and diluted to a final volume of 2.5 ml with 0.2 N sodium citrate buffer pH 2.6. Tyrosine and phenylalanine levels were determined on a JEOL model JLC-5AH amino acid analyzer.

Enzyme half-life determination: Blood samples were removed by orbital bleeding [11] into pre-chilled heparinized tubes. Each sample was centrifuged at 4 °C and the plasma levels of tyrosine phenol-lyase and phenylalanine ammonia-lyase determined.

Tumor implantation and measurements: B-16 melanoma was obtained through the courtesy of Dr. V. RILEY. Transplantation and tumor volume measurements were performed as described by RILEY et al. [16]. Tumor diameters were measured with calipers.

## Results and Discussion

The influence of tyrosine phenol-lyase administration on plasma tyrosine and phenylalanine levels is shown in table I. A single dose of 160 IU/kg significantly reduced plasma tyrosine levels at 7 h after injection. At 26 h after injection, tyrosine levels had returned to approximately nor-

Table I. Plasma tyrosine and phenylalanine levels after administration of tyrosine phenol-lyase

| Treatment | Time, hours after treatment | Tyrosine, nM/ml | | Phenylalanine, nM/ml | |
|---|---|---|---|---|---|
| | | group 1 | group 2 | group 1 | group 2 |
| 0.9% NaCl solution | 0 | 64 | 92 | 60 | 74 |
| | 7 | 85 | 60 | 81 | 73 |
| Tyrosine phenol-lyase | 0 | 87 | 129 | 81 | 113 |
| | 7 | 34 | 32 | 73 | 84 |
| | 26 | 67 | 75 | 101 | 91 |

A single injection of tyrosine phenol-lyase (160 IU/kg) was given to 2 groups of 3 mice. Two groups of 3 additional mice receiving 0.9% NaCl solution served as controls. All mice were bled at the indicated times.

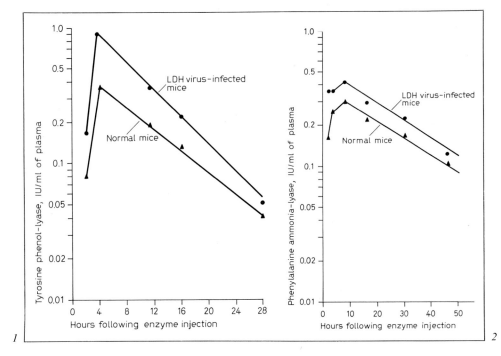

*Fig. 1.* Influence of the LDH virus on plasma clearance of tyrosine phenol-lyase. A group of mice was injected with the LDH virus 4 days prior to injection of enzyme. Mice not injected with the virus were kept isolated from the infected group. At day zero, 240 IU/kg of partially purified tyrosine phenol-lyase (specific activity = 0.63) was injected i.p. in all mice. At the indicated times, 3 mice from each group were bled, and the pooled plasma enzyme levels determined.

*Fig. 2.* Influence of the LDH virus on plasma clearance of phenylalanine ammonia-lyase. A group of mice was injected with the LDH virus 4 days prior to injection of enzyme. Non-infected mice were kept isolated from the infected group. At day zero, 60 IU/kg of phenylalanine ammonia-lyase was injected i.p. in all mice. At the indicated times, 3 mice from each group were bled, and the pooled plasma enzyme levels determined.

mal. The enzyme had a negligible effect on reducing phenylalanine. This is expected because the enzyme has no activity *in vitro* on this amino acid [8].

Data shown in figures 1 and 2 demonstrate that infection with the LDH virus has no significant influence on clearance of phenylalanine ammonia-lyase and tyrosine phenol-lyase. Infection was confirmed in mice

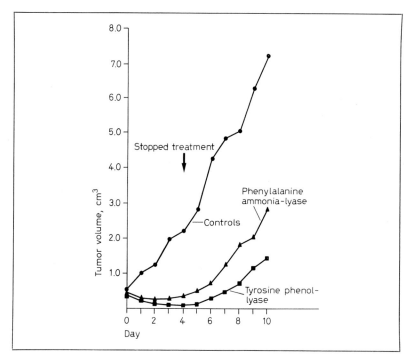

*Fig. 3.* Influence of tyrosine phenol-lyase and phenylalanine ammonia-lyase on growth of B-16 melanoma. Mice were treated starting at day zero with 100 IU/kg of tyrosine phenol-lyase (4 mice) or phenylalanine ammonia-lyase (9 mice) every 12 h for a total of 8 doses. Control mice (10 mice) were tumor-bearing mice which were similarly injected with a 0.9% NaCl solution. The tumor volumes of the treated mice were significantly different (p<0.005) from the control mice from day 2 through day 9.

injected with the virus by measuring plasma lactate dehydrogenase several days after virus administration. In the presence of the virus, plasma lactate dehydrogenase levels are substantially elevated [13]. Plasma from randomly selected normal mice gave lactate dehydrogenase values of $508 \pm 101$ U, while plasma from mice previously injected with the virus gave values of $4{,}208 \pm 1{,}310$ U. The lack of influence of the virus is in marked contrast to results reported for asparaginase EC-2 [15] and glutaminase asparaginase GA: 1.2 [16]. In these studies, mice infected with the virus showed a 5- to 10-fold increase in plasma half-life values over normal mice. The plasma half-life values calculated from data in figures 1 and 2 are approximately 6–7 h for tyrosine phenol-lyase, and about 24 h for phenylalanine ammonia-lyase.

The LDH virus has been reported to cause immunologic and other alterations in the host, in addition to its ability to prolong the clearance time of certain enzymes [14]. RILEY [12] has pointed out that this virus can be an unwanted variable when working with many transplantable mouse tumors since these tumors are often contaminated with the virus. Although the virus apparently has no influence on clearance of tyrosine phenol-lyase and phenylalanine ammonia-lyase, all tumor-bearing mice were purposefully infected with the virus 4 days prior to treatment in order to avoid these variabilities. The influence of short-term administration of tyrosine phenol-lyase and phenylalanine ammonia-lyase on the growth of transplanted B-16 melanoma is demonstrated in figure 3. Results show that both enzymes have rapid and potent activity. Tumor volumes in treated mice were significantly smaller than in untreated mice from day 2 to day 9 (p <0.005). Treatment was stopped after 4 days because of exhaustion of enzyme supply. T/C values calculated at this time were 0.03 for tyrosine phenol-lyase and 0.17 for phenylalanine ammonia-lyase. No toxic signs were noted in the treated mice. Weight changes essentially paralleled the growth or shrinkage of the tumors; the maximum weight decrease observed was 1.6 g after 3 days of treatment in the tyrosine phenol-lyase group.

Dietary studies in which phenylalanine- and tyrosine-depleted diets were fed have been shown to be beneficial in the treatment of malignant melanoma [4, 5, 7, 10]. In these studies, 4–6 weeks of dietary treatment was necessary to appreciably lower plasma levels of the two amino acids. Results of this investigation demonstrate that tyrosine phenol-lyase rapidly reduces plasma tyrosine when injected (160 IU/kg) into normal mice. Phenylalanine ammonia-lyase has previously been shown to reduce plasma phenylalanine and tyrosine in mice [2]. Considering the half-life values of 6–7 h for tyrosine phenol-lyase and 24 h for phenylalanine ammonia-lyase, a dosage schedule of 100 IU/kg every 12 h presumably kept tyrosine or phenylalanine levels in the experimental mice reduced throughout the treatment period. Both enzymes have relatively rapid and potent activity against B-16 melanoma with this dosage regimen. No attempt was made to restrict dietary intake of the amino acids in these experiments. A more thorough evaluation of the therapeutic potential of these enzymes will be offered by studies involving the concurrent restriction of dietary intake of tyrosine and phenylalanine, and long-term administration of the enzymes.

## Summary

In order to evaluate the effect of depleting serum tyrosine and phenylalanine levels on malignant melanoma, two enzymes that degrade these amino acids were purified and evaluated for activity in $BDF_1$ mice. The serum half-life values of tyrosine phenol-lyase and phenylalanine ammonia-lyase were found to be 6–7 and 24 h, respectively. Unlike results reported with glutaminase and asparaginase preparations, the lactate dehydrogenase-elevating virus (LDH virus) had no significant influence on serum clearance of phenylalanine ammonia-lyase and tyrosine phenol-lyase. Both enzymes showed potent activity against B-16 melanoma. T/C values calculated from tumor volume data at four days of treatment were 0.03 for tyrosine phenol-lyase and 0.17 for phenylalanine ammonia-lyase.

## References

1 ABELL, C. W.; HODGINS, D. S., and STITH, W. J.: An *in vivo* evaluation of the chemotherapeutic potency of phenylalanine ammonia lyase. Cancer Res. *33:* 2529–2532 (1973).

2 ABELL, C. W.; STITH, W. J., and HODGINS, D. S.: The effects of phenylalanine ammonia-lyase on leukemic lymphocytes *in vitro*. Cancer Res. *32:* 285–290 (1972).

3 BERGMEYER, H.-U.; BERNT, E., and HESS, B.: Lactic dehydrogenase; in BERGMEYER Methods of enzymatic analysis, pp. 736–740 (Academic Press, New York 1965).

4 DEMOPOULOS, H. B.: Effect of low phenylalanine-tyrosine diets on S-91 mouse melanomas, J. natn. Cancer Inst. *37:* 185–190 (1966).

5 DEMOPOULOS, H. B.: Effects of reducing the phenylalanine-tyrosine intake of patients with advanced malignant melanoma. Cancer *19:* 657–664 (1966).

6 HODGINS, D. S.: Yeast phenylalanine ammonia-lyase. Purification and identification of catalytically essential dehydroalanine. J. biol. Chem. *246:* 2977–2985 (1971).

7 JENSEN, O. A.; EGEBERG, J., and EDMUND, J.: The effect of a phenylalanine-tyrosine low diet on the growth and morphology of transplantable malignant melanomas of the Syrian golden hamster *(Mesocricetus auratus)*. Acta path. microbiol. scand. A *81:* 559–658 (1973).

8 KUMAGAI, H.; KASHIMA, N.; TORII, H.; YAMADA, H.; ENEI, H., and OKUMURA, S.: Purification, crystallization, and properties of tyrosine phenol lyase from *Erwinia herbicola*. Agric. Biol. Chem. *36:* 472–482 (1972).

9 KUMAGAI, H.; YAMADA, H.; MATSUI, H.; OHKISHI, H., and OGATA, K.: Tyrosine

phenol lyase. I. Purification, crystallization, and properties. J. biol. Chem. *245:* 1767–1772 (1970).

10 Lorincz, A. B.; Kuttner, R. E., and Brandt, M. B.: Tumor response to phenylalanine-tyrosine limited diets. J. Am. diet. Ass. *54:* 198–205 (1969).

11 Riley, V.: Adaptation of orbital bleeding technique to rapid serial blood studies. Proc. Soc. exp. Biol. Med. *104:* 751–754 (1970).

12 Riley, V.: Biological contaminants and scientific misinterpretations. Cancer Res. *34:* 1752–1754 (1974).

13 Riley, V.: Virus-tumor synergism. Science *134:* 666–668 (1961).

14 Riley, V.: Erroneous interpretation of valid experimental observations through interference by the LDH-virus. J. natn. Cancer Inst. *52:* 1673–1677 (1974).

15 Riley, V.: Lactate dehydrogenase in the normal and malignant state in mice and the influence of a benign enzyme-elevating virus; in Busch Methods in cancer research, vol. 4, pp. 493–618 (Academic Press, New York 1968).

16 Riley, V.; Spackman, D.; Fitzmaurice, M. A.; Roberts, J.; Holcenberg, J. S., and Dolowy, W. C.: Therapeutic properties of a new glutaminase-asparaginase preparation and the influence of the lactate dehydrogenase-elevating virus. Cancer Res. *34:* 429–438 (1974).

17 Wroblewski, F. and Due, J. S. La: Lactic dehydrogenase activity in blood. Proc. Soc. exp. Biol. Med. *90:* 210–213 (1955).

Dr. Gary W. Elmer, Department of Pharmaceutical Sciences, School of Pharmacy, University of Washington, *Seattle, WA 98195* (USA)

Pigment Cell, vol. 2, pp. 347–364 (Karger, Basel 1976)

# Manipulation of Free Radicals in Pigmented Melanomas

*Effects on Metabolism and Growth*

HARRY B. DEMOPOULOS, RICHARD G. POSER, W. BARRIE G. JONES, BEVERLY B. LAVIETES, PETER S. COLEMAN and MYRON L. SELIGMAN

Tumor Metabolism Unit, Division II, New York University Cancer Research Center, New York, N.Y.

## Introduction

The *in vivo* growth of pigmented S-91 and human melanomas has been inhibited with a variety of regimens [8, 17, 18]. Some of these were specifically designed to interfere with a vital bioenergetic pathway that depends on tyrosinase [8, 17]. This pathway has been shown to account for approximately one half of the ATP generated by melanotic S-91 tumors [22].

Some antioxidants and analogues of hydroquinones are effective inhibitors of active melanin synthesis, and sometimes of melanocyte growth [3, 5, 23]. A mechanism of action of these inhibitors against pigmented melanoma *in vivo* has not been clearly demonstrated although several have been proposed [5, 6, 23]. Some antioxidants and hydroquinone analogues inhibit tyrosinase activity in *other* melanocyte populations [5]. This suggests that tyrosinase inhibition might be one of the mechanisms of action of these agents against melanotic S-91 melanomas.

D-Penicillamine ($\beta,\beta'$-dimethylcysteine) has been used to inhibit S-91 melanoma growth *in vivo*, because it chelates copper and tyrosinase is copper-dependent [17]. However, D-penicillamine is also an antioxidant or radical scavenger which could be important when it is used in combination with other agents termed antioxidants [6].

The structural variety of the antioxidants which affect melanomas rules out an inhibitory effect on tyrosinase based on substrate analogy. These so-called 'antioxidants' are more accurately termed 'radical modulating agents'. All antioxidants function through a radical configuration.

However, depending on the properties and relative redox potentials of the other biomolecules in the immediate environment of the 'antioxidant', there may be radical initiation and/or chain reaction promotion. Ascorbic acid is a classical example of an antioxidant which can actually induce pathologic free radical reactions in fatty acids, as found in membrane phospholipids [6, 14].

In the present work, a broad spectrum of radical modulating agents, including D-penicillamine, were used to treat S-91 melanoma-bearing mice. Single and combination regimens were employed, and three major parameters were investigated: growth *in vivo*, tyrosinase activity, and free radical content. Electron paramagnetic resonance (e.p.r.) spectroscopy was used to study the S-91 melanomas' free radicals. These e.p.r. signals have been described in previous work [9, 12]. An amelanotic mouse melanoma line was used as one type of control. This tumor lacks measurable tyrosinase activity [16], and would therefore not have a tyrosinase-dependent bioenergetic pathway. In addition, a non-melanoma mouse tumor line, the sarcoma-180, was used as a further control. Preliminary studies of L-PAM were also made.

## Materials and Methods

### Tumor Source

S-91 melanomas, originally obtained from Dr. MARK WOODS (National Cancer Institute, NIH, Bethesda Md.) were transplanted into male DBA/2 mice, weighing about 10 g each. Successive transplantation at frequent intervals has maintained this tumor uniformly, and heavily pigmented. This line of S-91 was used for the present studies. It was generally a rapidly growing line of the S-91 tumor, killing the host in six weeks, rather than the usual twelve weeks. Viable, heavily pigmented tumor bits, 2 mm³, were implanted subcutaneously in the posterior axillary fold with the use of an 18-gauge hypodermic needle and needle stylet, used in trochar fashion. The mice for the present study were obtained from the Roscoe B. Jackson Memorial laboratories in Bar Habor, Maine.

Amelanotic B-16 melanomas were obtained from Dr. ALFRED KOPF, of the Department of Dermatology, N.Y.U. Medical Center, N.Y., N.Y. The palest portions were selectively transplanted through four generations, by which time an almost pure amelanotic line was established. The host-killing time for this tumor was four weeks; C-57/Bl male mice, from the Jackson Laboratories, were transplanted as above, in the posterior axillary fold. The mice weighed 20 g at this time.

Sarcoma-180 obtained from the Roscoe B. Jackson Laboratories, Bar Harbor, Maine, was maintained in BALB/c male mice as described above. The host-killing time was 2–3 weeks.

*Chemicals*

The chemicals used were obtained from the following sources: $\beta,\beta'$-dimethyl cysteine (D-penicillamine) from Calbiochem, San Diego, Calif.; $N,N'$-diphenyl-par-aphenylenediamine (DPPD) from Polysciences, Inc. Rydal, Pa.; p-ethoxy-phenol (EOP) from Eastman Organic Chemicals, Rochester, N.Y.; 3,3',4',5,7-pentahy-droxyflavone (Quercitin) from K&K Laboratories, Inc. Plainview, N.Y.; dihydrous 2',3,4',5,7-pentahydroxyflavone (Morin Dihydrate) from Aldrich Chemical Co., Mil-waukee, Wisc.; p-(benzyloxy) phenol (MBQ) from Eastman Organic Chemicals, Rochester, N.Y.; p-hydroxypropiophenone (PHP) from Aldrich Chemical Co., Inc., Milwaukee, Wisc.; dimethyl sulfoxide (DMSO) from Malinckrodt Chemical Works, St. Louis, Mo.

*Treatment Regimens*

Treatment against the S-91 tumors was begun either at one or three weeks af-ter transplantation to determine whether the effects of the drugs might differ with the growth rate of the tumor. Treatment of the B-16 and sarcoma-180-bearing mice was begun one week after transplantation since these tumors grow at 3 times the rate of the S-91 melanoma.

In each series involving the 3-week-old tumors, the mice were divided into ex-perimental groups such that the initial average tumor size and tumor ranges were approximately equal for each group. This method of equalization is necessary in this type of study because equal inocula of tumor transplanted into genetically identical hosts at the same time may grow to varying sizes [17].

In the groups where treatment was initiated one week post-transplantation, the equalization included mice whose tumors were not yet palpable. The latter com-prised approximately 20% of each group. The effective transplantation rate for S-91 tumors in these studies was 95%.

The treatment regimens were as follows. Tumor-bearing mice were divided into the groups indicated in table I. Solutions were prepared just before use and all injections were subcutaneous, far from the tumor site. The chemicals and their dose are detailed in table I. Injections were administered daily, 5 days/week, weekends skipped, for 2 weeks. Injection volumes were 0.1 ml for agents in DMSO. D-Penicil-lamine was in $H_2O$, with an injection volume of 0.5 ml. In the combination drug treatments, the following precautions were taken: the two different injections were given at least 3 h apart, at different sites, and far from the tumor, in order to elimi-nate the possibility of local interaction.

The volumes of the tumors were determined twice each week. The greatest di-ameter of the tumor was measured with skin calipers. Volume was calculated by the formula $V = 0.523 (d)^3$, where d is diameter in centimeters. As animals died in the course of the experiments, their tumor sizes and weights were recorded on the day of discovery, and excluded from subsequent calculations. The tumor sizes were aver-aged, and significant differences between the groups were determined by Student's *t*-test.

The toxicity of the drugs employed was evaluated in these studies by compar-ing weights of treated and untreated mice. Weights were recorded twice each week. Further, the conditions of the animals' coats, the amount of activity (especially when being handled for the injections every day), and the appearance of ulcerations

*Table I.* Treatment groups (numbers of mice per group)

| Chemical[1] | S-91 tumors[2] | | Sarcoma-180 | B-16 amelanotic |
|---|---|---|---|---|
| | 1-week | 3-week | | |
| EOP | 44 | 20 | | 34 |
| DPPD | 35 | 20 | | 33 |
| MBQ | | 20 | 19 | |
| PHP | | 20 | 19 | |
| Q | 24 | | | |
| MDH | 24 | | | |
| DMSO | 49 | 20 | 20 | 33 |
| EOP+PA | 24 | | | |
| DPPD+PA | 24 | | | |
| DPPD+H₂O | 25 | | | |

1 EOP=$p$-ethoxy phenol, 50 mg/kg; DPPD=diphenylparaphenylenediamine, 200 mg/kg; MBQ=$p$-(benzyloxy)-phenol, 100 mg/kg; PHP=$p$-hydroxypropiophone, 100 mg/kg; Q=3,3′,4′,5,7-pentahydroxyflavone (quercitin), 100 mg/kg; MDH= dihydrous 2′,3,4′,5,7-pentahydroxyflavone (morin dihydrate), 100 mg/kg; DMSO= dimethylsulfoxide, pure, 0.1 ml; PA=$\beta$-$\beta'$-dimethylcysteine (D-penicillamine), 500 mg/kg. All chemicals, except PA, dissolved in pure DMSO. Injection volume was 0.1 ml. PA in H₂O, 0.5 ml volume, pH adjusted to 7.0 with 0.1 N HCl.
2 Time post-transplantation is indicated. Regimens initiated at these times.

or other skin lesions locally at the injection sites were noted. Lethality studies were not conducted with these regimens since prior studies have indicated the range of doses for most of these agents [3].

Portions of skin from treated and untreated DBA mice were processed for histologic examination. The sections were stained with hematoxylin-eosin and with Fontana stains, the latter to outline the melanocytes in the skin.

*Tyrosinase Assay*

At the conclusion of treatment, 5 mice with representative tumor sizes were selected from each experimental group. These mice were sacrificed by cervical dislocation. The excised tumor tissue was washed in cold 0.25 M sucrose, and the necrotic portions separated from the viable areas. The tumor tissue was pooled for each group and weighed. 2 ml of 0.25 M sucrose was added for each gram wet weight of tumor and the tissue homogenized in a Potter-Elvejhem homogenizer for 3 min (12 strokes/min) at 0–5 °C. The homogenate was spun at 2,000 $g$ for 5 min at 0 °C in a Sorvall Model RC-3 centrifuge with an SS-34 angle rotor. The supernate, a cleared cytoplasmic fraction, was used in the manometric assay previously described [8]. Each flask contained L-tyrosine, 1.5 mg/ml; L-3,4-dihydroxyphenylalanine, 0.15 mg/ml; and cleared homogenate, 0.5 ml. The other components of the incubating medium, which totalled 2 ml, were identical to those used for succinoxidase assays [27]. Flasks were incubated 20 min. Longer runs result in product feedback inhibition when tyrosine is the substrate. The activity was normalized to protein content, determined by the method of LOWRY *et al.* [19]. Mice sacrificed for tyrosinase assays received their daily scheduled injection(s) 1 h before sacrifice, to maximize blood and tissue levels of drug. Assays were not done on MBQ and PHP groups, B-16 or S-180 groups.

### Electron Paramagnetic Resonance Spectroscopy

Undiluted, cytoplasmic homogenates of treated and untreated S-91 melanoma were used for e.p.r. spectroscopy. The effects of the various regimens on the 2 signals in the S-91 tumor were determined as previously described [9].

The amplitude of the e.p.r. signals was normalized readily because the homogenates were prepared by standardized procedures. The e.p.r. cell holds a fixed amount of material and therefore variation in the amplitude of the signals, which is an indirect measure of *relative* concentrations of free radicals in the samples, reflected valid differences in the treated and non-treated melanomas.

In addition to determining the relative radical contents of the tumors, e.p.r. spectroscopy was employed to study some of the agents used in the study, since these 'radical modulating agents' generally assume a radical configuration in the presence of other redox substances. All of the chemicals listed in table I were studied by e.p.r. using freshly prepared solutions as they were employed in the animal studies.

Solutions of DPPD were found to display a multiline spectrum, in DMSO, this being a free radical intermediate in the oxidation of DPPD. DMSO is a pro-oxidant and can induce the oxidation of substances like DPPD and ascorbic acid. DMSO increases the spin concentration of some radicals, permitting a more detailed study. The other agents did not display any signal in DMSO. In addition, D-penicillamine was used against solutions of DPPD to determine the effects on the DPPD free radical, with direct additions being made just before taking a spectrum, at concentrations of 1 and 10 mg/ml of the DPPD solutions. Timed spectra were recorded.

D-Penicillamine, as the chromatographically pure base, was used at varying concentrations, to confirm its effects on the melanoma signals in untreated S-91 tumors, as previously described. This drug was used in concentrations of 1 and 10 mg/ml of cytoplasmic homogenate, added just before placing the aqueous sample cell in the e.p.r. spectrometer. Spectra were taken at timed intervals following the addition, with the e.p.r. parameters set so as to detect the 2 melanoma signals previously described [9, 12], the broad singlet and the narrower doublet.

The pH of the various solutions to which D-penicillamine were added was measured before and after the addition, in a Beckman Expanded Scale meter.

A final e.p.r. study involved adding DMSO to cytoplasmic S-91 homogenate, in one-to-one ratios, by volume, in order to examine the doublet. Previous work had shown that DMSO increased the spin concentration of the species that was responsible for the doublet in S-91 homogenates. The modulation amplitude was decreased to 0.08 G, scan range to 5 G, microwave power to 5 mW, with the receiver gain at $3.3 \times 10^6$. This was done to try to split the doublet into a pair of triplets in order to confirm the identity of the doublet as the ascorbyl radical.

*Table II.* Effects of EOP and DPPD single regimens on S-91 melanoma growth[1] starting one week post-transplantation

| Measurement period[2] | Solvent control[3] | EOP | DPPD |
|---|---|---|---|
| I | 0.22±0.0009 (7) | 0.04±0.0002 (24) | 0.12±0.0005 (15) |
| II | 0.98±0.0012 (4) | 0.31±0.0004 (11) | 0.45±0.0006 (7) |
| III | 3.55±0.0029 (2) | 1.16±0.0011 (8) | 1.74±0.0013 (3) |
| | | $p<0.01 - <0.005$ | $p<0.10 - <0.05$ |

1 Injections started one week post-transplantation. All mice in this study were transplanted at the same time from a common pool of donor fragments. 24 mice in control, 44 in EOP, and 35 in DPPD group. EOP is *p*-ethoxy phenol. DPPD is diphenyl paraphenylenediamine.

2 Periods of measurement were 3 days apart. The first one was taken seven days after the start of treatment. Total treatment time shown was two weeks.

3 Average tumor volumes and standard errors of the means are in milliliters. Mice without palpable tumors in parentheses.

The values of significance, p, were derived by comparing EOP and DPPD to DMSO controls separately.

## Results

### In vivo *Growth Studies*

The positive inhibition data are shown in table II and figure 1. Single regimens of EOP, DPPD, PHP, and MBQ significantly inhibited growth of pigmented S-91 melanoma.

The precise volumes, and the statistical evaluation of the differences are given in table II. The general degree of inhibition was approximately 50%. The time of initiation of treatment did not influence the efficacy of EOP, or DPPD. These two drugs were equally effective against 3- and 1-week-old tumors.

The PHP and MBQ were used only against 3 week-old tumors. MBQ was constantly superior to PHP, while EOP was approximately equal to MBQ in its inhibitory activity. This data, however, must also be considered in light of the toxic effects of these drugs. MBQ was markedly toxic against DBA and BALB/c mice; 60% of the mice with or without tumors died after 10 days of treatment with MBQ. The mice were young at the time of starting the regimens, and all groups, except those treated with MBQ, gained somatic weight.

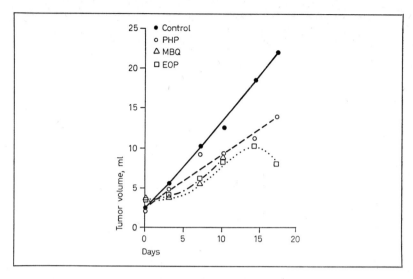

*Fig. 1.* The volumes of pigmented S-91 tumors, treated and untreated, starting *three* weeks after transplantation. The black solid circles are the solvent controls, receiving DMSO. Each point represents the averages of all the tumors in that group. The standard error of all the means for the points displayed did not exceed ± 0.004 in any case. The MBQ curve is not shown beyond 10 days because its high toxicity led to a loss of too many mice, resulting in a sample size that was too small to determine significance.

Combining EOP with D-penicillamine, and DPPD with D-penicillamine, negated the inhibitory properties of EOP and DPPD on S-91 melanoma growth *in vivo*. Quercitin, and Morin dihydrate, had no effect on the growth of S-91 tumors.

Single regimen treatment with EOP or DPPD had no effect on growth of amelanotic B-16 melanomas or sarcoma 180. Since the combination regimens had no effect on S-91 tumors, they were not tested against the B-16 melanomas or S-180 tumors.

### Tyrosinase Activity

Tyrosinase activity was markedly decreased in the tumor from the DPPD and EOP treatment groups. The results are shown in figure 2. Tyrosinase activity in tumors from the combination regimens was not affected. The data in figure 2 is expressed as oxygen consumption per 0.5 ml of

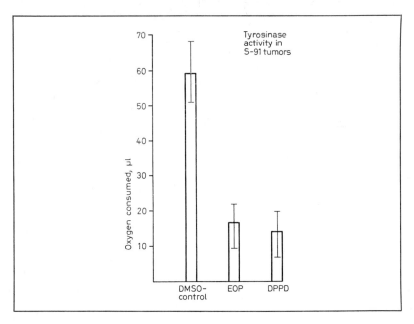

*Fig. 2.* The microliters of oxygen consumed by tumor preparations, with L-ty-rosine as substrate, *after* subtracting endogenous respiration and autoxidation con-trol vessels are shown. The bars represent the average oxygen consumption, and the range of values is shown by the single vertical line in each bar. Each run was done with triplicate vessels, using material from 5 tumors for a run. The data shown is from mice carrying 3-week-old tumors at the start of treatment.

cytoplasmic homogenate, normalized to protein content. The results were similar, regardless of the age of the tumor at the time of initiating treat-ment.

### Electron Paramagnetic Resonance Spectroscopy

In the S-91 tumor preparations that showed inhibition by EOP, DPPD, PHP, and MBQ, the melanin and doublet signals were diminished by 80–100%. The regimens with no effect on tumor growth had no signif-icant effect on e.p.r. signals. Figures are not presented for each drug; the results are analogous to the D-penicillamine figures shown below (fig. 3–6).

The effects of D-penicillamine on free radicals in melanoma homo-

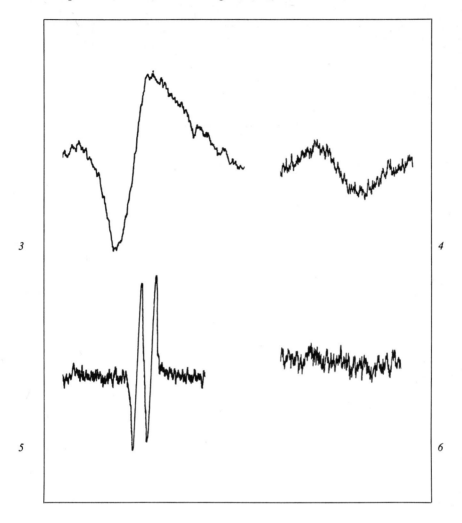

*Fig. 3.* The broad e.p.r. signal, 4.5 gauss wide, attributable to 'semiquinones that are trapped within the melanin polymer'. No penicillamine.

*Fig. 4.* The amplitude of the broad signal is decreased 6 min after the addition of 10 mg of D-penicillamine per ml of homogenate. The instrument parameters are identical to those in figure 3. Non-specific decay of the signal is ruled out by timed controls that are not shown here.

*Fig. 5.* The narrow, doublet signal, 1.7 gauss wide, also found in S-91 melanoma homogenates, is shown without D-penicillamine.

*Fig. 6.* Addition of 10 mg/ml D-penicillamine to homogenate results in complete eradication of the doublet after 6 min. Power saturation, and non-specific decay were ruled out by control runs not shown here.

genates *in vitro,* were striking and rapidly induced. Within 6 min after addition of this drug, the narrow doublet signal disappeared, and the broad melanin line was diminished approximately 80%. Figures 3, 4, 5, and 6 show results with 10 mg/ml concentration of D-penicillamine. The effects of the lower dose, 1 mg/ml, were similar but took 15 min to become evident.

D-Penicillamine completely obliterated the DPPD free radical signal within the same time period. This data is not shown. The pH of the solutions was not affected by the addition of D-penicillamine.

The addition of DMSO to control S-91 homogenate permitted splitting of the doublet into the characteristic pair of triplets with relative line intensities of (1; 2; 1) (1; 2; 1). This supports the identity of the S-91 doublet as an ascorbyl radical, with matching of splitting, line numbers, and G-values.

### Evaluation of Toxicity of Regimens

Except for those receiving MBQ, the drug-treated groups gained as much somatic weight as the non-treated tumor-bearing mice. The mice used in all of the studies were young and showed weight gains of approximately 8 g/mouse/2 weeks.

The mice in all the groups except MBQ, displayed no differences in coat characteristics, activity, or injection site lesions. The drugs did not produce severe lesions locally at the doses employed. Occasional small ulcerations did appear randomly among the various treatment groups, but these did not correlate with the observed inhibition of tumor growth. The ineffective agents and the combination regimens produced as many of these small ulcerations as the effective, single regimens. These ulcers were probably due to the animal scratching at the site rather than an inherent dermal necrotogenic effect of the drugs.

Autopsies were performed routinely on all mice. Those treated with Quercitin and Morin dihydrate showed large amounts of pale yellow precipitate at the injection sites, most likely representing an inability on the part of the subcutaneous tissue and blood to absorb and transport these 2 drugs.

At no time during treatment did the mice exhibit any loss of pigment from the integument or the retinae. Histologic examination of the DBA skin from treated groups failed to reveal evidence of melanocyte destruction. The melanocytes in the treated and untreated DBA skins appeared similar in terms of dendritic processes and pigment content.

*Discussion*

The present studies show that radical modulating agents can selectively inhibit growth of pigmented melanoma *in vivo*. They depressed the melanoma-free radical signals; moreover, the inhibitory effects were eliminated by another radical scavenging agent, D-penicillamine, when it was used concurrently with EOP and DPPD. There were no discernible effects on the growth of amelanotic B-16 melanomas, or sarcoma 180 tumors by these substances. Except for MBQ, minimal toxicity was evident with these regimens. The multiple inhibitory effects on growth *in vivo*, tyrosinase activity, and relative spin concentrations of two indicator-free radicals suggest a correlated adverse effect on bioenergetic pathways and radical-mediated reactions.

The effective agents, EOP, DPPD, PHP, and MBQ, have different structures and, therefore, could not have exerted their anti-tyrosinase effects by substrate analogy to tyrosine or 3,4-dopa. The inhibitors are most appropriately termed 'radical-modulating agents', meaning they can inhibit, or accelerate, radical reactions. As antioxidants, they quench radical species and reactions, and this may indeed be one of the possible ways that these substances selectively inhibited the S-91 tumors. The tyrosinase-dependent segment of respiration in these tumors is thought to have radical intermediates, such as dopa semiquinones [9, 12]. Eliminating them could be detrimental and could possibly explain all of the selective effects. When tyrosinase is functioning optimally, there may be few radical semiquinones, as these are but fleeting intermediates. Other radical species that are thought to accompany tyrosinase activity include the superoxide radical, $\cdot O_2^-$. This is probably produced during the hydroxylation of tyrosine to 3,4-dopa, as is usual in all biologic hydroxylations [28]. The superoxide radical is dysmutated by a specific enzyme superoxide dysmutase, into $H_2O_2$, and this in turn is acted upon by catalase or substances with peroxidase activity. The chemicals employed may become free radicals themselves as they are undergoing oxidation as classical antioxidants, e.g. DPPD. In such a configuration they interact with other free radicals, by radical-radical termination reactions. A free radical is a moiety which has an unpaired electron in an outer orbital. Two free radicals of diverse chemical nature may therefore establish a new, covalent, two-electron bond, ending their free radical state, and forming a relatively stable product.

The chemicals used are preferentially soluble in non-polar environments and will, for example, seek out the hydrophobic zones of membranes, and other macromolecular complexes that constitute the non-polar regions in a living cell. If these radical-modulating agents (antioxidants) are converted into free radicals while they are in cell membranes or within macromolecular hydrophobic aggregates, a series of damaging radical chain reactions may occur among the lipid and protein constituents of the various membranes and non-polar structures [7, 10, 25].

Antioxidants, or radical modulators, vary in the ease with which they become free radicals, as a function of their structure and the chemical environment. The presence of metals, such as copper and iron, or other free radicals, may initiate a radical configuration in the antioxidant. These aspects of radical modulating agents offer possible mechanisms of action of S-91 inhibitors in the present study.

Radical modulating agent, X, in the presence of endogenous radicals, Y·, which include oxygen radicals, may undergo the following general reaction:

$$X + Y \cdot \rightarrow X \cdot + Y,$$

with the transfer of the lone electron (·). In pigmented melanomas there are several endogenous free radicals: (1) the physico-chemical structure responsible for the melanin signal; (2) ascorbyl; (3) intermediates in prostaglandin synthesis [15], and (4) $\cdot O_2^-$ arising from hydroxylation reactions, and flavin enzymes [28]. Of these, only the first is exclusive to pigmented S-91 melanomas. Ascorbyl radicals are present or can be made to appear in a variety of tissues. Prostaglandin intermediates and $\cdot O_2^-$ are likewise not distinctive. Furthermore, the melanin radical is the only one present in a relatively high steady state concentration. The others (ascorbyl, prostaglandin intermediates, and $\cdot O_2^-$) are coupled to active metabolic pathways and generally would not be as available as the melanin species.

Melanin is a semiconductor and can transfer energy [21]. It is also hydrophobic and would thus attract the various substances used in the present study. In addition, melanin is juxtaposed to tyrosinase within melanosomes. In melanosomes that are not yet fully melanized, there will be significant tyrosinase activity, as well as melanin deposits. Studies dealing with tyrosinase extraction and purification have demonstrated its intense particulate attachment, which is due to lipids; however, it is still not clear where tyrosinase is bound within the melanosome. The two possibilities are the internal filamentous matrix, or the limiting membrane of the melanosome [4].

It is possible that the presently employed inhibitors may have concentrated in the non-polar melieu afforded by the macromolecular lipo-
protein complexes that contain tyrosinase. In this location, the inhibitors
may have been converted into free radicals by energy exchange with melanin. Subsequently, the inhibitors as radicals could initiate uncontrolled
pathological chain reactions among lipids and proteins, thereby affecting
tyrosinase structure and activity.

The cellular changes and lethality of abnormal radical reactions induced by $CCl_4$, ionizing radiation, ozone, UV light and other agents have
been substantiated and form the basis for the field of free radical pathology, which has focused on membrane lipids, membrane proteins, and
membrane-associated nucleic acids [7, 10, 25]. The present study suggests that the inhibitors are acting within the realms of free radical pathology, although it is impossible to detail the precise radicals and kinetics
that might be involved. The fact, that DPPD, as injected into the mice,
contained detectable radicals, and that D-penicillamine could obliterate
them *in vitro,* demonstrate the potentials of these substances. By extra-
polation, the ability of D-penicillamine to negate the *in vivo* growth inhibition of DPPD and EOP suggests that pathologic radical mechanisms might
be involved in the inhibitory actions of DPPD and EOP.

In terms of 'classical' free radical pathology, unsaturated lipids, which
are most susceptible to pathological radical reactions, are damaged first.
By chain reactions, or as a result of structural alteration, lipid associated
proteins are inactivated [7, 10]. Model systems for these processes have
been proven with Na-K ATPase, and suggested for adenyl cyclase, the
prostaglandin synthetase system, Ca-Mg ATPase, succinic dehydrogenase,
and other membrane-bound enzymes [2, 7]. Tyrosinase has been shown
to be vital in the bioenergetics of pigmented S-91 tumors. Its inhibition by
radical modulating agents could explain the observed growth inhibition.

Of interest are the reports of others which show that antioxidants
(radical modulating agents) have adverse effects on glycolytic and other
pathways in tumors [26]. Hence, shutting down the tyrosinase bioenergetic pathway in pigmented tumors (which accounts for about 50% of ATP
production), plus inhibiting glycolytically derived ATP, may be a fortun-
ate coincident series of effects produced by the general class of compounds under discussion.

Not all of the agents used in the present study were effective as single
regimens, but this may have been caused by their precipitation and inacti-
vation at the sites of subcutaneous injection.

The lack of general somatic depigmentation by the tumor inhibitors may be accounted for in several ways. The time course of treatment was only two weeks and this may be shorter than the turnover time of integumentary and ocular melanin. If somatic depigmentation were to occur at a slower rate, the necessity to sacrifice the experimental animals in the present study precluded an opportunity to study such a possibility. Further, tyrosinase activity is far greater in the pigmented malignant melanocyte and there are attendant bioenergetic aspects. Normal, adult melanocytes differ from the S-91 cells in both respects.

In conclusion, it is essential to emphasize that D-penicillamine alone has been shown in previous studies to be an effective inhibitor of S-91 pigmented melanoma growth [17]. Its copper-chelating properties and the copper dependence of tyrosinase were thought to be related to its selective antimelanoma effects. However, in this and in prior work, D-penicillamine has also been shown to be capable of scavenging melanoma radicals [6]. Metal-chelating properties often accompany antioxidant effects. In the present work, D-penicillamine, administered concurrently with DPPD and EOP, resulted in no inhibition of S-91 growth, possibly because the radicals of these agents interacted and terminated with each other.

The marked diminution of melanoma radicals following single regimens with DPPD, EOP, PHP, and MBQ shows that there was an effect on the melanoma radicals. The concurrent blocking of tyrosinase suggests a relationship between these two parameters. Whether these effects were direct, and causally related, or whether they were secondary and due to another as yet, non-defined, property of the antioxidants cannot be determined from the present work.

There are many more requisite investigations that must be performed before the selective effects of the presently employed agents can be fully understood. As but one example, the presence of what appears to be significant levels of ascorbic acid in the S-91 tumor needs to be investigated. The doublet, with a 1.7-G splitting, was further split into the typical pair of triplets indicating its identity as the ascorbyl radical [1]. The effect that this substance might have on the metabolism and growth of S-91 tumors requires study in view of the known property of ascorbic acid in facillitating hydroxylation reactions, such as tyrosine. Since the metabolism of tyrosine and of dopa provide energy which is used for growth in this tumor, the precise role(s) of any substance which modulates this metabolism becomes important.

## Appendix: L-PAM

Of practical therapeutic interest is the question of whether two clinically useful antimelanoma drugs, p-di-(2-chloroethyl)-amino-L-phenylalanine (L-PAM), and 5-(3,3-dimethyl-1-triazeno)-imidazole-4-carboxamide (DTIC) have properties that might affect radical-related parameters in melanomas. Preliminary studies were conducted with L-PAM as follows.

L-PAM, in concentrations of 5 mg/0.5 ml (Burroughs Wellcome Co.) was used elsewhere [27]. L-PAM was used in doses of 1 mg versus 0.5-ml aliquots of melanosomal and mitochondrial S-91 fractions, melanin-formation, and the e.p.r. spectra of S-91 cytoplasmic homogenates.

Tissue respiration was assayed as in previous studies, using 50 mg of non-manipulated, pigmented S-91 tissue in 3 ml of medium [8], which contained 11 mM tyrosine and 5 mg of L-PAM. Triplicate determinations revealed an immediate 51% decrease in oxygen consumption. Over a time course of 1 h, the respiratory inhibition fluctuated between 75 and 35%, indicating that the drug was not simply killing the tumor cells on contact.

Succinoxidase activity in melanosomal and mitochondrial fractions, prepared from S-91 tumors as previously described [13], was assayed using methods defined elsewhere [27]. L-PAM was used in dose of 1 mg versus 0.5-ml aliquotes of melanosome and mitochondrial fractions, separately, in 3 ml of media with 15 min of pre-incubation [11]. The succinoxidase activity of the melanosomal fraction was inhibited by 80%, whereas that of the mitochondrial fraction prepared from the same S-91 tumor homogenate was not affected.

The melanosome fractions, with and without L-PAM, were subsequently allowed to incubate for 10 h to determine overall melaninzation, measured spectrophotometrically. The degree of melanin formation in the melanosomes containing L-PAM was diminished to 20% of controls.

In e.p.r. studies, L-PAM decreased both the melanin and doublet signals after 30 min of incubation, using homogenates of S-91 tumor as in the present studies. 5 mg of L-PAM in 0.5 ml solution were added to 5 ml of cytoplasmic homogenate to produce this effect.

These pilot studies suggest that L-PAM may function in a manner different from other alkylating agents, or may function to alkylate a greater variety of biomolecules, other than DNA, in pigmented melanomas.

Others have suggested that L-PAM may not function like other alkylating agents [20]. Of some curiosity is the observation that '... a fair-skinned red headed person is more likely to develop a burn of the extremity from drug (PAM) action than a dark skinned person...' [20]. This suggests that PAM interacts with integumentary melanin, the melanin 'muting' some of the toxic potential of the drug. This is analogous to the ability of melanin to absorb UV light and thus protect the skin against 'burns'. In pigmented malignant melanomas, an interaction between PAM and melanin, or between PAM and melanoma radicals, may initiate a chain of free radical pathologic reactions in proximity to essential enzymes.

Whether L-PAM exerts all, or some of its antimelanoma effects by interacting with melanin radicals and subsequently modulating radicals in proximity to tyrosinase, analogous to the other agents described in this work, cannot be determined from the present preliminary data. However, it appears to be worthy of further investigations, especially since another clinically useful antimelanoma drug, DTIC, may also have radical-modulating properties. Examination of the structure of DTIC, and its recently described metabolites [24], reveal that some of the moieties have a radical configuration, and/or have gone through a pathway wherein the intermediates had to assume a free radical configuration.

## Summary

Physiologic preparations of pigmented melanomas contain two readily detectable free radical signals, the melanin signal attributable to trapped semiquinones, and a doublet due to a nontrapped semiquinone, possibly ascorbyl. Irradiation with light in the blue spectrum, minus UV and red, alters these signals, and the metabolism and *in vitro* growth of melanotic S-91 mouse melanomas. These results are thought to be due to detrimental effects on tyrosinase, an enzyme which plays a vital respiratory role in pigmented melanomas.

Chemical means have been sought which would interact specifically with pigmented melanomas on the basis of free radical interactions, and might subsequently produce inhibition of the tyrosinase-dependent respiration and growth. A variety of antioxidants were employed *in vivo*, including diphenylparaphenylenediamine, ethoxyphenol, among others. There were selective inhibitory effects on growth of pigmented tumors *in vivo*, their tyrosinase activity, and the free radical content. In addition, a chemotherapeutic agent, L-phenylalanine mustard (PAM), was tested for its effects on tyrosinase and radical content of melanomas. It has been shown to have some efficacy with respect to growth inhibition in patients. PAM has been shown to inhibit tyrosinase activity, melanosomal succinoxidase activity, and to reduce the free radical content of S-91 mouse melanomas.

## References

1   BIELSKI, B. H. J. and GEBICKI, J. M.: Atlas of electron spin resonance spectra, p. 51 (Academic Press, New York 1967).

2   BRODY, P. M.; AKERA, T.; BASKIN, S. I.; GUBITZ, I., and LEE, C. Y.: Interaction of Na-K ATPase with chlorpromazine. Ann. N.Y. Acad. Sci. *242:* 527–542 (1974).

3   CHAVIN, W. and SCHLESINGER, W.: Effects of melanin depigmentational agents upon normal pigment cells, melanoma, and tyrosinase activity; in MONTAGNA and HU Advances in biology of the skin, vol. 8, pp. 421–445 (Pergamon Press, Oxford 1967).

4   CHEN, Y. M.: Solubilization and activation of mammalian melanoma particulate tyrosinase by lipase digestion. Cancer Res. *34:* 3192–3196 (1974).

5   CHEN, Y. M. and CHAVIN, W.: Effects of depigmentary agents and related compounds upon *in vitro* tyrosinase activity; in RILEY Pigmentation: its genesis

and biologic control, pp. 593–606 (Appleton, Century Crofts, New York 1972).

6 DEMOPOULOS, H. B.: Control of free radicals in biologic systems. Fed. Proc. Fed. Am. Socs exp. Biol. *32:* 1903–1908 (1973).

7 DEMOPOULOS, H. B.: The basis of free radical pathology. Fed. Proc. Fed. Am. Socs exp. Biol. *32:* 1859–1861 (1973).

8 DEMOPOULOS, H. B. and KALEY, G.: Selective inhibition of respiration of pigmented S-91 mouse melanoma by phenyl lactate and the possible related effects on growth. J. natn. Cancer Inst. *30:* 611–633 (1963).

9 DEMOPOULOS, H. B.; LANDGRAF, W.; DUKE, P. S., and TAI, H.: Light-induced alterations in melanoma related free radicals, and the consequences on respiration and growth. Lab. Invest. *15:* 1652–1658 (1966).

10 DEMOPOULOS, H. B.; MILVY, P.; KAKARI, S., and RANSOHOFF, J.: Molecular aspects of membrane structure in cerebral edema; in REULEN and SCHURMANN Steroids and brain edema, pp. 29–39 (Springer, Berlin 1972).

11 DEMOPOULOS, H. B.; SABATINI, M. T.; MAVROMATIS, M. I.; DAVIS, L., and SCHWARZ, R.: Succinoxidase activity in melanosomes of pigmented mouse melanomas. Yale J. Biol. Med. *46:* 706 (1973).

12 DUKE, P. S.; LANDGRAF, W.; MITAMURA, A., and DEMOPOULOS, H. B.: Study of S-91 mouse melanomas by electron paramagnetic resonance spectroscopy and tissue culture. I. The effect of cysteine on the blue light signals and on growth *in vitro.* J. natn. Cancer Inst. *37:* 191–198 (1966).

13 FIERMAN, H. and DEMOPOULOS, H. B.: Preparation of fractions of premelanosomes and melanosomes from pigmented S-91 melanomas; in RILEY Pigmentation: its genesis and biologic control, pp. 515–524 (Appleton Century Crofts, New York 1972).

14 FUJITA, T.: Lipid peroxide content in rat liver microsomes and soluble fraction after administration of ascorbic acid and ferrous ion. J. pharm. Soc. Jap. *94:* 215–220 (1974).

15 HAMBERG, M. and SAMUELSSON, B.: Prostaglandin endoperoxides. Novel transformations of arachidonic acid in human platelets. Proc. natn. Acad. Sci. *71:* 3400–3404 (1974).

16 HESSELBACH, M. L.: On the participation of two enzyme systems in melanin production *in vitro* by melanotic and amelanotic tumors of mice. J. natn. Canc. Inst. *12:* 337–360 (1951).

17 HOURANI, B. T. and DEMOPOULOS, H. B.: Inhibition of S-91 mouse melanoma metastases and growth by D-penicillamine. Lab. Invest. *21:* 434–438 (1969).

18 JENSEN, O. A.; EGEBERG, J., and EDMUND, J.: The effect of a phenylalanine-tyrosine low diet on the growth and morphology of transplantable malignant melanomas of the Syrian golden hamster. Acta path. microbiol. scand. *81:* 559–568 (1973).

19 LOWRY, O. H.; ROSEBROUGH, N. J.; FARR, A. L., and RANDALL, R. J.: Protein measurement with the folin phenol reagent. J. biol. Chem. *193:* 265–275 (1951).

20 McBRIDE, C. M. and CLARK, R. L.: Experience with 1-phenylalanine mustard dihydrochloride in isolation-perfusion of extremities for malignant melanoma. Cancer *28:* 1293–1296 (1971).

21 McGinness, J.; Corry, P., and Proctor, P.: Amorphous semiconductor switching in melanins. Science *193:* 853–855 (1974).

22 Regan, M. A. G.; Regan, D., and Demopoulos, H. B.: The vital respiratory role of tyrosinase in pigmented S-91 melanomas; in Riley Pigmentation: its genesis and biologic control, pp. 543–549 (Appleton Century Crofts, New York 1972).

23 Riley, P. A.: Mechanism of pigment-cell toxicity produced by hydroxy anisole. J. Path. Bact. *101:* 163–169 (1970).

24 Saunders, P. P. and Chao, L. Y.: Fate of ring moiety of 5-(3,3-dimethyl-1-triazeno) imidazole-4-carboxamide in mammalian cells. Cancer Res. *34:* 2464–2469 (1974).

25 Seligman, M. L. and Demopoulos, H. B.: Spin-probe analysis of membrane pertubations produced by chemical and physical agents. Ann. N.Y. Acad. Sci. *222:* 640–667 (1973).

26 Suolinna, E. M.; Lang, D. R., and Racher, E.: Quercetin, an artificial regulator of the high aerobic glycolysis of tumor cells. J. natn. Cancer Inst. *53:* 1515–1519 (1974).

27 Umbreit, W. W.; Burris, R. H., and Stauffer, J. F.: Manometric techniques, p. 174 (Burgess, Minneapolis 1957).

28 White, A.; Handler, P., and Smith, E. L.: Principles of biochemistry, p. 404 (McGraw-Hill, New York 1973).

Dr. H. B. Demopoulos, New York University, Medical Center, School of Medicine, Department of Pathology, 550 First Avenue, *New York, NY 10016* (USA)

Pigment Cell, vol. 2, pp. 365–378 (Karger, Basel 1976)

# The Evolution of Therapy for Malignant Melanoma at The University of Texas M. D. Anderson Hospital and Tumor Institute 1950 to 1975

R. Lee Clark

The University of Texas System Cancer Center, Houston, Tex.

The therapeutic philosophy for malignant melanoma and the research investigational approaches have undergone many changes during the past 25 years at the Anderson Hospital. Knowledge has been accumulated regarding the biology, pathology, metastatic routes, hereditary aspects, and the immunology of melanoma, and this progressively acquired information has been utilized to instigate changes in therapy for local, regional, and systemic disease. The therapeutic modalities have included surgery, radiation therapy, chemotherapy, and immunotherapy.

Through unremitting efforts at communication with practicing physicians and the general public, many more people are aware of the potentially fatal prognosis resulting from neglect of a newly appearing, rapidly growing mole or a long-standing mole which suddenly manifests changes. In addition, knowledge regarding the hereditary aspects of the disease contributes to a more efficient means of prevention.

With gradual improvement in the control of local primary and recurrent disease, survival has been significantly extended, functional limbs have been salvaged, and more active attempts are being made to rehabilitate melanoma patients following therapy.

## Basic Science

*Biological behavior.* In the late 1950s, what was known about the biological behavior of melanoma was summarized by Russell [27] of our institution: (1) metastases may occur within a very brief period of time or as late as 32 years later; (2) the best hope of improved 5-year survival lies in better control of the metastatic process; (3) lymphatic spread and extension are the most frequent means of metastases, although vascular dissemination occurs also; (4) in some cases no history of a primary lesion or site can ever be determined; (5) some melanomas remain superficial for 8–9 years; (6) occasionally spontaneous regression occurs and only a flat blue coloration may be found at the site; (7) the proof of the existence of particular mechanisms of spread still remains to be elucidated.

Since the 1950s, progressively more sophisticated biochemical and molecular studies have revealed additional facts.

In 1963, members of the Anderson department of pathology confirmed previous studies indicating that a majority of melanomas are tyrosinase-positive as determined by quantitative radiochemical or autoradiographic techniques [6]. Although other types of pigmented cells, as pigmented basal cell carcinoma, junctional, compound, intradermal and blue nevi cells, etc. also have tyrosinase activity, the levels appear higher in patients with melanoma, and especially in those with disseminated disease. This test was considered adjunctive to other diagnostic procedures, but it was believed that no unequivocal diagnosis of melanoma could be made on the basis of this test.

*Staging.* The attempts at classification and staging of melanoma were undergoing periodic changes from 1958, and by 1965 the classification, based on clinical and microscopic evidence at the time of therapy, was essentially as it remains today [30]:

*Stage 0.* Superficial lesions.

*Stage I.* No metastases (clinically or in nodes examined after regional lymphadenectomy): (A) primary intact; (B) primary removed (diagnosed clinically, histologically, following incisional biopsy), and (C) multiple primaries.

*Stage II.* Local metastases (not more than 3 cm from the primary lesion or excisional scar – cutaneous, subcutaneous, or both – satellitosis).

*Stage III.* Regional metastases: (A) skin and subcutaneous tissue more than 3 cm from primary or scar (intransit metastases); (B) regional lymph node(s) (axilla, epitrochlear region or groin), and (AB) skin and regional lymph node(s) (no metastases outside the extremity detected).

*Stage IV.* Distant metastases (spread outside the extremity with or without invasion of the regional lymph nodes); primary tumor in the upper extremity (excluding shoulder) with metastases to supraclavicular nodes; lower extremity metastases to iliac or obturator nodes or both).

Conclusions in this 1965 report regarding the biological behavior of melanoma of an extremity were that: (1) of the primary stage I melanomas that metastasized, three fourths spread via the regional lymphatics, and one quarter spread via the bloodstream, and those patients with no lymph nodes involved lived twice as long as those with positive nodes; (2) of those local recurrences (stage II) which metastasized, half spread via the regional lymphatics, and the other half where no regional lymph nodes were involved apparently metastasized via the bloodstream. These patients lived a much shorter period of time than those with stage I tumors that metastasized. Therefore, local recurrence is probably the first manifestation of disseminated disease; (3) those patients with stage IIIB disease treated with lymphadenectomy and perfusion who died, lived a very short time following surgery; (4) the possibility of explosive disease should be considered in any patient who, at the time of diagnosis, has a rapidly enlarging lymph node or local recurrence – this patient may develop fulminating disease rapidly and consideration should be given to the possibility that local or regional tumor may inhibit the growth of occult disease; (5) metastases to the supraclavicular, iliac, and/or obturator nodes (exclusive of the shoulder or gluteal regions) indicate a grave prognosis, and radical surgery for cure was *not* advocated, although lymph nodes might be removed for palliation; (6) melanoma can be unique and totally unpredictable.

Considerable controversy still existed in 1967 regarding the correct diagnosis of the disease in its early and superficial phases, and even more controversy existed regarding what constituted proper initial therapy. If two criteria and only two were observed in studying survivals, namely, if the study was based upon a sufficiently large number of patients whose disease was adequately staged, and if all patients without regard to status of disease were included, there was very little difference in survival rates in a majority of the reports [31]. Because of this similarity, it was speculated that the single most important factor in the biologic behavior of melanoma might be its aggressiveness relative to the resistance of the patient.

*Hereditary aspects.* The first familial occurrence of melanoma were reported in 1952 by CAWLEY [5] and by VON GREIFELT [35], and a review of the literature in 1967 [1] revealed that familial occurrence was generally not known or not considered important. For the average population melanoma occurs in 1 person in 100,000, but the average occurrence of hereditary melanoma is 3 members per family. Statistical chances of this happening in non-hereditary melanoma are $1.5 \times 10^{-7}$. Of approximately 1,000 melanoma patients seen at Anderson Hospital by 1967, 28 patients (3%) studied by Drs. ANDERSON, LESLIE SMITH, and McBRIDE were found to have a family history of melanoma. Only 22 patients could be sufficiently documented for publication. In those 22 kindreds, 67 individuals were reliably reported to have melanoma, 48 (72%) of whom were verified histologically or by physician, hospital or laboratory reports.

The genetic basis appeared to be inheritance through autosomes rather than through sex chromosomes, and dominance was involved, but not the usual type of dominance, because the distribution of the affected members did not follow the classical hereditary pattern. The development of melanoma in these patients was characterized by a relatively early age at first diagnosis and an increased number of multiple primary lesions. A high number of these primaries were located on parts of the body generally exposed to sunlight.

Because of these findings, it was recommended that intensive regular examinations of family members be conducted, especially of those with light complexion and eyes and sandy or light hair, and removal of any suspicious lesions plus careful inspection of all other moles. The majority of melanoma lesions had developed from preexisting nevi with junctional activity.

By August of 1971, a total of 37 kindred with hereditary malignant melanoma had been studied (one with ocular melanoma) [7]. Additional facts that had been revealed were: (1) these patients have a significantly higher survival rate, probably because their lesions tend to be more superficial and, therefore, more amenable to therapy; (2) there appear to be several autosomal gene loci involved; and (3) there appears to be an extranuclear component which has not yet been identified.

*Origin of melanosomes – ultrastructural investigations.* In 1968, the origin of melanosomes in human melanoma was reinvestigated *in vitro* by MAUL [23], who used an established melanoma cell line. By means of 3-dimensional reconstruction of serial sections, it was found that most premelanosomes are contained in and develop within a tubular smooth endoplasmic reticulum (SER) which is connected with the Golgi apparatus during melanogenesis. With increasing melanization, the frequency with which there are connections between melanosomes and SER decreases. It was concluded, therefore, that the connection is resolved before melanization is completed. These observations were made on melanoma cells. Whether they could be reproduced with normal melanocytes remained open for speculation and further investigation.

*Cytokinetic studies.* Antitumor drugs are divided into two groups: those that affect proliferating cells only and those that affect both proliferating and non-proliferating cells. Thus, the choice of single or combinations of drugs, the duration of administration, dose scheduling, the total duration of treatment, and the interpretation of the response should ideally be predicated on the basis of cytokinetic information regarding tumor and normal cells, particularly the rapidly proliferating cells.

In 1969, members of the departments of developmental therapeutics and experimental radiotherapy attempted to determine the cytokinetics of subcutaneous metastatic melanoma cells [28]. Multiple simultaneous biopsies and sequential biopsies following pulse labeling with tritiated thymidine (a precursor specific for DNA) in three patients were studied. Computer analysis of the mitotic indexes revealed that the median $G_2$ period was 5.3 h and the median S period was 21 h. The generation time was highly variable with a median of 3 days.

In addition, intermittent or continuous tritiated thymidine was administered over a 10- to 20-day period to 2 patients. Computer analysis of labeling index curves indicated a growth fraction of 20–30%. The potential tumor doubling time calculated from the generation time and the growth fraction was much shorter than the actual doubling time, indicating that cell loss was approximately 70% of the rate of cell production. It has been suggested that cell loss can be explained by exfoliation, metastases, or cell death. Cell loss is a significant factor in determining growth rate in relatively small tumors. In experimental solid tumors, the rate of cell loss increases as the tumor size increases. In the human tumors examined, the labeling and mitotic indexes in the center of the large tumors were one third less than at the periphery, and there was no morphological evidence of necrosis in the tumor center. The periphery of the large tumors had labeling and mitotic indexes comparable to those of small tumors.

*Immunological and virological studies.* As a result of studies conducted in 1969 [25] and 1970 [26] by members of the department of surgery, initiated by reports by MORTON et al. [24] and LEWIS et al. [14], indicating that indirect immunofluorescence testing had revealed that a majority of melanoma tumors contain an antigen or antigens against which antibodies were directed in some patients, the members of the departments of virology, surgery, and developmental therapeutics initiated a project to determine whether there is a viral etiology for melanoma [3, 4, 7]. Their studies using a number of immunological methods revealed that the sera of some melanoma patients contain antibodies that react with antigen associated with autologous or homologous tumor cell nucleoli; that 40–50% of patients tested have antigen but do not produce antibodies to react against the antigen; that the nucleolar antigen was not melanoma-specific (as a few non-melanoma lesions tested were weakly positive); that the nucleolar antigen appears to be a protein complexed in some manner with nuclear RNA but not with DNA; and that there is a striking correlation between the presence of the nucleolar antigen and the clinical status of the patient. Electron microscopic studies did not reveal any virus particles or unusual structural components associated with the nucleolar antigens.

*Biochemical studies.* (1) Reverse-phase chromatographic elution patterns indicate that transfer RNAs of melanoma tissue differ from those of normal tissue [7]. (2) Two human tumors (malignant melanoma and breast cancer) were tested for altered transfer RNAs and revealed a third peak on reverse-phase chromatographic studies which appears in virally induced hamster liver tumors, but does not appear in normal hamster liver tissue or in experimentally induced liver tumors of chemical origin. These findings may have some direct relationship to viral oncogenesis of malignant melanoma.

The elaboration of melanin through its various biochemical stages has been done by various researchers in the hope that it would show a specificity with regard to chemotherapeutic control.

*Histochemical studies.* There is usually little difficulty in establishing a diagnosis of primary melanoma, but many patients present with recurrent disease, no primary lesion can be located or has previously been removed, and the histological appearance of metastatic melanoma can be quite variable. In these instances, histochemical procedures used in the department of anatomical pathology in conjunction with electron microscopic technique have been helpful in clarifying the diagnosis [7].

Other studies in the pathology department indicate that the degree of chronic inflammatory response invoked by the primary lesion probably reflects the host-tumor immune relationship and is probably responsible for the differences in the biological behavior of lesions [7]. The inflammatory response is the histological feature of importance in tumor regression and is related to tumor cell degeneration. Continuing studies are attempting to determine whether the degree of inflammation can predict the future behavior of melanoma in individual cases. Efforts are being aimed at the establishment of a workable and uniformly applicable staging classification to correlate macroscopic morphology with biological behavior.

These are only some of the studies that have been and are being conducted in the institution in an attempt to better define and, therefore, to offer more comprehensive therapy for malignant melanoma.

*Therapy*

*Radical surgery.* Prior to World War II, therapy for malignant melanoma was solely surgical excision, but because of the marked tendency for metastases and invasion of the lymphatics, mortality rates were very discouraging. Following World War II, antibiotics became widely available, and with the advent of better transfusions, better control of hemorrhage and shock, and better surgical techniques, extreme radical surgery (hemipelvectomy, hip disarticulation or interscapulothoracic amputation) for the treatment of melanoma of the extremities became the primary therapeutic approach for approximately 10 years.

There have been a total of 3,249 melanoma patients treated at Anderson Hospital from 1944 through August 1974. Of these, 1,314 have been treated by surgery alone.

In 1950, hemipelvectomy was believed to give a 4-fold increased chance of survival over the more conservative hip disarticulation with an iliofemoral lymph node dissection [33]. In 1958, Anderson Hospital reported 24 hemipelvectomies and only one postoperative death [13]. For anorectal lesions, an abdominoperineal resection was performed with a subsequent bilateral node dissection, done one side at a time [22]. Beginning in 1952, a routine neck dissection was performed for all primary melanomas of the head and neck, and exenteration, not enucleation, was performed for melanoma of the eye [17]. A total of 479 patients with melanoma of all sites had been seen at Anderson from March 1, 1944, to December 31, 1956, 77% of whom had received previous therapy. The absolute 5-year survival for all of these patients was 24.3% [18].

Therapy for melanoma of the head and neck region has remained essentially surgical with the initial effort directed toward local control of the primary lesion [2]. Elective neck dissection is considered if the primary is more than superficial, and the value of this procedure has been established for positive nodes, because of the reduction of points at which metastases can spread to the circulatory system.

*Chemotherapy*

*Systemic.* The synthesis of *l*-phenylalanine mustard was accomplished in 1953 [19]. Poor results achieved by excision of the primary lesion in an extremity plus regional lymph node dissection, and the demon-

*Table I.* Major treatment regimes

| Name | Regimen | Dates |
|---|---|---|
| 1. DIC | DIC, 250 mg/m² i.v., for 5 days every 21 days | 3/67–8/69 |
| 2. BVD | BCNU, 150 mg/m² i.v., on day 1 every 28–42 days; Vincristine, 2 mg i.v., on days 1 and 5 every 28–42 days; DIC, 150 mg/m² i.v., for 5 days every 28–42 days | 8/69–8/71 |
| 3. DIC-procarbazine | DIC, 250 mg/m² i.v., for 5 days every 28 days Procarbazine, 100 mg/m² p.o., for 10 days every 28 days | 8/71–3/72 |
| 4. DIC-BCG | DIC, 250 mg/m² i.v., for 5 days every 21 days BCG (6 × 10⁸ organisms by scarification on days 7, 12, and 17 of each treatment course) every 21 days | 3/72–3/73 |

stration in 1956 by LUCK [16] that $p$[di(2-chloroethyl)]-amino-$l$-phenyl-alanine was effective in inducing remission of melanomas in Harding-Passey mice, stimulated the use of systemic chemotherapy at Anderson Hospital.

For 7 years (1955–1962), many compounds were tried for the systemic therapy of melanoma. Beginning in 1959, clinical trials were conducted with $l$-phenylalanine mustard, meta-phenylalanine mustard, PA-144 (mithramycin) and actinomycin-D, used singly and in various combinations on 44 patients with disseminated melanoma. None of the agents produced 'good' objective responses, whether used singly or in combination, which was judged by a measurable decrease in the size of the tumor or more than half of the multiple nodules for a period of 90 days or longer. There were subjective responses, such as relief of pain or discomfort, especially of metastatic bone pain, for 30–60 days in approximately 20% of patients.

*Systemic chemotherapy (recent).* Even though systemic chemotherapy gave disappointing results in the past, the development or discovery of more active antitumor drugs encouraged further attempts to control disseminated melanoma. In 1972, many drugs were undergoing clinical trials at Anderson. As shown in table I, from March 1967 to August 1969 dimethyl triazeno imidazole carboxamide (DTIC) was used singly and produced objective responses in 19 and 86 evaluable patients [10]. This encouraged trials with a combination of 1,3-bis(2-chloroethyl)-1-nitrosourea

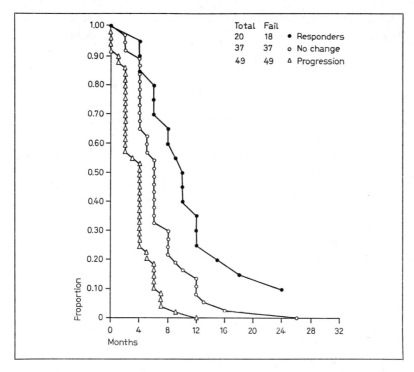

*Fig. 1.* Survival of melanoma patients, indicating those with progression, no change, and objective response, from administration of BVD to death.

(BCNU) and vincristine which produced objective responses in 8 of 18 patients. This led to a combination of the three drugs, DTIC, BCNU, and vincristine (BVD) from August 1969 to August 1971. Objective responses were obtained in 20 of 84 evaluable patients (24%). From August 1971 to March 1972, DTIC was combined with procarbazine and objective responses were obtained in 11 of 45 evaluable patients (24%). The most recent regimen has been with DTIC and bacille Calmette-Guérin (BCG) [12].

Therefore, between March 1967 and March 1973, there was a total of 426 patients treated with various regimens of chemotherapy for disseminated melanoma. There was a total of 75 objective responses for a total response rate of 18% for all patients and of 23% for evaluable patients. The median survival from onset of chemotherapy to death for all patients was only 4.7 months, but as shown in figure 1, responders clearly live longer than those in whom the drug has no effect. While it is obvious that the presently available chemotherapeutic agents are not yet producing major improvements, and survival data remain disappointing, it is hoped that a combination of chemotherapy plus immunotherapy will improve survival for metastatic disease.

Another study was done on 17 patients with advanced regional malignant melanoma, who were treated with intra-arterial infusion therapy with 5-(3,3-dimethyl-1-triazeno) imidazole-4-carboxamide for isolated inoperable lesions [9]. There were 6 partial objective responses and one complete remission for an overall response rate of 41%. Toxicity was less than that usually seen with systemic chemotherapy with DTIC, and the local response rate was higher.

*Regional isolation perfusion.* The work of CREECH et al. [8] inspired the use of regional isolation perfusion with *l*-phenylalanine mustard (*l*-PAM) prepared in prophylene glycol for melanoma of the extremity in 1958 at ANDERSON [29], which was used until 1962 when water-soluble *l*-phenylalanine mustard dihydrochloride became available [19], to reduce the incidence of local recurrence and lymph node metastases. Annual reports were published of the results of, first, the single [15, 30–32] and, later, a triple drug [20, 21] (*l*-PAM, actinomycin-D, and mechlorethamine hydrochloride ($HN_2$)) regional isolation perfusion as compared with standard surgical therapy [20]. Gradually, the results revealed that perfusion: (1) materially reduced the incidence of recurrence in extremities, particularly the lower; (2) if there were recurrences in a limb following lymphadenectomy and perfusion, the perfusion seemed to forestall their appearance until systemic disease became overwhelming; (3) perfusion reduced significantly the necessity for radical amputation; (4) it was decreasing the need for skin grafts; (5) the 5-year survival was at least equal to that achieved with conventional surgical therapy and eventually proved to be up to 11% higher [7]; (6) operative mortality was less than 1%; and (7) the average hospital stay was 8 days.

At the Anderson Hospital, 709 patients have received a total of 880 perfusions for the treatment of malignant melanoma of the extremity from January 1958 through September 1974 [21]. L-PAM dihydrochloride alone was given to 282 patients, 100 of whom have had a 10-year follow-up; 193 patients were treated with the 3-drug regimen, and there is a 5-year follow-up for 100 of these patients. These patients have been compared with 150 controls who received surgery only for their melanoma prior to the availability of perfusion therapy. There is a 10-year follow-up on all of these patients.

The results for these patients range from:

|  | 5-year survival, % | 10-year survival, % |
|---|---|---|
| *Stage I* |  |  |
| Controls | 73 | 61 |
| L-PAM dihydrochloride | 86 | 76 |
| *Stage IV* |  |  |
| Controls | 7 | 4 |
| L-PAM dihydrochloride | 13 | 0 (numbers too small to be significant) |

There is evidence that the single-drug regimen is satisfactory for stages I and II, but not for the later stages.

All three regimens are compared for 2- and 5-year survivals for stage IIIA disease of the extremities:

|  | 2-year survival, % | 5-year survival, % |
|---|---|---|
| *Stage IIIA* |  |  |
| Controls | 63 | 12 |
| L-PAM dihydrochloride | 71 | 29 |
| 3-Drug regimen | 80 | 43 |

Some patients on the 3-drug regimen have lived more than 7 years with no evidence of recurrence. The secondary immunological effects must be the determining factor, because we do not expect 100% cell kill with perfusion. For some patients, the drugs are effective, but for some the drugs do nothing and the downhill course is rather rapid, no matter what stage disease they have.

*Radiation therapy.* Although it has been taught traditionally that melanoma is radioresistant, it has been our finding that there is a significant response rate to radiotherapy, but the responses are usually of short duration [11]. There were 47 patients in whom central nervous system metastases were discovered prior to chemotherapy. Of these patients, 26 received whole brain radiotherapy and most received concomitant dexamethasone. An objective response was seen in 8 of these patients, and the median survival was 5 months [10].

*Rehabilitation.* Since amputation has been largely avoided through therapy with regional isolation perfusion, the need for artifical limbs has been reduced and physical medicine, as it pertains to soft tissues, and physiatric rehabilitation have become more important. The melanoma patients who have been treated with regional isolation perfusion generally can be divided into two groups, those who are considered uncomplicated cases (minimal to moderate edema) and the complicated cases (moderate to massive edema). Edema is the primary problem in the rehabilitation of these patients, and if allowed to exist on a long-term basis, muscle loss and neurological deficit can occur [34].

The primary therapy for uncomplicated cases is proper positioning to avoid neurological deficit and the establishment of a full range of motion for the limb. It is not necessary to aim for initial full weight support on the damaged lower limb, but ambulation is important.

For the complicated cases, if edema is massive, even passive movement is restricted, but exercises are very important so that edema will not restrict blood circulation. Neurological deficit is usually not caused by the perfusion itself, but by improper positioning and lack of exercise.

The data included in this presentation indicate that, although we have achieved progressively better results in the treatment of malignant melanoma, continued efforts are needed to acquire better antitumor drugs and earlier diagnosis for truly adequate control of non-disseminated melanoma. Disseminated malignant melanoma will await prevention or control based on a better understanding of causation, host resistance, and chemical ablation.

## Summary

The clinical philosophy for treatment of malignant melanoma patients and the research investigational approaches on melanoma have undergone many changes during the past 25 years at the M. D. Anderson Hospital and Tumor Institute. Investigations have revealed additional information regarding the biology, pathology, metastatic processes, heredity, and immunology of malignant melanoma. This new knowledge has been reflected in the changes in therapy for regional and systemic disease, which includes surgery, chemotherapy, and immunotherapy. In addition, more knowledge is available to use in the prevention of the disease, particularly with regard to familial incidence and, with the increased survival of patients with melanoma, more active attempts are being made to assist with the rehabilitation of patients who have had their disease brought under control.

## References

1  ANDERSON, D. E.; SMITH, J. L., jr., and MCBRIDE, C. M.: Hereditary aspects of malignant melanoma. J. Am. med. Ass. *200:* 741–746 (1967).

2  BALLANTYNE, A. J.: Malignant melanoma of the skin of the head and neck. An analysis of 405 cases. Am. J. Surg. *120:* 425–431 (1970).

3  BOWEN, J. M.; ANGERMANN, J.; McBRIDE, C. M.; MILLER, M. F.; HERSH, E., and DMOCHOWSKI, L.: Anti-nucleolar antibodies in sera of patients with melanoma. Proc. Am. Ass. Cancer Res. *12:* 85 (1971).

4  BOWEN, J. M.; McBRIDE, C. M.; HERSH, E.; MILLER, M. F., and DMOCHOWSKI, L.: Nuclear antigens in tumor cells of patients with malignant melanoma; in Immunological aspects of neoplasia. The University of Texas M. D. Anderson Hospital and Tumor Institute 26th Ann. Symp. Fundamental Cancer Research, 1973 (Williams & Wilkins, Baltimore, in press).

5  CAWLEY, E. P.: Genetic aspects of malignant melanoma. Archs Derm. *65:* 440–450 (1952).

6  CHANG, J. P.; RUSSELL, W. O.; STEHLIN, J. S., jr., and SMITH, J. L., jr.: Chemical and histochemical analysis of tyrosinase activity in melanoma and related lesions. Ann. N.Y. Acad. Sci. *100:* 951–964 (1963).

7  CLARK, R. L.: The research and clinical approach to melanoma at The University of Texas M. D. Anderson Hospital and Tumor Institute. Pigment Cell, vol. 1 (Karger, Basel 1973).

8  CREECH, O., jr.; KREMENTZ, E. T.; RYAN, R. F., and WINBLAD, J. N.: Chemotherapy of cancer; regional perfusion utilizing extracorporeal circuit. Ann. Surg. *148:* 616–632 (1958).

9  EINHORN, L. H.; McBRIDE, C. M.; LUCE, J. K.; CAOILI, E., and GOTTLIEB, J. A.: Intra-arterial infusion therapy with 5-(3,3-dimethyl-1-triazeno) imidazole-4-carboxamide (NSC 45388) for malignant melanoma. Cancer *32:* 749–755 (1973).

10  EINHORN, L. H.; BURGESS, M. A.; VALLEJOS, C.; BODEY, G. P., sr.; GUTTERMAN, J.; MAVLIGIT, G.; HERSH, E. M.; LUCE, J. K.; FREI, E., III; FREIREICH, E. J., and GOTTLIEB, J. A.: Prognostic correlations and response to treatment in advanced metastatic malignant melanoma. Cancer Res. *34:* 1995–2004 (1974).

11  GOTTLIEB, J. A.; FREI, E., III, and LUCE, J. K.: An evaluation of the management of patients with cerebral metastases from malignant melanoma. Cancer *29:* 704–705 (1972).

12  GUTTERMAN, J. U.; MAVLIGIT, G.; GOTTLIEB, J. A.; BURGESS, M. A.; McBRIDE, C. M.; EINHORN, L.; FREIREICH, E. J., and HERSH, E. M.: Chemoimmunotherapy of disseminated malignant melanoma with dimethyl triazeno imidazole carboxamide and bacillus Calmette-Guérin. New Engl. J. Med. *291:* 592–597 (1974).

13  Hemipelvectomy. Cancer Bull. *10:* 22–23 (1958).

14  LEWIS, M. C., *et al.*: Tumor-specific antibodies in human malignant melanoma and their relationship to the extent of disease. Br. med. J. *iii:* 547–552 (1969).

15  LONSDALE, D.; BERRY, D. J.; HOLCOMB, T. M.; NORA, A. H.; SULLIVAN, M. P.; THURMAN, W. G., and VIETTI, T. J.: Chemotherapeutic trials in patients with metastatic retinoblastoma. Cancer Chemother. Rep. *52:* 631–634 (1968).

16  LUCK, J. M.: Action of $p$[di(2-chloroethyl)]-amino-$l$-phenylalanine on Harding-Passey mouse melanoma. Science *123:* 984 (1956).

17  MacCOMB, W. S.: Abstr. The University of Texas M. D. Anderson Hospital and Tumor Institute 2nd Ann. Clinical Conf. Melanoma, 1957. Cancer Bull. *10:* 26–27 (1958).

18  MacDonald, E. J.: Abstr. The University of Texas M. D. Anderson Hospital and Tumor Institute 2nd Ann. Clinical Conf. Melanoma, 1957. Cancer Bull. *10:* 27 (1958).

19  McBride, C. M. and Clark, R. L.: Experience with 1-phenylalanine mustard dihydrochloride in isolation perfusion of extremities for malignant melanoma. Cancer *28:* 1293–1296 (1971).

20  McBride, C. M.: Advanced melanoma of the extremities. Treatment by isolation-perfusion with a triple drug combination. Archs Surg. *101:* 122–126 (1970).

21  McBride, C. M.: Management of malignant melanoma. Adv. Surg. *8:* 129–150 (1974).

22  Martin, R. G.: Abstr. The University of Texas M. D. Anderson Hospital and Tumor Institute 2nd Ann. Clinical Conf. Melanoma, 1957. Cancer Bull. *10:* 26 (1958).

23  Maul, G. G.: Golgi-melanosome relationship in human melanoma *in vitro*. J. Ultrastruct. Res. *26:* 163–176 (1969).

24  Morton, D. L., *et al.*: Demonstration of antibodies against human malignant melanoma by immunofluorescence. Surgery, St Louis *64:* 233–240 (1968).

25  Romsdahl, M. M. and Cox, I. S.: Immunofluorescent studies of antibodies against human malignant melanoma. Surg. Forum *20:* 126–128 (1969).

26  Romsdahl, M. M. and Cox, I. S.: Human malignant melanoma antibodies demonstrated by immunofluorescence. Archs Surg., Chicago *100:* 491–497 (1970).

27  Russell, W. O.: Abstr. 2nd Ann. Clinical Conf. Melanoma, 1957. Cancer Bull. *10:* 6 (1958).

28  Shirakawa, S.; Luce, J. K.; Tannock, I., and Frei, E., III: Cell proliferation in human melanoma. J. clin. Invest. *49:* 1188–1199 (1970).

29  Stehlin, J. S., jr.; Clark, R. L., jr.; Smith, J. L., jr., and White, E. C.: Malignant melanoma of the extremities: experiences with conventional therapy; a new surgical and chemotherapeutic approach with regional perfusion. Cancer *13:* 55–66 (1960).

30  Stehlin, J. S., jr. and Clark, R. L.: Melanoma of the extremities: experiences with conventional treatment and perfusion in 339 cases. Am. J. Surg. *110:* 366–383 (1965).

31  Stehlin, J. S., jr.; Hills, W. J., and Rufino, C.: Disseminated melanoma: biologic behavior and treatment. Archs Surg., Chicago *94:* 495–501 (1967).

32  Tapley, N. duV: Bilateral retinoblastoma, combined treatment with irradiation and chemotherapy; in Vaeth Frontiers of radiation therapy and oncology. 4th Ann. San Francisco Cancer Symp., San Francisco 1968, vol. 4 (Karger, Basel 1969).

33  Tumor Clinic Conf.: Cancer Bull. *2:* 67 (1950).

34  Villanueva, R.: Pathophysiology of the disabilities in the patient with cancer and his rehabilitation. Proc. 2nd World Congr. Ass. Rehab. Med. (in press).

35  Greifelt, A. von: Malignes Melanom: Beziehungen zu Schwangerschaft. Pubertät. Kindheit: Familiäre maligne Melanome. Ärztl. Wschr. *7:* 676–679 (1952).

R. Lee Clark, MD, The University of Texas System Cancer Center, M. D. Anderson Hospital and Tumor Institute, 6723 Bertner Avenue, *Houston, TX 77030* (USA)

Pigment Cell, vol. 2, pp. 379–385 (Karger, Basel 1976)

# Mayo Clinic Experience with Isolated Limb Perfusion for Invasive Malignant Melanoma of the Extremities

## A Retrospective Study of Long-Term Results and Complications

Claude D. Davis, John C. Ivins and Edward H. Soule

Mayo Clinic and Mayo Foundation, Rochester, Minn.

The action of the chloroethyl amines and synthesis of phenylalanine mustard was first reported in 1955 [8]. Animal experiments demonstrated the antisarcoma activity of this agent, especially against melanin-producing tumors [8]. In 1956, it was first suggested that the action of phenylalanine mustard might be due to its active deposition by the melanocyte, since phenylalanine mustard is a derivative of phenylalanine, an ultimate precursor of melanin [9]. Experiments with the Harding-Passey melanoma paved the way for subsequent human clinical trials [9].

In 1958, the technique of isolation perfusion of regional arteries with phenylalanine mustard was first reported for various sarcomas [6]. Some of the best responses occurred in cases of malignant melanoma [6]. Refinements in the original technique ensured more complete isolation of the limb and perfusate from the systemic circulation, thus reducing systemic toxic effects of the agent [6]. Subsequent reports added further refinements in technique and detailed the results of treatment and the complications encountered [2, 7, 10, 11, 16–18].

In 1962, several groups performing isolated limb perfusion changed from *l*-phenylalanine mustard (melphalan; PAM) (free bases requiring preparation in propylene glycol) to the water-soluble product, *l*-phenylalanine mustard dihydrochloride. This modification apparently reduced the number of complications to an acceptable level in some series.

Many series of isolated limb perfusion for malignant melanoma have been reported. Generally, most workers indicate a significant increase in survival of patients with deeply invasive stage I disease and stage II disease and some increase in survival of patients with stage III disease. Meaningful comparison of these series to each other or to conventional surgical therapy is futile without sufficient control groups or uniform classification of patients and results.

A clinically meaningful histopathologic classification of the primary lesion in malignant melanoma has been developed and refined by several authors [4, 12–15]. As the depth of invasion bears a direct correlation to results of treatment, it is essential to provide this information in any clinical series [3, 4, 12, 13].

The present study is a report of the experience with isolated limb perfusion from 1960 to 1968 at the Mayo Clinic. Long-term results and complications were evaluated. An attempt was made to review all pathologic material and to reclassify it in the light of present concepts.

## Materials and Method

From 1960 to 1968, 141 of 269 patients with malignant melanoma of the extremities were selected for perfusion. Reasons for exclusion included advanced age, medical contraindications, *in situ* lesions, advanced metastatic disease, and peripheral vascular disease. All medical charts were reviewed and the patients were reexamined or follow-up was obtained by a detailed questionnaire completed by the patient or his physician. The clinical stage of disease was classified at the time of the patient's initial perfusion as follows: stage I, primary lesion only (intact or previously biopsied); stage II, regional recurrence in the limb (no nodal or distant involvement); stage III, regional nodes involved, with or without regional recurrence; stage IV, distant cutaneous or visceral disease.

All original obtainable biopsy material was reviewed and reclassified as to tumor type (superficial spreading, nodular, lentigo maligna melanoma) and depth of invasion according to the criteria of CLARK et al. [4] and McGOVERN et al. [12, 13]. Levels of invasion were defined as follows: level I, epidermis only; level II, invasion into papillary layer but not to reticular layer of dermis; level III, tumor fills papillary layer to reticular layer; level IV, invasion into reticular layer; level V, invasion of subcutaneous fat.

Briefly, the technique of isolated limb perfusion, which has been well described in previous papers [5–7, 10, 11, 16–18], was as follows (fig. 1):

With the patient surgically prepared and anesthetized, the regional artery and vein were exposed and the patient was given 500 ml of whole blood and was heparinized. A pump-oxygenator[1] was primed with 2 units of whole blood. The limb was isolated from the systemic circulation by a proximal tourniquet. The artery and vein were cannulated with polyethylene cannulas[2] and connected to the pump-oxygenator to allow continuous perfusion of the limb with warmed (38.5–41.0 °C) blood, and the appropriate dose of PAM (0.5–1.5 mg/kg), dissolved in propylene glycol, was

1   Travenol Perfuso-pak.
2   Travenol Plexitron.

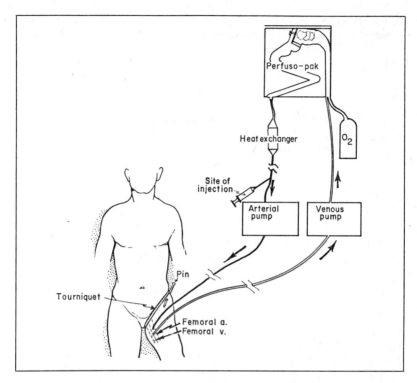

*Fig. 1.* Schematic representation of perfusion circuit and apparatus for common femoral perfusion.

administered in two divided doses 10 min apart. The artery was perfused at a flow rate of 200–400 ml/min. After 60–80 min of perfusion, the limb was flushed with 500 ml of Dextran and 500 ml of whole blood. The artery and vein were repaired, the action of heparin was reversed, and the tourniquet was released.

Wide excision of the primary lesion or biopsy site and regional node dissection were performed at the time of perfusion in 68 patients, prior to perfusion in 32 patients and after perfusion in 10 patients. Regional nodes were not excised in one patient.

### Group Characteristics

Sufficient data for inclusion in the study were available on 111 patients; follow-up of at least 4 years was obtained on survival and long-term complications, and adequate pathologic specimens for review were obtained from the initial biopsy.

Of the 141 patients perfused, 112 had initial biopsy tissue available for review. Classification included depth of invasion in 103 and tumor type in 96. In 29, primary lesions were not identifiable or original tissue was not available. There were 74 females and 37 males. The average age was 43 years with a range from 16 to 68 years. The time from initial biopsy establishing the diagnosis to perfusion was highly variable with a mean of 340 days and median of 37 days (range, 0 to 15.9 years). Of 111 patients, 75 underwent perfusion within 3 months of their initial biopsy. The distribution of the 111 primary lesions was as follows: leg, 49; foot, 20; thigh, 13; hand, 10; forearm, 10, and arm, 9. Follow-up from perfusion to death or last examination averaged 6.7 years with a range of 4–13 years.

## Results

Of the 111 patients with identifiable primary lesions, 78 survived at time of follow-up. One survivor had evidence of recurrent stage II disease 5 years after initial perfusion. Of the 33 who died, 3 died of causes not related to their melanoma or treatment (breast carcinoma 7 years 5 months after perfusion, stroke 7 years 10 months after perfusion, suicide 5 years 4 months after perfusion). Two of these three had evidence of recurrent melanoma at the time of death. The most significant correlations were between survival and stage at perfusion and between depth of invasion of initial lesion and survival. No significant differences were noted between nodular and superficial spreading lesions when correlated with depth of invasion or survival.

The survival rates by stage at perfusion and by depth of invasion of the primary lesion are shown in tables I and II. Survival times are calculated from *time of perfusion* to follow-up or death, rather than from time of original biopsy.

Recurrences developed after perfusion in 35 patients. The mean length of time to recurrence was 2 years with a range up to 9 years from the date of perfusion. Only 23 of 35 recurrences (66%) occurred during the first 2 years.

## Complications

A review of the medical records, questionnaires, and follow-up examinations revealed a relatively high complication rate. Some of the complications, such as wound slough and edema may be related to the associated surgical treatment (wide local excision and regional node dissec-

*Table I.* Survival by stage at perfusion (111 patients)

| Stage at perfusion | Length of follow-up, years | Patients | | Survival, % |
|---|---|---|---|---|
| | | total number | number alive | |
| I | 4–13 | 72 | 65 | 90 |
| II | 5–13 | 9 | 6 | 67 |
| III | 5–13 | 30 | 7 | 23 |

*Table II.* Survival by depth of invasion of primary lesion (103 patients)

| Level of invasion[1] | Patients | | Survival, % |
|---|---|---|---|
| | total number | number alive | |
| II | 3 | 3 | 100 |
| III | 23 | 19 | 83 |
| IV | 74 | 49 | 66 |
| V | 3 | 1 | 33 |

1 No patient had level I invasion.

tion). Five amputations were the direct result of complications of perfusion. An additional five patients had significant loss of limb function due to muscle contractures or sympathetic dystrophy. Transient complications developed in 60 patients; long-term complications developed in 34. No patient had bone marrow depression severe enough to produce secondary infection or bleeding difficulties. Nonhemolytic anemia requiring multiple blood transfusions developed in one patient. 18 further major surgical procedures (excluding amputations) were necessary to deal with the complications. There was no evidence that complications were dose-related.

*Discussion and Conclusions*

Several conclusions seem warranted. For deeply invasive (levels III, IV, and V) primary malignant melanoma (stage I disease), adjunctive perfusion therapy may offer significantly better results than similar lesions treated with standard surgical therapy alone [1, 7, 14].

The number of patients with level II invasion is too small to warrant any conclusions, but we would agree with other authors that conventional surgical treatment alone affords a high rate of cure [1, 7, 12, 14].

Although only nine patients had stage II disease, the survival of six for 5 years or more warrants further prospective investigation. Perfusion therapy may offer significantly improved results for these patients [7, 17, 18]. KREMENTZ and RYAN [7] cite a 5-year survival rate of 28% for patients with satellitosis and a rate of 77% for patients with isolated limb recurrences when treated with perfusion.

The survival rate of patients with stage III disease showed little improvement over that of groups treated by standard surgical measures [1, 7, 14].

The high complication rate may well be reduced by several modifications now available. The use of water-soluble *l*-phenylalanine mustard should afford the most dramatic improvement [11]. Monitoring systemic leakage with $^{131}$I or fluorescein prior to introduction of PAM into the perfusion circuit should further reduce systemic toxicity [5, 11]. Stricter exclusion of patients with evidence of peripheral vascular disease should decrease the incidence of vascular complications. Newer therapeutic agents under investigation may further reduce local and systemic complications [10].

## Summary

From 1960 through 1968, 141 patients with invasive malignant melanoma of the extremities were treated at the Mayo Clinic with isolated limb perfusion with phenylalanine mustard. Clinical follow-up and available pathologic tissue were analyzed in 111 cases. Of the 111 patients, 78 survived 4–13 years after their initial perfusion. Complications developed in 94 patients and were permanent in 34. Survival was correlated with both depth of invasion of the primary lesion and stage of disease at the time of perfusion. Results indicate the need for a well-controlled, prospective study of isolation perfusion in the treatment of patients with invasive malignant melanoma of the extremities.

## References

1  BOOHER, R. J.: Recognition and treatment of melanoma. Surg. Clins N. Am. 49: 389–405 (1969).

2  CAVALIERE, R.; CIOCATTO, E. C.; GIOVANELLA, B. C.; HEIDELBERGER, C.; JOHNSON, R. O.; MARGOTTINI, M.; MONDOVI, B.; MORICCA, G., and ROSSI-FANELLI,

A.: Selective heat sensitivity of cancer cells: biochemical and clinical studies. Cancer *20:* 1351–1381 (1967).

3 CLARK, W. H., jr.: A classification of malignant melanoma in man correlated with histogenesis and biologic behavior; in Advances in biology of the skin, vol. 8, pp. 621–647 (Pergamon Press, Oxford 1967).

4 CLARK, W. H., jr.; FROM, L.; BERNARDINO, E. A., and MIHM, M. C.: The histogenesis and biologic behavior of primary malignant melanomas of the skin. Cancer Res. *29:* 705–727 (1969).

5 CREECH, O., jr. and KREMENTZ, E.: Techniques of regional perfusion. Surgery *60:* 938–947 (1966).

6 CREECH, O., jr.; KREMENTZ, E. T.; RYAN, R. F., and WINBLAD, J. N.: Chemotherapy of cancer: regional perfusion utilizing an extracorporeal circuit. Ann. Surg. *148:* 616–632 (1958).

7 KREMENTZ, E. T. and RYAN, R. F.: Chemotherapy of melanoma of the extremites by perfusion: fourteen years clinical experience. Ann. Surg. *175:* 900–915 (1972).

8 LARIONOV, L. F.; SHKODINSKAJA, E. N.; TROOSHEIKINA, V. I.; KHOKHLOV, A. S.; VASINA, O. S., and NOVIKOVA, M. A.: Studies on the anti-tumour activity of *p*-di-(2-chloroethyl) aminophenylalanine (sarcolysine). Lancet *i:* 169–171 (1955).

9 LUCK, J. M.: Action of *p*-[di-(2-chloroethyl)]-amino-L-phenylalanine on Harding-Passey mouse melanoma. Science *123:* 984–985 (1956).

10 McBRIDE, C. M.: Perfusion treatment for malignant melanoma of the extremity. Archs Chir. Neerl. *22:* 91–95 (1970).

11 McBRIDE, C. M. and CLARK, R. L.: Experience with *1*-phenylalanine mustard dihydrochloride in isolation-perfusion of extremities for malignant melanoma. Cancer *28:* 1293–1296 (1971).

12 McGOVERN, V. J.: The classification of melanoma and its relationship with prognosis. Pathology *2:* 85–98 (1970).

13 McGOVERN, V. J.; MIHM, M. C., jr.; BAILLY, C.; BOOTH, J. C.; CLARK, W. H., jr.; COCHRAN, A. J.; HARDY, E. G.; HICKS, J. D.; LEVENE, A.; LEWIS, M. G.; LITTLE, J. H., and MILTON, G. W.: The classification of malignant melanoma and its histologic reporting. Cancer *32:* 1446–1457 (1973).

14 MEHNERT, J. H. and HEARD, J. L.: Staging of malignant melanomas by depth of invasion. Am. J. Surg. *110:* 168–175 (1965).

15 MIHM, M. C., jr.; CLARK, W. H., jr., and FROM, L.: The clinical diagnosis, classification and histogenetic concepts of the early stages of cutaneous malignant melanomas. New Engl. J. Med. *284:* 1078–1082 (1971).

16 ROCHLIN, D. B. and SMART, C. R.: Treatment of malignant melanoma by regional perfusion. Cancer *18:* 1544–1550 (1965).

17 SHINGLETON, W. W.: Perfusion chemotherapy for recurrent melanoma of extremity: a progress report. Ann. Surg. *169:* 969–972 (1969).

18 STEHLIN, J. S., jr. and CLARK, R. L.: Melanoma of the extremities: experiences with conventional treatment and perfusion in 339 cases. Am. J. Surg. *110:* 366–383 (1965).

Dr. J. C. IVINS, Mayo Clinic, 200 First Street SW, *Rochester, MN 55901* (USA)

Pigment Cell, vol. 2, pp. 386–393 (Karger, Basel 1976)

# Role and Results of Treating Malignant Melanoma Intralymphatically with Radioactive Isotopes[1]

Irving M. Ariel

The Pack Medical Foundation and the Department of Surgery,
New York Medical College, New York, N.Y.

## Introduction

The proper method of treating malignant melanoma has not been devised, although the surgical extirpation of this form of cancer is the best method at present. When a malignant melanoma is located juxtaposed to the primary chain of lymph nodes draining that region, the best method is to perform a monobloc resection of the primary cancer, the intervening lymphatics, and the lymph nodes to which the melanoma may spread. The problem arises when a melanoma is located at a great distance from the lymph node basin to which metastases may occur. For example, if a malignant melanoma is located on the foot or lower leg, the question of how to treat the lymph node-bearing area remains problematical. The problem becomes more complex when metastases to the lymph node region are not clinically evident. Several surgical courses are available: the surgeon may either ignore such lymph nodes and adopt a policy of watchful waiting to see if these nodes become involved by cancer at some later date, or he may elect to perform a discontinuous operation.

A natural development from diagnostic lymphadenography was the administration of chemotherapeutic agents and/or radioactive isotopes into the lymphatic vessels as a means of delivering a large dose of radia-

1    Assisted by Grants-in-Aid from the Mr. and Mrs. Arnold Rosen Cancer Research Fund, and the Foundation of Clinical Research, New York, New York.
Published with alterations and additions from an article published in Surgery Gynecol. Obstet. *139:* 726–730 (1974) with permission of the publisher (originally published under the title: Results of treating malignant melanoma intralymphatically with radioactive isotopes).

tion to the lymph nodes, described by ARIEL *et al.* [3], CHIAPPA *et al.* [6], and FISCHER [9].

This is a report of our policies and results to date in the overall treatment, using endolymphatic isotopes for patients with malignant melanoma whose primary melanoma is distant from the chain of lymph nodes draining the site of the malignant melanoma.

## Technic

The technic of KINMOTH and TAYLOR [12] was utilized, and the isotope used in this investigation was $^{131}$I-ethiodol – a special preparation of radioactive ethiodol in oil which contains 37% iodine in organic combination with ethyl esters of the fatty acids of poppy seed oil. Other radioactive nuclides which have been utilized are radioactive $^{198}$gold [11, 16], $^{90}$yttrium microspheres [5], chromic phosphates, and $^{32}$P-Lipiodol.

The radiation factors, including distribution of the isotope, radiation doses, excretion, etc., have been described [9]. The results herein presented were those obtained by $^{131}$I-ethiodol. *We are now using $^{32}$P-lipiodol. It is more readily obtained, has a more desirable radiation spectrum, and its use permits comparative evaluation with the studies being performed in England by EDWARDS [7, 8] and his group.* These results shall be reported later; to date, they are encouraging.

### Treatment Policies
Indication for Endolymphatic Isotope Therapy

The treatment policies and the results are best described by presenting the data according to the clinical staging of malignant melanoma. All melanomas were of the invasive type.

Stage I melanomas indicate that the regional lymph nodes are clinically and roentgenographically negative for evidence of metastases. Stage II indicates patients whose regional nodes contain metastases. Stage III means that satellites, i.e. deposits of melanoma throughout the skin of the involved extremity, have formed, or there is other evidence of melanoma involving the extremity, such as subcutaneous or deeper nodules. Stage IV indicates distant metastases.

### Stage I Melanomas
The treatment policy for this grade of cancer consists of a wide, tridimensional resection of the primary melanoma. If the melanoma is adjacent to a lymph node draining area, an enbloc surgical dissection of the melanoma, the intervening lymphatics, and the first echelon of lymph nodes is performed, and no isotopes are administered. If an en bloc dissection cannot be performed, i.e. where the lymph nodes are distant from the primary melanoma, only the primary lesion is radically excised.

Unlike EDWARDS [7, 8] and his group, who do not resect the deep fascia, we firmly believe that the deep fascia should be resected and that the dissection should extend to naked muscle. We cannot accept the claims of OLSEN [13] that the resection of the deep fascia has certain disadvantages. It is close to this deep fascia that the lymphatics traverse (we have found melanoma deposits in close approximation to the fascia), and we routinely remove a much larger amount of the deep fascia than of the overlying skin.

Within 3–4 weeks after the resection of the primary melanoma, a therapeutic lymphadenogram is performed. Immediately after administering the radioactive $^{131}$I-ethiodol into the lymphatics and again 24 h later, diagnostic roentgenograms were made. When possible, the lymphatic vessel isolated is just proximal to the line of resection. In a few instances, we have injected in different areas to assure filling all lymphatic vessels. The injections in the posterolateral aspects of the foot permit filling of the popliteal chain of lymph nodes.

If the roentgenograms of the lymph nodes is considered negative for evidence of metastases, no further treatments are given, but the patient is followed carefully. If a defect which might be considered a metastasis exists within the lymph nodes, the patient is subjected to a dissection of the lymph node-bearing region; if metastases are discovered, he is placed in the category of stage II.

### Dosage and Volume

The dose of $^{131}$I-ethiodol varied from 40 to 50 mCi in 4 ml for the lower limb and 30 to 40 mCi in 2 ml for the upper limb. We gave 5–6 mCi $^{32}$P-lipiodol for the lower extremities and 2–3 mCi $^{32}$P-lipiodol for the upper extremities. Measurements performed on the nodes regarding the radioactivity have revealed that such dosages will deliver from 50,000 to 100,000 rads beta to the lymph nodes. Repeated scannings have revealed that any spillover of this isotope into the lungs is eliminated. Long-term studies, including pulmonary function tests, to date, have demonstrated no untoward pulmonary reactions [1].

### Stage II Melanomas

In these patients, the primary melanoma was treated in the same way as with stage I. Staging is determined either by clinical examination of the patient or by the lymphogram, if it reveals a space-occupying defect in one of the lymph nodes; the node is then excised for histologic study. The overall treatment policy consists of a wide resection of the primary melanoma just as for stage I, endolymphatic isotope, and 3–4 weeks later, a bloc dissection of the lymph nodes is performed. The delay before performing the surgical resection of the lymph nodes permits deterioration of the isotope; this results in a beneficial radiation effect to the tissues and allows the isotope to reach a dose safe for the operating team. The Atomic Energy Commission recommends a dose of 5 mCi to be safe for the operating team, and inasmuch as the biologic half-life of $^{131}$I-ethiodol is approximately 6 days, a delay from 3 to 4 weeks permits maximum irradiation to the tissues and maximum protection to the operating team. We have encountered no unusual surgical difficulties or complications resulting from the preoperative internal irradiation [2].

### Stage III Melanomas

We have treated ten patients suffering from satellitoses of their extremities by the endolymphatic administration of radioactive isotopes. Each of these patients had been treated previously by resection of the lymph nodes, and the satellitoses developed subsequently. The mechanism for this is believed to be a regurgitation of lymph-carrying cancer cells as a result of blockage caused either by tumor or by the surgical procedure, described by ARIEL and RESNICK [1]. Two of these patients have demonstrated complete disappearance of the satellites, and one patient remains clinically free of melanoma 5 years after such treatment. In 2 patients, the nodes involving the inner aspects of the thigh, i.e. the distribution of the lymphatic vessels, disappeared, whereas those involving the lateral aspect of the thigh did not change in appearance. The remaining patients manifested no benefit.

### Stage IV Melanomas

No beneficial clinical response was observed in ten patients treated by [131]I-ethiodol delivered via the lymphatics of the feet. Metastases to the lungs, liver, or other sites existed, and irradiation to the pelvic and periaortic lymph nodes had no demonstrable clinical effect. All patients died from disseminated melanoma. We have abandoned endolymphatic isotopes for this group of patients.


## Results

We have previously described marked shrinkage of lymph nodes [4] and destruction of malignant melanoma following [131]I-ethiodol administration endolymphatically [12].

In our series of 120 patients treated by this technic, 22 patients in clinical stage I were treated over 5 years ago. A survival rate (free of melanoma) of 82% was obtained (table I). A 5-year survival rate of 28.5% for the 11 patients in clinical stage II was obtained.

Table I compares the clinical accomplishments of endolymphatic isotope therapy with surgical excision in treating malignant melanoma. The data for those patients treated by surgical resection alone, reported by PACK et al. [15] represent patients treated by the same technic and for the most part by the same group of surgeons. An index of improvement was noted in those patients who received [131]I-ethiodol endolymphatically.


## Discussion

As a means of determining the reliability of endolymphatic isotope therapy, EDWARDS [8] and his co-workers described experimental work performed on VX2 tumor in a host animal – the rabbit. They analyzed their results according to the lymphographic appearance of the lymph nodes, microscopic findings on autopsy, and survival time of the animals.

*Table I.* Comparison of survival rates of patients with malignant melanoma treated by surgery alone or surgery with endolymphatic radioactive isotopes (Pack Medical Foundation, New York)

| Stage | Treated with surgical excision alone (wide local excision and node dissection)[1] | | Treated with endolymphatic radioactive isotopes and surgical excision | |
|-------|----------------------|----------------------|----------------------|----------------------|
|       | number of patients | 5-year survival rate, % | number of patients | 5-year survival rate, % |
| I     | 37                 | 40.5                 | 22                 | 82.0                 |
| II    | 199                | 14.1                 | 11                 | 28.5                 |

1 From PACK and ARIEL [14].

*Table II.* Melanoma 5-year survival of patients as indicated by EDWARDS [7]

| Stage | Number of cases | Females | Males | Deaths | Survival rate, % |
|-------|-----------------|---------|-------|--------|------------------|
| *Surgical excision* | | | | | |
| I     | 51              | 30      | 21    | 21     | 58.9             |
| II    | 8               | 4       | 4     | 7      | 12.5             |
| *Endolymphatic therapy* | | | | | |
| I     | 45              | 36      | 9     | 9      | 80.0             |
| II    | 28              | 16      | 12    | 12     | 21.4             |

There was a marked increase in survival times of the treated animals. Only in the animals with nodes involved with microscopic metastases was the survival markedly increased, and 25% of these rabbits were cured. Other treated animals eventually died, but far outlived those rabbits who were treated as controls.

EDWARDS obtained a 5-year survival rate of 80% for 45 patients with stage I melanoma and a 28.5% 5-year survival for patients in stage II classification treated for malignant melanoma by similar technics (surgical excision and endolymphatic isotope therapy). The only significant difference in technics is that EDWARDS used $^{32}$P-lipiodol whereas we used $^{131}$I-ethiodol. EDWARDS (table II) evaluated the results from *surgical ablation alone* at the St. Thomas Hospital, London, where he performed his investigations, and he was able to show that, in stage I cancer, the 5-year survival rate was 58.9%, and in stage II, the survival rate was 12.5%. He further believes that a more relevant comparison of the efficiency of the endolymphatic form of therapy in comparison to surgery alone is the recurrence rate in lymph nodes. In 31 patients treated by surgical resection and endolymphatic therapy, 9.7% developed recurrences in the region of the lymph nodes and eventually died. In those treated by surgical excision alone, of 42 patients, 15 developed recurrences in the lymph node region, and 14 died.

We have observed that approximately 40% of the patients in clinical stage I eventually develop metastases to the lymph nodes. We are accordingly convinced that the policy of watchful waiting is not justified.

If the melanoma is in juxtaposition to the lymph node-bearing region, a dissection of the primary melanoma, the intervening lymphatics, and the lymph nodes in continuity is considered the procedure of choice. If, however, the melanoma is distant from the lymph nodes and an *en bloc* dissection is not technically feasible, a discontinuous operation (removal of the primary melanoma followed by a groin or axillary dissection) ignores the intervening lymphatics possibly harboring melanoma cells in transit. ARIEL and RESNICK [1] have demonstrated that the discontinuous operation is not without hazard. Following the groin or axillary dissection, there is a sealing off of the severed lymphatics with resultant increase in lymphatic pressure which enhances the lodgement and growth of melanoma cells in transit. The resultant development of collateral lymphatic circulation may convey melanoma cells to unusual and unpredictable locations. If the collateral circulation is inadequate, lymphatic regurgitation occurs with the functional development of the dermal network of lymphatic vessels, which is the mechanism whereby melanoma cells are transported to the tiny superficial lymphatics where they lodge and grow producing satellitosis.

*Comparison of Complications from a Nodal Resection with those Resulting from Endolymphatic Isotope Injection*

FORTNER et al. [10] described complications following groin dissections for melanoma. Three patients had serious complications – cardiac arrest with death, a severed ureter and bladder, and a tear in a major vein. Local complications consisted of necrosis of skin flaps necessitating skin grafts. Moreover, a significant number of patients had swelling of the affected limb, severe at times. The incidence of satellitoses varied from 9 to 25%.

The complications following isotope therapy have been minimal. We have an 8% failure rate to administer a proper therapeutic dose due to technical problems. At first, we had difficulty with the healing of the incision site, but pouring a liter of saline solution over the wound after the removal of the catheter and before the wound is sutured closed has completely eliminated this complication. One patient developed a transient rash, possibly due to a sensitivity to iodine. 5% of the patients had a mild cough for 1–3 days. No pulmonary complications have been observed.

When given in the dose range described herein, internal irradiation therapy apparently exerts no demonstrable effect upon lymphatic dynamics. It does not cause blockage of lymphatic flow, nor does it result in the formation of collateral lymphatic channels for unpredictable dissemination of cancer cells throughout the body. Even after the administration of therapeutic doses of irradiation, the filtration stability of the residual lymph nodes remains intact.

The continued application of these clinical investigations, adhering to the principles of therapy described above, is warranted.

*Summary*

The treatment of malignant melanoma by a combination of surgery and endolymphatic isotopic therapy is based on experimental evidence that the dose of irradiation delivered by this route will destroy microscopic deposits of cancer. This has been accomplished with no demonstrable interference to lymph flow due to marked differences in sensitivity to irradiation of the lymph nodes and the lymphatic vessels. The lymph nodes are radiosensitive, and the lymphatic vessels are radioresistant.

Endolymphatically administered $^{131}$I-ethiodol and $^{32}$P-lipiodol deliver sufficient irradiation to the lymph nodes in humans to destroy microscopic deposits of melanoma cells lodged within the nodes. The primary melanoma is treated by orthodox surgical technics. Patients classified as clinical stage I receive no additional surgical intervention, but receive $^{131}$I or $^{32}$P endolymphatically and are thus spared the trauma of a radical axillary or groin dissection and their ensuing complications. A 5-year survival rate without evidence of residual or recurrent melanoma by *18* of the 22 patients (82%) followed five years or longer is encouraging.

Patients with stage II melanoma are treated by a combination of endolymphatic isotopes and surgical removal of the primary melanoma and the lymph nodes. The penetration of the irradiation from the administered isotope is not sufficient to destroy the cancer. In such instances, irradiation of lymph nodes outside the field of surgery, irradiation of any nodes inadvertently left behind, and irradiation to cancer cells within the lymphatics offer an additional dimension in the treatment of these patients. A 5-year survival rate of 28.5% in a small group of patients is better than that obtained with surgical excision alone.

Several patients with satellitoses have markedly benefited from endolymphatic isotopic therapy.

Patients with distant metastases so treated have shown no improvement, and endolymphatic isotopes are not indicated for such patients.

## References

1  ARIEL, I. M. and RESNICK, M. I.: Altered dynamics following groin and axillary dissection; its relationship to treatment policies for malignant melanoma. Surgery, St Louis *61:* 210 (1967).

2  ARIEL, I. M. and RESNICK, M. I.: Altered lymphatic dynamics by cancer metastases. Archs. Surg., Lond. *94:* 117 (1967).

3  ARIEL, I. M.; RESNICK, M. I., and GALEY, D.: The intralymphatic administration of radioactive isotopes and cancer chemotherapeutic drugs. Surgery, St Louis *55:* 355 (1964).

4  ARIEL, I. M.; RESNICK, M. I., and ORPEZA, R.: Effects of irradiation (external and internal) on lymphatic dynamics. Am. J. Roentg. *99:* 404 (1967).

5  ARIEL, I. M.; RESNICK, M. I., and ORPEZA, R.: The intralymphatic administration of radioactive isotopes for treating malignant melanoma. Surgery Gynec. Obstet. *124:* 25 (1967).

6  CHIAPPA, S.; GALLI, G., and PALMIA, C.: Observations on lymphatic radiotherapy and general chemotherapy. Clin. Radiol. *15:* 202 (1964).

7  EDWARDS, J. M.: Malignant melanoma endolymphatic therapy. Melanoma and skin cancer. Proc. Int. Cancer Conf., Sidney 1972.

8  EDWARDS, J. M.: Malignant melanoma. Treatment by endolymphatic radio-isotope infusion. Ann. R. Coll. Surg. *44:* 237 (1969).

9  FISCHER, H. W.: Intralymphatic therapy for lymph-node metastases of carcinoma of the cervix. Cancer *18:* 1059 (1965).

10  FORTNER, J. G.; BOOHER, R. J., and PACK, G. T.: Results of groin dissection for malignant melanoma in 220 patients. Surgery, St Louis *55:* 485 (1964).

11  JANTET, G. H.; EDWARDS, J. M.; GOUGH, M. H., *et al.:* Endolymphatic therapy with radioactive gold for malignant melanoma. Br. med. J. *ii:* 904 (1964).

12  KINMOTH, J. B.: Lymphangiography in man. A method of outlining lymphatic trunks at operation. Clin. Sci. *11:* 13 (1952).

13  OLSEN, G.: Removal of fascia – cause of more frequent metastases of malignant melanoma of the skin to the region? Cancer *17:* 1159 (1964).

14  PACK, G. T. and ARIEL, I. M.: Treatment of malignant melanoma by adequate (radical) surgical resection and radical amputation when indicated; in MULHOLLAND, ELLISON and FREISON Current surgical management, pp. 438–446 (Saunders, Philadelphia 1957).

15  PACK, G. T.; SCHARNAGEL, I., and MORFITT, M.: The principle of excision and dissection in continuity for primary and metastatic melanoma of the skin. Surgery, St Louis *17:* 849 (1945).

16  SCHWARTZ, S. I.; GREENLAW, R. H.; ROB, C., *et al.:* Intralymphatic injection of radioactive gold. Cancer *15:* 623 (1962).

IRVING M. ARIEL, MD, The Pack Medical Foundation and the Department of Surgery, New York Medical College, 137 East 36 Street, *New York, NY 10016* (USA)

Pigment Cell, vol. 2, pp. 394–406 (Karger, Basel 1976)

# Thermal Neutron Capture Treatment of Malignant Melanoma using $^{10}B$-Dopa and $^{n}B_{12}$-Chlorpromazine Compounds[1]

YUTAKA MISHIMA and TATSUYA SHIMAKAGE

Departments of Dermatology, Kobe University School of Medicine, Kobe, and Wakayama Medical University, Wakayama

In 1972, the new development [1–3] of thermal neutron capture treatment of malignant melanoma using a molecular hybrid compound of one $^{10}B$ atom and chlorpromazine which has a selective affinity to melanin, was reported. Since then, we have synthesized newer compounds, chlorpromazine having 10 or 12 atoms of non-radioactive natural boron per molecule, and also $^{10}B$-dopa borate, a molecular hybrid of $^{10}B$ with a substrate for melanin. In addition, we have better collimation methods of thermal neutron reducing secondary gamma rays, detection and quantitation methods of (n, $\alpha$) reaction occurring in the unit area of various tissue, and the trial method of combination treatment controlling cell cycles, during $^{10}B$ compound administration increasing the efficiency of neutron capture treatment.

Thermal neutrons are shown to be well absorbed by the non-radioactive $^{10}B$ isotope [4, 5] and this absorption is known to induce the emission of $\alpha$-particles and Li atoms sharing between them an energy of 2.79 MeV transferred totally to tissue:

$$^{10}B + n \begin{cases} \rightarrow {}^{7}Li + \alpha + 2.79 \text{ MeV } (6.1\%) \\ \rightarrow {}^{7}Li + \alpha + 2.31 \text{ MeV } (93.9\%) \\ \hookrightarrow {}^{7}Li + \gamma + 0.48 \text{ MeV} \end{cases}$$

Due to the relatively large size of these particles, the primary radiation injury is confined within a distance of 10–14 $\mu$m from the point of the neutron activated boron atom. This distance of 10–14 $\mu$m is equal to the di-

1 Supported by a Grant-in-Aid for Cancer Research 1975 No. 101049 from the Ministry of Education, Science and Culture, Japan.

ameter of individual melanoma cells. Malignant melanoma is the cancer-
ous growth of cells having a specific function to synthesize melanin; malignant transformation in these pigment cells usually accentuates their melanin-synthesizing ability. Consequently melanoma cells usually contain
numerous melanized melanosomes. We thought that biological and nonsurgical eradication of malignant melanoma might be achieved if we
could synthesize molecular hybrid compounds with $^{10}$B which selectively
accumulate in melanoma cells, utilizing this specific melanin synthesizing
ability.

BLOIS [6] showed that $^{35}$S-labeled chlorpromazine binds selectively
with melanin and is presumed to form a charge transfer complex as a result of the $\pi$-electron interaction between an indole nucleus on the surface of melanin particles and a molecule of chlorpromazine. It was shown
that 3 days after systemic administration of chlorpromazine, melanin-containing melanoma tissue and the eyes have a chlorpromazine concentration 19–15 times that of other tissue; this selective localization can still be
seen even after 7 days. Thus, in cooperation with Dr. T. NAKAGAWA, a
boron chemist, we synthesized $^{10}$B-chlorpromazine borane, which was
effective in significantly depressing the growth rate of malignant melanoma as compared with a control group and a group with only neutron irradiation [1].

Since then we have continued to work on improving the effectiveness
of neutron capture treatment toward the eradication of malignant melanoma. One advancement is success in synthesizing newer boron compounds having more than one boron atom in each chlorpromazine molecule. Compared to the previous chlorpromazine compound containing
only one $^{10}$B non-radioactive isotope, our two new water-soluble compounds have 10 and 12 boron atoms per molecule [10], respectively, although these are natural boron, 20% being $^{10}$B atoms at present (fig. 1).
Condensation and purification of $^{10}$B from natural boron has been
achieved but is still not an easy procedure. Thus, in cooperation with a
nuclear chemist, Prof. H. KAKIHANA of Tokyo Technological University,
we have been working on the development of less difficult purification
methods. Once we succeed in doing this, the synthesis of large amounts of
chlorpromazine having 10 or 12 atoms of $^{10}$B per molecule, with at least
five times greater effect will be possible.

In the course of the study it seemed necessary to create a compound
which would specifically accumulate even in melanoma cells which are
non-pigmented or scarcely melanin-containing but which have tyrosinase

activity. Thus, we have synthesized $^{10}$B-dopa borate (fig. 2) with the specific aim to eradicate the newly divided young melanoma cells, which appeared during the administration of $^{10}$B-chlorpromazine compounds, as well.

The distribution of irradiation energy in the human body has been studied by Dr. T. SATO of our group, using a human body phantom [1, 7]. Figure 3 is an acrylic phantom model of a human thigh containing an acrylic cube-shaped model of melanoma at a depth equivalent to the subcutaneous level. Rossi's tissue equivalent solution composed of carbon, hydrogen, oxygen and other elements similar to those contained in the soft tissue of the human body, was put into the thigh phantom model. In a melanoma model $5\times5\times5$ cm, $^{10}$B of 70 $\mu$g/g concentration was added to the Rossi's solution. Figure 4 is an iso-dose distribution curve of irradiation energy measured after irradiation with the Kyoto University Thermal Column of Nuclear Reactor Heavy Water Facility (KUR) operated at 1,000 kW for 30 min which has a flux of $5\times10^8$n/cm$^2$/sec on the surface of the phantom using a $10\times10$ cm size collimator. It is clearly revealed that the irradiation energy is highly concentrated within this melanoma model in the range of 40–60 times that of the surrounding normal tissue equivalent solution (fig. 4).

In order to establish optimum administration methods of $^{10}$B compounds for thermal neutron capture therapy, we have studied the actual distribution and population density of released $\alpha$-particles following neutron irradiation inside and outside of melanoma lesions. Figure 5 shows a total body cryotome section of a Greene's malignant melanoma-bearing Syrian golden hamster, into which 13.9 mg of $^n$B$_{12}$-chlorpromazine, equivalent to 1,000 $\mu$g of $^{10}$B, was injected intraperitoneally, as in neutron capture treatment. An (n, $\alpha$) reaction, releasing $\alpha$-particles and $^7$Li

---

*Fig. 1.* Chemical structure of our previous and current synthesized chlorpromazine boron hybrids [10]. *A* Chlorpromazine borane. *B* Chlorpromazine nonahydrodecaborate. *C* Chlorpromazine undecahydrododecaborate.

*Fig. 2.* Chemical structure of $^{10}$B-dopa borate synthesized in cooperation with N. TAKEMOTO.

*Fig. 3.* Acrylic phantom model of a human thigh with a cube-shaped model of melanoma (M) at a depth equivalent to the subcutaneous tissue level. Within the thigh model at different depth levels, gold thermal neutron detectors and TLD gamma ray detectors are placed.

*Fig. 4.* Iso-dose distribution curve of irradiation energy in phantom models of a human thigh and melanoma when RBE of (n, $\alpha$) reaction and of (n, p) reaction is considered to be 10.

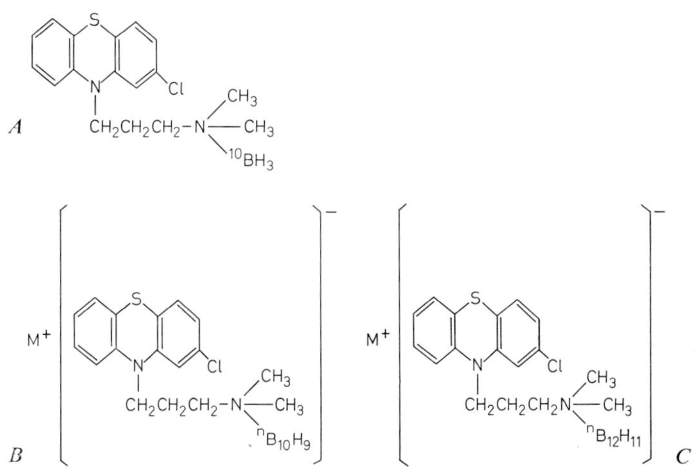
A
S
N
Cl
CH2CH2CH2-N
CH3
CH3
10BH3
M+
S
N
Cl
CH2CH2CH2-N
CH3
CH3
nB10H9
B
M+
S
N
Cl
CH2CH2CH2N
CH3
CH3
nB12H11
C

1

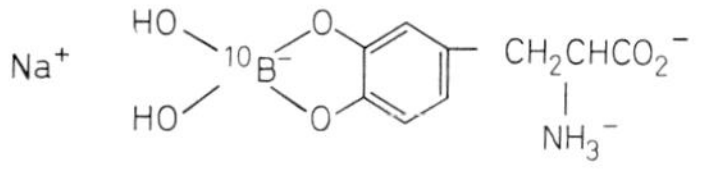
Na+
HO
HO
10B-
O
O
CH2CHCO2-
NH3-

2

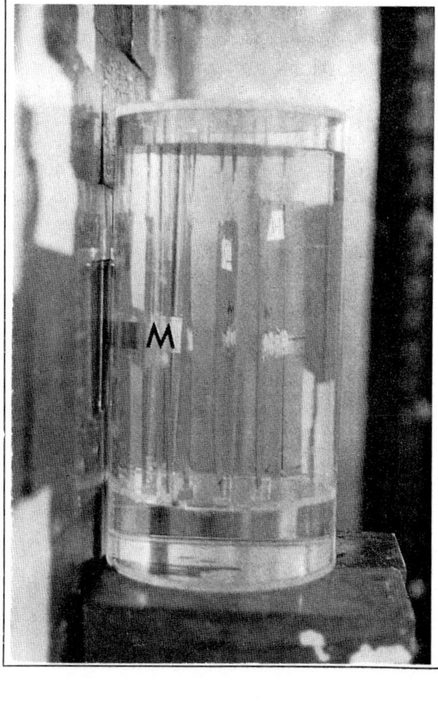
M

3

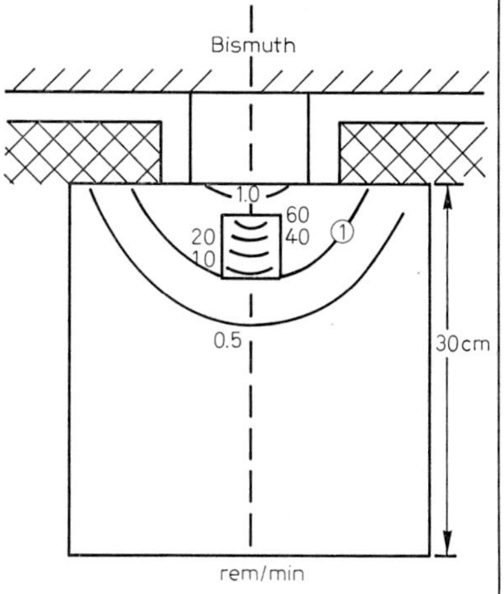
Bismuth
1.0
60
40
20
10
1
0.5
30cm
rem/min

4

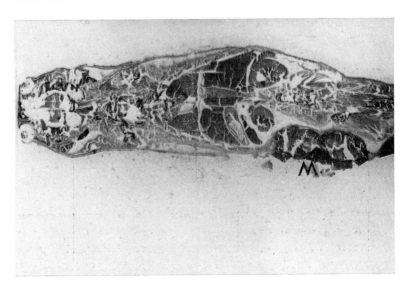

*Fig. 5.* A total body cryotome section of a Greene's malignant melanoma (M) bearing hamster into which a $^{10}$B compound was injected intraperitoneally. $\times$ 0.9.

with a relatively large amount of energy from the $^{10}$B activated by thermal neutron irradiation, can be revealed as $\alpha$-particle etch pits occurring on a cellulose nitrate film covering malignant melanoma tissue by the use of an $\alpha$-track method (fig. 6A). This Greene's melanoma-bearing Syrian golden hamster received a total dosage of 13.0 mg of $^{n}$B$_{12}$-chlorpromazine divided into three subcutaneous administrations. A high magnification (fig. 6B) of $\alpha$-particle etch pits actually occurring on a special cellulose nitrate film placed on a melanoma cryo-section induced by thermal neutron irradiation clearly exhibits trace lines of the particles.

Using the $\alpha$-track method, we have quantitated the population density of $\alpha$-particles occurring inside and outside of melanoma lesions. Figure 7 shows a sampling method for such determination of population density of $\alpha$-track etch pits in melanoma as compared with surrounding normal tissue. Figure 8A is one of the results revealing markedly greater density of $\alpha$-particles induced by the (n, $\alpha$) reaction occurring within melanoma. However, the population density obtained by the counting of etch pits represents a portion of the total (n, $\alpha$) reaction due to several factors limiting detecting efficiency. Figure 8B shows two of these factors presently being investigated with Dr. T. TSURUTA, a nuclear chemist, for the final

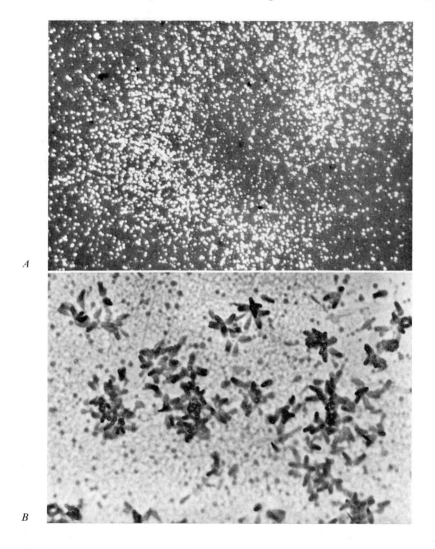

*Fig. 6.* α-Track method revealing the distribution and population density of α-particles and ⁷Li released by an (n, α) reaction resulting from thermal neutron irradiation on tissue treated with a ¹⁰B compound. *A* Low magnification using Kodak LR115, type II film. × 120. *B* Higher magnification using Kodak CA80-15 film clearly revealing trace lines of α-particles. × 1,225.

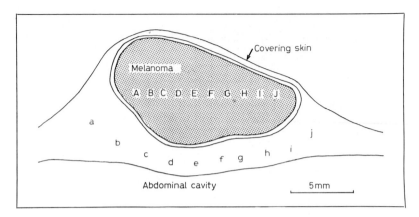

*Fig. 7.* Counting area for the population density of $\alpha$-track etch pits occurring in melanoma and surrounding normal tissue, using a total body cryotome section.

establishment of an (n, $\alpha$) reaction assay method. One of the factors is that due to the limitation of the traveling distance of $\alpha$-particles, they can be detected as etch pits on the film only if they have traveled within the critical angle toward the surface. Another factor shown is that due to the difference of surface etching speed G and pit etching speed T, we cannot detect $\alpha$-particles entering at an angle less than the critical angle $\Theta c$, and such geometrical determining efficiency $f_G$ can be expressed by the equation shown in the last line. With clarification of various factors limiting the detecting efficiency, the density distribution of the (n, $\alpha$) reaction or of $^{10}B$ molecules and the absolute amount of $^{10}B$ per unit of melanoma or other organ tissue can be obtained for finding optimum methods of thermal neutron capture treatment. The last factor limiting detection efficiency is that the absorption dose related to the energy rate, should be above the critical level to induce etch pits on a cellulose nitrate film (fig. 8C).

Based on the above findings, we have carried out 22 thermal neutron capture experiments irradiating Fortner's and Greene's melanotic melanoma subcutaneously proliferating in Syrian golden hamsters using a KUR Thermal Column of Nuclear Reactor with and without administration of $^{10}B$ compounds. Growth curves of control and irradiated melanotic malignant melanoma are expressed by individual tumor volume calculated by VAN WOERT and PALMER's [8] equation based on the actual three dimensional measurement of melanoma diameters every 24 h. In cooperation with Dr. K. KANDA and Prof. S. SHIBATA, nuclear physicists, we have

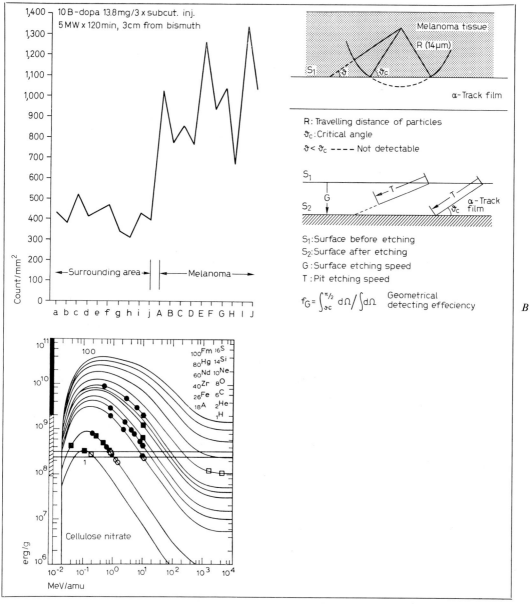

*Fig. 8. A* Population density of α-track etch pits occurring in melanoma lesions and surrounding normal subcutaneous tissue after thermal neutron irradiation. *B* Factors limiting the detecting efficiency of (n, α) reaction in counting α-particles and ⁷Li etch pits using the α-track method. *C* Absorption doses inducing etch on cellulose nitrate [KATZ, R. and KOBETICH, E. J.: Phys. Rev. *170:* 401–405 (1968)].

found that a dosage on the surface of the skin covering the melanoma, of $1.2 \times 10^{13}$ nvt to $1.9 \times 10^{13}$ nvt, which equals 5 MW for 90–120 min, is the range of optimum dosage in the present experimental system. Melanoma-bearing hamsters were held without anesthesia within a specially designed acrylic cage. These were placed directly in front of a bismuth plate in order to avoid an increase of gamma rays and to maintain constant high neutron dosage using a newer method of collimation [9], which employs not only a boron-containing polyethylene plate and a lead block, but also an LiF-containing collimator placed on the innermost layer, minimizing the secondary gamma rays.

One of the representative results of the experiments (fig. 9) shows that, as compared with a growth curve for a control melanoma group and for a melanoma group treated only by neutrons, a melanoma growth curve of thermal neutron-irradiated Greene's melanoma combined with $^{n}B_{12}$-chlorpromazine administration has resulted in maximum suppressive effect on the melanoma growth. One of the current results in the recent use of $^{10}B$-dopa borate is shown in (fig. 10).

The growth curves of both control melanoma groups show a steep linear increase in tumor volume 2–4 days after the irradiation date of the other groups. This is equivalent to 13–15 days after subcutaneous implantation of the melanoma. The growth curves of melanoma treated only by thermal neutron irradiation for 120 min at 5 MW show a suppressive effect, which however tends to be lost 6–7 days after irradiation; a linear increase again occurs as in the control groups. As compared with these two groups, the growth curves of melanoma treated with a combination of thermal neutron and $^{10}B$-compounds, particularly 12 mg of $^{n}B_{12}$-chlorpromazine (fig. 9), show a maximum and continuously longer suppressive effect.

Although neutron capture treatment with the present $^{10}B$ compounds is found to be a maximally effective method of melanoma treatment, the complete eradication of melanoma with a single neutron irradiation has not yet been achieved. One of the possible reasons for this is the uneven labelling of melanoma cells by $^{10}B$ compounds mostly due to the cell cycle of proliferating melanoma cells. In order to prevent non-labelling of new-

---

*Fig. 9.* Melanoma growth curves seen in Experiment No. 20 using 12 mg of $^{n}B_{12}$-chlorpromazine, equivalent to 3,000 $\mu$g of $^{10}B$.

*Fig. 10.* Melanoma growth curves seen in Experiment No. 18 using 27.6 mg of $^{10}B$-dopa, equivalent to 1,000 $\mu$g of $^{10}B$.

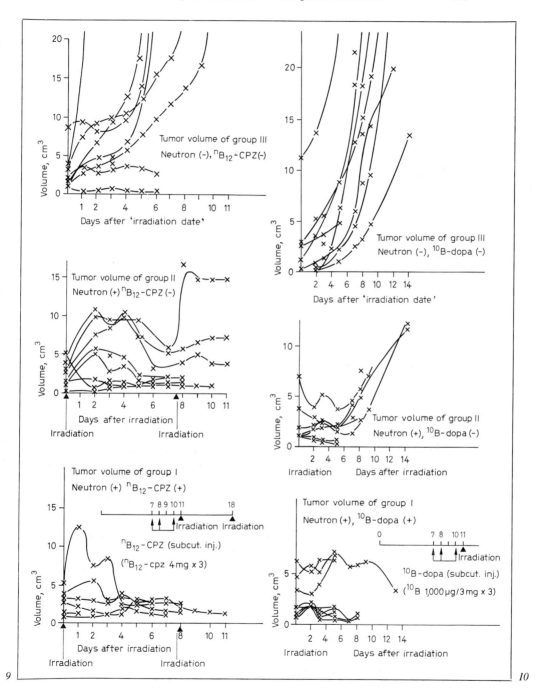

9

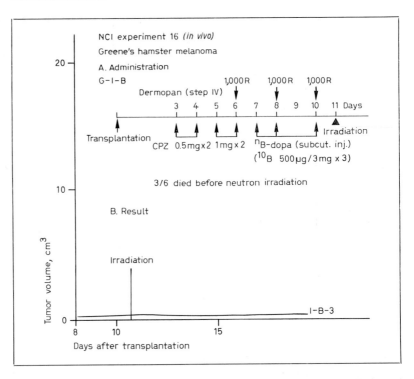

*Fig. 11.* Thermal neutron capture treatment using nB-dopa, with inhibition of cell mitosis by X-ray irradiation before and during its administration.

ly born post-mitotic melanoma cells with $^{10}$B, as shown in figure 11, we have treated melanoma with superficial X-ray to inhibit cell mitosis before and during the administration of $^{10}$B-dopa, and then thermal neutron capture treatment has been performed. Even though this is only a preliminary result, the greater and longer suppressive effect seen with this combination treatment suggests that the control of cell cycles, melanogenesis and other biological activities of melanoma cells, together with neutron capture treatment, can increase the efficiency of this new therapeutic modality.

The remaining foreseen problems can be divided into four major areas: (1) better collimation methods of thermal neutron beams with minimal occurrence of secondary gamma rays; (2) synthesis and condensation of $^{10}$B and of its better hybrid compounds with clarification of their metabolic pathways in the body; (3) the distribution of irradiation energy and induced $\alpha$-particles in relation to radiation damage of melanoma cells; and (4) the establishment of optimum methods of boron administration for various types of human melanoma lesions, leading to uniform distribution of $^{10}B$ atoms among melanoma cells. Our cooperative study groups are working presently on these problems with aid from the Japan Ministry of Education, Science and Culture to achieve the eradication of malignant melanoma.

## Summary

The absorption of thermal neutrons by the nonradioactive boron-10 isotope results in the emission of alpha particles and lithium atoms which share between them a relatively large energy transferred totally to tissue as shown in the following equation:

$$^{10}B + n \begin{cases} \rightarrow\, ^{7}Li + a + 2.79 \text{ MeV } (6.1\%) \\ \rightarrow\, ^{7}Li + a + 2.31 \text{ MeV } (93.9\%) \\ \rightarrow\, ^{7}Li + a + 0.48 \text{ MeV} \end{cases}$$

Since these particles have a relatively large size, the primary radiation injury is confined within a distance of 14 $\mu$m from the point of the activated boron atom. Melanin synthesis is specifically accentuated in most malignant melanoma cells. Therefore, by synthesizing molecular hybrid compounds between $^{10}B$ and chemicals which bind selectively with melanin, neutron capture treatment for melanoma has been developed. Since our last report, we have further developed $^{n}B_{10}$-chlorpromazine borane and $^{n}B_{12}$-chlorpromazine borane. For the eradication of relatively less pigmented but actively melanin-synthesizing post-mitotic or younger melanoma cells, we have also made $^{10}B$-dopa. Fortner's melanotic melanoma subcutaneously transplanted in hamsters and B-16 mouse melanoma have been irradiated by a Thermal Column of Nuclear Reactor at a dosage of $1.2 \times 10^{13}$ nvt/cm² on the skin surface covering the melanoma with and without administration of $^{10}B$-compounds. Findings show that neutron irradiation in addition to the compounds, most strongly depressed the growth rate of malignant melanoma, as compared with the control group and the group with only neutron irradiation.

## References

1    MISHIMA, Y.: Neutron capture treatment of malignant melanoma using $^{10}B$-chlorpromazine compound; in McGovern and Rusell Mechanisms in pigmentation. Proc. 8th Pigment Cell Conf., Sydney 1972. Pigment Cell, vol. 1, pp. 215–221 (Karger, Basel 1973).
2    MISHIMA, Y.: The effect of neutron capture treatment using $^{10}B$-chlorproma-

zine compound on malignant melanoma; in Proc. 2nd Meet. Biomed. Use of Nuclear Reactors, pp. 52–60 (University of Kyoto Press, Kumatori 1971).

3   Mishima, Y.: Precancerosis of pigment cells; in Okinaka Proc. 18th General Assembly Japan Medical Congress, Tokyo 1971, pp. 94–101 (Jap. Med. Ass., Tokyo 1972).

4   Entzian, W.; Soloway, A. H.; Raju, R.; Sweet, W. H., and Brownell, G. L.: Effect of neutron capture irradiation upon malignant brain tumors in mice. Acta radiol. 5: 95–100 (1966).

5   Hatanaka, H.; Soloway, A. H., and Sweet, W. H.: Incorporation of pyrimidines and boron analogues into brain tumor and brain tissue of mice. Neurochirurgia 10: 87–95 (1967).

6   Blois, M. S.: On chlorpromazine binding in vivo. J. Invest. Derm. 45: 475–481 (1965).

7   Sato, T.; Ono, K.; Kanda, K.; Shibata, S., and Mishima, Y.: Treatment of malignant melanoma by a nuclear reactor. II. Reactor radiation dosimetry in man-phantom. The 32nd Ann. Meet. Japanese Cancer Association, Tokyo 1973, p. 332.

8   Van Woert, M. H., and Palmer, S. H.: Inhibition of the growth of mouse melanoma by chlorpromazine. Cancer Res. 29: 1952–1955 (1969).

9   Kanda, K.; Kobayashi, T.; Ono, K.; Sato, T.; Shibata, S., and Mishima, Y.: Treatment of malignant melanoma by a nuclear reactor. I. Neutron irradiation and reactor physics. 32nd Ann. Meet. Japanese Cancer Association, Tokyo 1973, p. 331.

10  Nakagawa, T. and Aono, K.: Syntheses of chlorpromazine undecahydrododecaborate and nonahydrodecaborate – prosmising agents for neutron capture therapy of malignant melanoma. Chem. Pharm. Bull. 24: 778–781 (1976).

Prof. Dr. Yutaka Mishima, Department of Dermatology, Kobe University School of Medicine, 12 Kusuniki-cho 7-chome, Ikuta-ku, Kobe 650 (Japan)

Pigment Cell, vol. 2, pp. 407–413 (Karger, Basel 1976)

# Therapy of Malignant Melanoma with DTIC, Methyl CCNU, or BCG

*Progress Report*

L. Nathanson, M. Costanza, J. Wolter, J. Colsky, W. Regelson, N. Sedransk and T. Cunningham

Tufts New England Medical Center Hospital, Boston, Mass.

The majority of medically treated patients with metastatic and inoperable melanoma fail to show a dramatic clinical improvement with treatment [1]. In an attempt to improve the effectiveness of treatment, the Eastern Cooperative Oncology Group completed a large trial (EST, 1672) in which patients were randomized to receive either DTIC alone (200 mg/M2, i.v., q.d., × 5) or MeCCNU (200 mg/M2, p.o., × 1) or DTIC 150 mg/M2, i.v., q.d., × 5) plus MeCCNU (130 mg/M2 on day 2). The doses of MeCCNU were repeated every six weeks and those of DTIC every three weeks.

Separately randomized were patients with metastatic intradermal melanoma, with or without local or regional lymphoadenopathy, who had no clinically demonstrable evidence of visceral metastases. These patients with 'superficial disease' were given either intralesional doses of Tice BCG (approximately $3 \times 10^6$ CFU) or multipuncture intradermal Tice BCG (approximately $3 \times 10^7$ CFU) [2]. This paper is a progress report of the study as of November 1, 1974.

## Methods

Minimum requirements for admission to the trial included an expected survival greater than two months, a white blood count greater than 5000, a platelet count of 100,000 or greater, and a normal BUN. All patients had to have incurable, measurable, biopsy-proven, malignant melanoma. Base line studies included complete blood count, liver function tests, chest roentgenogram, metastatic skeletal survey, liver scan, chest laminograms, urinary melanogens, and tumor measurements. Drug dose modifications were stipulated if white count or platelet count fell below baseline minimum. No drug was given if the white count was below 3,000 or the platelet count 75,000.

Response to therapy was defined as follows: completed response – disappearance of all measurable disease for at least two observation periods for a minimum of at least two weeks. Partial response – 50% or greater decrease in the sum of the products of the diameters of all measurable lesions. Progression – documented increase in the size of measurable lesions, or appearance of new lesions.

## Results

270 patients were evaluable in the study as of November 1, 1974. Of these 85, 81, and 78 patients were randomized to DTIC, MeCCNU and the combination of the two agents, respectively, for a total of 244 patients in the 'internal disease' group. In the 'superficial disease' 14 and 12 patients, of the total 26 patients in this group, were randomized respectively to intralesional or multipuncture BCG.

Table I compares the characteristics of the patients on the three drug regimens, of the internal disease group. These are essentially similar with the single exception that the mean performance status appeared to be somewhat better for the MeCCNU group ($p < 0.01$). The majority of patients had visceral, bone and/or central nervous system metastases although a significant number had soft tissue (including lymph node) metastases only. It should be noted that the treatment given in this study was usually the first type of nonsurgical treatment which these patients had received.

In table II, toxicity with combination therapy (MeCCNU plus DTIC) is demonstrated. 'Toxicity index' is a measure of the average severity of each of any given toxic manifestation for the entire group of patients. Two patients died following drug treatment and their deaths may have been drug-related. One of these underwent severe bone marrow suppression, the other, severe hepatotoxicity. However, these were the only reported deaths. Toxicity indices for the three groups of patients in the 'internal disease' group were 1.13, 1.51, and 1.96, respectively, for DTIC, MeCCNU, and the combination-treated patients. Combination treatment therefore was shown to be slightly more toxic ($p < 0.01$) than any of the single drug programs, although the toxicity encountered was considered to be within tolerable limits.

12 of 79 (15.2%), 12 of 77 (15.6%), and 14 of 74 (18.9%), of patients receiving DTIC, MeCCNU, and combination therapy, respectively, demonstrated objective response. The slightly greater response for combination treatment was not statistically significantly different from that ob-

*Table I.* Patient characteristics

| | Number of 'internal disease' patients on treatment | | | |
| --- | --- | --- | --- | --- |
| | DTIC | MeCCNU | DTIC and MeCCNU | total |
| Extent of disease | | | | |
| Soft tissue only | 24 | 26 | 20 | 70 |
| Visceral, bone and/or CNS | 60 | 55 | 57 | 172 |
| Unknown | 1 | | 1 | 2 |
| Performance status | | | | |
| Ambulatory | 54 | 59 | 45 | 158 |
| Nonambulatory | 22 | 14 | 24 | 60 |
| Unknown | 9 | 8 | 9 | 26 |
| Mean performance status | (1.10) | (0.75) | (1.25) | (1.06) |
| Age, years | | | | |
| 10–29 | 9 | 9 | 17 | 35 |
| 30–49 | 30 | 34 | 23 | 87 |
| 50–69 | 36 | 30 | 39 | 105 |
| >70 | 9 | 6 | 9 | 24 |
| Unknown | 1 | 2 | 0 | 3 |
| Sex | | | | |
| Male | 48 | 49 | 42 | 139 |
| Female | 37 | 32 | 36 | 105 |
| Previous surgery | | | | |
| No | 17 | 16 | 10 | 43 |
| Yes | 68 | 65 | 68 | 201 |
| Previous irradiation | | | | |
| No | 71 | 66 | 70 | 207 |
| Yes | 14 | 15 | 8 | 37 |
| Previous chemotherapy | | | | |
| No | 78 | 75 | 67 | 220 |
| Yes | 7 | 6 | 11 | 24 |
| Urinary melanogen | | | | |
| Initially − | 17 | 7 | 17 | 41 |
| Initially + | 9 | 5 | 6 | 20 |
| Studies | | | | |
| Not done | 50 | 55 | 37 | 142 |
| Unknown | 9 | 14 | 18 | 41 |
| Studies repeated | 8 | 6 | 5 | 19 |

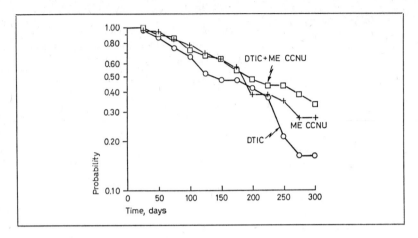

*Fig. 1.* Survival from start of therapy – 'internal disease' group.

*Table II.* Toxicity with combination therapy, MeCCNU, plus DTIC (number of 'internal disease' patients)

|  | Mild | Moderate | Severe | Life-thr. | Lethal | Toxicity index |
|---|---|---|---|---|---|---|
| Vomiting | 18 | 26 | 7 | 0 | 0 | 1.17 |
| Other GI (incl. diarrhea) | 3 | 3 | 0 | 0 | 0 | 0.12 |
| Skin | 1 | 0 | 1 | 0 | 0 | |
| Hematologic | 7 | 10 | 12 | 7 | 1 | 1.21 |
| Other | 4 | 2 | 0 | 0 | 1 | 0.17 |
| Worst toxicity | 15 | 25 | 18 | 6 | 2 | 1.96 |

served in patients treated with a single drug ($p < 0.1$). However, of great significance was the fact that 43% of patients undergoing objective response to combination treatment had a 'complete' response, whereas the same was true in only 17 and 25% of patients treated with DTIC, MeCCNU, respectively. 'Complete' response tends to be associated with a better quality of response than 'partial' response. Median duration for response ranged from 100 to 110 'plus' days. It was clearly demonstrated that patients who were considered 'nonambulatory' had an extremely short survival (none longer than 250 days) and may be assumed to have achieved no benefit from treatment. Figure 1 is a life table analysis of all ambulatory patients with internal disease in the treated groups. Patients

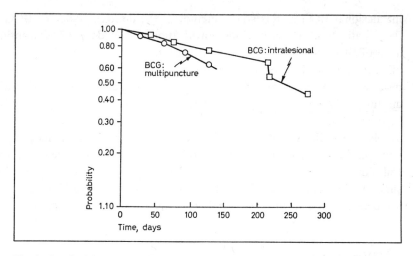

*Fig. 2.* Survival from start of therapy – 'superficial disease' group.

*Table III.* Toxicity with intra-lesional BCG (number of 'superficial disease' patients)

|  | Mild | Mode-rate | Severe | Life-thr. | Lethal | Toxicity index |
|---|---|---|---|---|---|---|
| Vomiting | 1 | 2 | 1 | 0 | 0 | 0.67 |
| Other GI (incl. diarrhea) | 0 | 1 | 0 | 0 | 0 | 0.17 |
| Infection | 1 | 0 | 1 | 0 | 0 | 0.33 |
| Skin | 2 | 0 | 1 | 0 | 0 | 0.42 |
| Hematologic | 0 | 2 | 0 | 0 | 0 | 0.33 |
| Liver | 0 | 1 | 1 | 0 | 0 | 0.42 |
| Other | 1 | 7 | 2 | 0 | 0 | 1.75 |
| Worst toxicity | 1 | 9 | 2 | 0 | 0 | 2.083 |

who underwent combination treatment appear to have a slightly better, but not statistically significantly different ($p < 0.1$), survival than those treated with single drug therapy.

The type of treatment with intralesional BCG, given to the superficial disease category of patients, has received a good deal of criticism because of significant toxicity. Table III summarizes the toxicity seen in intralesional treated patients; no patient suffered life-threatening or lethal toxicity. A significant number of patients did experience fever (listed under 'other' toxicity), local skin manifestations, nausea, vomiting, or anorexia. It should be noted that several important principles governed the use of intralesional BCG in this study, including: (1) discontinuance of BCG in those patients in whom obvious sensitization was evident; (2) discontinuance of BCG in patients in whom visceral metastases were noted; (3) termination of BCG in patients in whom obvious evidence of progressive disease took place. In any patient in whom fever persisted, treatment with antitubercular chemotherapy was carried out; all such therapy proved to be successful.

Figure 2 illustrates the survival curves of the small number of patients in the 'superficial disease' section of the study. The patients with intralesional treatment, although they seem to have a slightly greater initial survival than those treated with multipuncture intradermal BCG, have not been accrued in sufficient numbers to demonstrate any differences.

## Discussion

Although there were no significant differences noted in the three drug regimens used to treat patients with visceral metastases, some interesting observations may be made. First, in such patients with visceral metastases, who had ambulatory status at the time of onset of the study, a slight superiority of survival appears to be present in the patients given combination therapy. In addition, the response rate, and of greater importance, the percentage of responding patients who underwent complete response, was greater than for patients receiving single drug therapy. Toxicity was somewhat more severe in the combination treatment program, but appeared to be within acceptable limits.

Among the patients with intradermal metastases only, treated with BCG, there are too few patients to tell whether intralesional therapy may be superior to intradermal therapy. However, it would appear that intralesional therapy did not produce intolerable toxicity, when used with care. It is hoped that statistically significant data may be achieved in this latter category of patients in the near future.

## Summary

270 patients with metastatic malignant melanoma were separated into categories of 'internal disease' (visceral involvement) and 'superficial disease' (regional intradermal or lymph node metastases). Patients in the former group were treated

with either DTIC, Methyl CCNU or the combination of these two agents. Slightly, but not statistically significantly, superior survival was seen in the patients treated with the combination of the two agents. Toxicity was also slightly greater for the combination treatment regimen. Patients in the 'superficial disease' category were treated with either intralesional BCG, or intradermal BCG at an indifferent skin site. Both BCG immunotherapy programs appeared to be tolerable, but the number of patients on study was too few to determine whether a difference between survival in the two treatment categories was present.

## Acknowledgments

This paper is supported in part by the US Public Health Service Grant numbers CA 07190 (Tufts), CA 10948 (Rush-Presbyterian), CA 10572 (Medical College of Virginia), CA 06594 (Albany Medical College).

This is a publication of the Eastern Cooperative Oncology Group, PAUL P. CARBONE, MD, Chairman. Other investigators include: NEIL ABRAMSON, MD, University of Florida, Jacksonville; JOHN M. BENNETT, MD, University of Rochester School of Medicine and Dentistry; ISADOR BRODSKY, MD, Hahnemann Medical College Hospital; HARVEY S. BRODOVSKY, MD, Jefferson Medical College; S. FRED BRUNK, MD, University of Iowa; MARTIN COHEN, MD, National Cancer Institute; RICHARD A. COOPER, MD, University of Pennsylvania; FRANK J. CUMMINGS, MD, Brown University; RONALD DECONTI, MD, Springfield Hospital Medical Center; WILLIAM D. DEWYS, MD, Northwestern Medical Center; EDIZ Z. EZDINLI, MD, Chicago Medical School; BERNARD FISHER, MD, University of Pittsburgh; DAVID J. KLAASSEN, MD, University of Ottawa; RAYMOND E. LENHARD, MD, Johns Hopkins Hospital; HARVEY J. LERNER, MD, Pennsylvania Hospital; MARTIN LEVITT, MD, University of Manitoba; EDWARD G. MANSOUR, MD, Case Western Reserve University; ARNOLD MITTELMAN, MD, Roswell Park Memorial Institute; FRANCO MUGGIA, MD, Albert Einstein College of Medicine; RICHARD A. OBERFIELD, MD, Lahey Clinic Foundation; ALBERT SCHILLING, MD, Boston University Medical Center; BRUCE I. SHNIDER, MD, Georgetown University School of Medicine; ROBERT SILBER, MD, New York University Medical Center; ROLAND T. SKEEL, MD, Yale School of Medicine; MARK S. TOBIN, MD, Brookdale Hospital Center; STANLEY ZUCKER, MD, State University of New York.

## References

1   COSTANZA, M. E.; NATHANSON, L., et al.: Therapy of malignant melanoma with imidazole carboxamide and bis-chloroethyl nitrosourea. Cancer 30: 1457–1461 (1972).
2   NATHANSON, L.: Use of BCG in the treatment of human tumors. Sem. Oncol. 1: 337–350 (1974).

L. NATHANSON, MD, Tufts New England Medical Center Hospital, 171 Harrison Avenue, Boston, MA 02111 (USA)

Pigment Cell, vol. 2, pp. 414–420 (Karger, Basel 1976)

# The Current Rapid Increase in Incidence and Mortality from Malignant Melanoma in Developed Societies

J. A. H. LEE

Department of Epidemiology and International Health (SC-36), School of Public Health and Community Medicine, University of Washington, Seattle, Wash.

## Registry Data

In systems of cancer registration, the reported incidence of malignant melanoma has been rising rapidly in recent years. Table I shows the data for Connecticut [6] where the rate in males has gone from 24 per million in the early 1950s to 66 per million in the early 1970s. In females, the rate has gone from 30 per million to 54 per million in the same period. This is a typical finding. There is a similar increase between the Second [12] and Third [19] National Cancer Surveys and in Upper New York State [24] and Alameda County, Calif. [1]. Similar increases have been found in the experience of registries in the Scandinavian countries [5, 20], and in Britain [21]. Thus, the phenomenon appears to be a rather general one. Cancer registries can only record the data that are sent to them, and it is possible that such a rise could be largely the result of the diagnosis being made more frequently or recorded better [9]. The diagnosis is essentially a microscopic one, and there has been a large increase in the number of such examinations of tissue in recent years.

## Mortality Data

The death rate certified to malignant melanoma has also risen rapidly in recent years. For example, the rates for malignant melanoma and for other skin tumors for Canada for males are shown in table II [23]. Similar data are shown for England and Wales in table III [22]. The

Table I. Incidence of malignant melanoma[1], all sites combined (Connecticut 1950–1972)

| | 1950–54 | 1955–59 | 1960–64 | 1965–69 | 1970–72 | Annual % change 1950–54 to 1970–72 |
|---|---|---|---|---|---|---|
| Male | 24.0 | 38.3 | 43.2 | 43.1 | 66.1 | +9 |
| Female | 29.8 | 35.9 | 40.7 | 47.7 | 54.3 | +4 |

1 All rates in tables I–IV are per million per year, and are age adjusted to the standard UICC European population. Differences in the age distributions of the different geographical populations referred to, between males and females, and within the broad age groups compared have thus been eliminated.

Table II. Death rates for primary skin tumors by type and sex (Canada 1951–1955 and 1966–1970[1])

| | 1951–55 | 1966–60 | Annual % change |
|---|---|---|---|
| *Male* | | | |
| Melanoma | 7.1 | 13.7 | +6 |
| Other | 19.6 | 14.9 | −2 |
| All primary skin | 26.7 | 28.6 | +1 |
| *Female* | | | |
| Melanoma | 5.9 | 12.2 | +7 |
| Other | 11.3 | 7.0 | −3 |
| All primary skin | 17.2 | 19.2 | +1 |

1 The time periods used for the mortality tables II, III, and IV conform to the British series from 1911 [4]. The Connecticut time periods are those used by the Registry. US melanoma mortality data have only been tabulated by age since 1967 [16].

Table III. Death rates from primary skin tumors by type and sex (England and Wales 1951–1970)

| | 1951–55 | 1966–70 | Annual % change |
|---|---|---|---|
| *Male* | | | |
| Melanoma | 6.8 | 10.6 | +4 |
| Other | 21.8 | 12.2 | −3 |
| All primary skin | 28.6 | 22.2 | −1 |
| *Female* | | | |
| Melanoma | 7.2 | 10.8 | +3 |
| Other | 11.9 | 6.4 | −3 |
| All primary skin | 19.1 | 17.2 | −1 |

rise in the melanoma rate in Canada has more than compensated for the decline in the mortality certified to other skin tumors so that the total mortality from all primary neoplasms of skin has risen over this period in Canada. There has been a bigger decline in the other skin tumors in Britain, so that the compensatory effect of the melanomas has not quite prevented a decline there (table III). The experience of the US white population has been intermediate between the Canadian and British, with a slightly larger decline in the rates for other skin cancers than a rise in the melanomas [15]. Certification of death to the squamous cell and basal cell carcinomas is, of course, highly unreliable [7].

Mortality data are important complements to registration data. The sources of error are different, and it is unlikely that many fatal terminations of the course of melanoma were not recorded 20 years ago in these countries. Thus, both incidence data from limited areas and mortality data from whole countries show the same rapid rise in the incidence of malignant melanoma in prosperous white populations.

### The Influence of Age

The change in the mortality from tumors of skin in Canada is selective by age. For the totality of primary tumors of skin (table IV), the young males have a remarkable rise which carries through to middle

Table IV. Death rates from all primary tumors of skin and percent change, by age and sex (Canada 1951–1955 and 1966–1970)

| Age years | 1951–55 | 1966–70 | Annual % change |
|-----------|---------|---------|-----------------|
| *Male* | | | |
| 15–44 | 5.2 | 7.9 | +3 |
| 45–64 | 25.2 | 34.5 | +2 |
| 65 and over | 164.5 | 151.4 | −1 |
| All ages | 26.7 | 28.6 | 0 |
| *Female* | | | |
| 15–44 | 4.8 | 7.9 | +4 |
| 45–64 | 18.8 | 26.2 | +3 |
| 65 and over | 97.2 | 83.6 | −1 |
| All ages | 17.2 | 19.2 | +1 |

age, and in the 65-year-olds and older, there has been an actual decline. A similar pattern is found for Canadian females. Lethal squamous cell tumors occur at a much greater average age than lethal melanomas. It is clear from both the actual certification and the age distribution that these changes are being produced by a change in the incidence of malignant melanoma. The pattern is similar in the US [15] and is of long duration [11, 12, 16].

These changes are the result of differences between successive birth cohorts in their long-term risk of dying of skin cancer [8, 12, 16]. There is no reason to suppose that any change in diagnosis or certification would produce a pattern that was ordered in terms of birth cohorts, and the age specificity of the changes in total mortality from all primary neoplasms of skin is further evidence for the biological reality of the reported rapid rise in the incidence of malignant melanoma.

### Trends by Site

Malignant melanoma behaves in a paradoxical way in that there is ample evidence that direct exposure to sunlight is important as an etiological factor (the high rates for exposed sites in the sex whose habits of dress or hairstyle produce this, i.e. lower limbs in females; ears, scalp, and neck in males [3, 14, 18], but, at the same time, there are factors which insure that the distribution by site of malignant melanoma is fairly independent of wide changes in the incidence [13, 17]. The incidence of malignant melanoma of the head and neck in males has approximately doubled in the last 20 years in Connecticut (table V), while the incidence in females has remained stable. In contrast, the incidence of melanomas of the trunk has increased 3-fold in males in the same period in Connecticut (table V), while showing a much smaller rise in females. Excess of tumors of the lower limb in females was present in the early 1950s (table V) and this has changed little, although the rates for the lower limb have risen drastically in both sexes. It could be thought that the excess of tumors of the lower limb in females might be due to a confusion with nevi removed for cosmetic reasons, although there is no excess in the reported incidence of melanoma on the female face. Mortality data are sufficiently well certified to site in Britain (table VI) for analysis and the excess mortality of females from melanomas of the lower limb are clearly shown (table VI).

*Table V.* Incidence of melanoma by site and sex (Connecticut 1950–1972)

|  | 1950–54 | 1955–59 | 1960–64 | 1965–69 | 1970–72 | Annual % change 1950–54 to 1970–72 |
|---|---|---|---|---|---|---|
| *Head and neck* | | | | | | |
| Male | 6.7 | 5.5 | 9.1 | 10.0 | 14.3 | +9 |
| Female | 7.1 | 4.9 | 7.4 | 7.5 | 7.3 | 0 |
| *Trunk* | | | | | | |
| Male | 8.9 | 10.5 | 16.7 | 17.5 | 27.4 | +11 |
| Female | 7.5 | 8.8 | 8.9 | 11.5 | 11.9 | +3 |
| *Upper limb* | | | | | | |
| Male | 1.8 | 3.6 | 6.3 | 10.1 | 14.6 | +37 |
| Female | 2.8 | 4.4 | 7.4 | 9.9 | 13.4 | +20 |
| *Lower limb* | | | | | | |
| Male | 2.7 | 5.3 | 6.4 | 8.3 | 8.5 | +11 |
| Female | 9.0 | 11.1 | 13.5 | 18.5 | 20.6 | +7 |
| *Site unspecified* | | | | | | |
| Male | 5.4 | 8.5 | 4.7 | 2.0 | 1.3 | −4 |
| Female | 3.4 | 6.6 | 3.6 | 0.3 | 1.1 | −4 |

*Table VI.* Death rates from malignant melanoma of the lower limb by sex (England and Wales, 1958–1972)

|  | 1958–62 | 1963–67 | 1968–72 | Annual % change |
|---|---|---|---|---|
| Male | 2.4 | 2.6 | 2.5 | 0 |
| Female | 5.6 | 7.5 | 10.7 | +9 |

## Conclusion

The incidence and mortality of malignant melanoma are rising. This rise is selective for particular age groups, and is interpretable in terms of differences between cohorts. It is selective for particular sites. The changes occur in a number of developed white populations, including the Australians [2]. It is clear that these are not, to any substantial extent, artifacts of certification.

Our ignorance of the factors in a patient's way of life which lead to the development of malignant melanoma is nearly total. We know that exposure to sunlight is important, but the tiny amount of evidence that is available suggests that occupational exposure is very much less important for malignant melanomas than it is for the squamous and basal cell carcinomas. There is need to divert a modest amount of medical effort and resources to establishing the place of leisure-time pursuits, vacations in the sun, and other factors relevant to the genesis of malignant melanoma. A pioneering study [10] appears to be a unique application of modern case-control methods. Even that was based on a total of only 79 patients and made no attempt at a division by site. We are, at the moment, unable to offer useful advice on the prevention of these tumors or of establishing, on any rational basis, the identification of groups at special risk who could be helped by information directed specifically to them.

## Summary

In the US white population, and in Canada and Britain, mortality from primary malignant tumors of skin is approximately stable, as the number of elderly people certified as dying from squamous cell carcinomas declines, the number of young people certified as dying of malignant melanoma rises. Melanoma incidence rates are also rising, and the trends are long-term. There seems no doubt that the changes observed in hospital, registry, and mortality experience are the result of a genuine and large rise in the incidence of malignant melanoma. The sites showing the greatest change are trunk in males and lower limb in females. The explanation of these changes must come from orderly clinical observations of cases and control subjects.

## References

1   Alameda, California: Unpublished data.
2   BEARDMORE, G. L.: The epidemiology of malignant melanoma in Australia, in McCARTHY Melanoma and skin diseases (Government Printer, Sydney 1972).
3   BODENHAM, D. C.: A study of 650 observed malignant melanomas in the South-West Region. Ann. R. Coll. Surg. 43: 218 (1968).
4   CASE, R. A. M. and PEARSON, J. T.: Cancer statistics for England and Wales 1901–1955 (HMSO, London 1957).
5   CLEMMESEN, J.: Statistical studies in the aetiology of malignant neoplasms. IV. Lung/bladder ratio, Denmark, 1943–1967 (Munksgaard, Copenhagen 1974).
6   Connecticut State Department of Health: Cancer in Connecticut, Incidence and rates 1935–1962 (1966); Cancer in Connecticut 1963 (n.d.); Cancer in Connecticut 1964 (n.d.); Cancer in Connecticut 1965 (n.d.); Cancer in Con-

necticut 1966–1968 (1971). Hartford, Connecticut, State Department of Health, 1966–1971, also unpublished tables.

7   DUNN, J. E.; LEVIN, E. A.; LINDEN, G., et al.: Skin cancer as a cause of death. Calif. Med. 102: 361–363 (1965).

8   ELWOOD, J. M. and LEE, J. A. H.: Trends in mortality from primary tumors of skin in Canada. Can. med. Ass. J. 110: 913–915 (1974).

9   End Results Group: End results in cancer, Report No. 4 (National Cancer Institute, USDHEW, Washington 1972).

10  GELLIN, G. A.; KOPF, A. W., and GARFINKL, L.: Malignant melanoma. A controlled study of possibly associated factors. Archs Derm. 99: 43–48 (1969).

11  GORDON, T.; CRITTENDEN, M., and HAENSZEL, W.: End results and mortality trends in cancer. National Cancer Institute Monogr. No. 6, pp. 262–267 (US-DHEW, Washington 1961).

12  HAENSZEL, W.: Variation in skin cancer incidence within the United States; in URBACH Conf. on Biology of Cutaneous Cancer. pp 225–243) National Cancer Institute Monogr. No. 10 (USDHEW, Washington 1963).

13  LANCASTER, H. O. and NELSON, J.: Sunlight as a cause of melanoma. A clinical survey. Med. J. Aust. i: 452 (1957).

14  LEE, J. A. H.: Fatal melanoma of the lower limbs and other sites. An epidemiologic study. J. natn. Cancer Inst. 44: 257–261 (1970).

15  LEE, J. A. H.: The Trend of mortality from primary malignant tumors of skin. J. Invest. Derm. 59: 445–448 (1973).

16  LEE, J. A. H. and CARTER, A. P.: Secular trends in mortality from malignant melanoma. J. natn. Cancer Inst. 45: 91–97 (1970).

17  LEE, J. A. H. and MERRILL, J. M.: Sunlight and the aetiology of malignant melanoma. A synthesis. Med. J. Aust. ii: 846–851 (1970).

18  LEE, J. A. H. and YONGCHAIYUDHA, S.: Incidence of and mortality from malignant melanoma by anatomical site. J. natn. Cancer Inst. 47: 253–263 (1971).

19  National Cancer Institute, Biometry Branch: Preliminary Report, Third National Cancer Survey, 1969 Incidence. Publication No. 72–128 (USDHEW, Washington 1971).

20  Norway Cancer Registry: Trends in cancer incidence in Norway 1955–1967 (Universitetsforlaget, Oslo 1972).

21  Registrar General: Statistical review of England and Wales. Tables, part I (HMSO, London 1953–1972).

22  Registrar General: Statistical review of England and Wales for the two years 1966–1967. Supplement on Cancer (HMSO, London 1972).

23  Statistics Canada: Causes of death: Canada.

24  Upper New York State: Unpublished data.

J. A. H. LEE, MD, Department of Epidemiology and International Health (SC-36), School of Public Health and Community Medicine, University of Washington, Seattle, WA 98195 (USA)

Pigment Cell, vol. 2, pp. 421–426 (Karger, Basel 1976)

# Familial Melanoma [1]

C. M. SUTHERLAND, H. W. KLOEPFER, P. W. A. MANSELL and
E. T. KREMENTZ

Tulane University School of Medicine, Department of Surgery,
New Orleans, La.

## Introduction

Over the past several years, 2 patients with malignant melanoma
have been referred to the Tulane Clinical Cancer Research Center, both
of whom had 3 similarly affected siblings. These 2 families have
prompted our investigation into the genetics of malignant melanoma of
the skin in man.

Familial occurrence of malignant melanoma of the skin was first reported by CAWLEY [4] in 1952. Numerous other families with malignant
occurrence have since been reported [3, 5, 7, 10–12], and large series of
patients have been analyzed for the occurrence of familial disease [2, 8,
9, 14, 15]. These surveys have shown that 1 to 7% of the total patients
have given information of relatives with malignant melanoma. Analyses
of familial patients indicate that these patients are younger, have a
greater tendency toward multiple primaries, and survive longer [1, 13].
It has not been established whether these observations are artifactual
based on the method of data collection or whether true differences exist.

A genetic evaluation of one of the families has been carried out and
is reported. The pedigree of this family is listed in figure 1. The second
family lives out of state and, since this investigation has not been completed, will not be reported.

1   This work has been supported by US Public Health Service Grant Nos.
CA05837-12 and CA05108-12, by the J. Douglas Eustis Fund for Cancer Research, and by the Ladies Auxialiary of the Veterans of Foreign Wars.

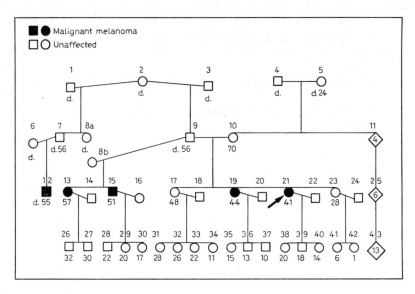

*Fig. 1.* Pedigree showing occurrence of malignant melanoma. The number above the symbol identifies the individual; the number below the symbol represents the age or age at death; number within a diamond-shaped symbol indicates the number of individuals. Males = □; females = O.

## Case Reports

Case No. 21 (J. G.) is a 41-year-old Caucasian female who developed a malignant melanoma of the left leg in 1968. She was treated with melphalan by a common femoral perfusion, wide excision of the primary, skin graft, and groin dissection. In 1972, she developed another primary malignant melanoma of the back and a separate new malignant melanoma of the left lateral thigh, both of which were widely excised. She developed a fourth primary of the right upper abdominal wall which was widely excised on Nov. 15, 1973. She has since remained free of disease after being treated for 4 separate primary melanomas.

Case No. 13 (C. A.) is a 57-year-old half-sister of J. G. In November 1973, at age 55, she developed a malignant melanoma of the right shoulder. She was treated by wide excision of the primary lesion, and remains free of disease to date.

Case No. 15 (A. M.) is a 51-year-old half-brother of J. G. This patient developed a malignant melanoma of the left shoulder in 1958, at the age of 33. He was treated by wide excision of the primary lesion and has since remained in good health.

Case No. 19 (D. H.) is a 44-year-old full-sister of J. G. In 1968, she developed a malignant melanoma of the dorsum of the middle of the left foot. She was treated by femoral perfusion with melphalan, groin dissection, and disarticulation of the third and fourth digits. She has remained well since.

Case No. 12 (J. R.) was a first cousin of J. G. This patient developed a malignant melanoma of the back in 1956, at the age of 45, which was treated by local excision. At age 47, he developed a second primary of the left forearm, which also was treated with local excision. During the next several years, he developed local recurrence and systemic disease. He died of metastatic disease in 1966.

## Materials and Methods

Since 1972, all newly referred patients have been interviewed by trained personnel utilizing a questionnaire designed to elicit basic data on all patients concerning possible pertinent features of historical, environmental, familial, and physical nature. These records have been examined for incidence of melanoma and other cancers from which the patient's relatives may have suffered. We presently maintain data, collected from 1972 to early 1974, on 193 patients in this group. Before 1972, records are available on approximately 800 patients seen at Tulane since 1957. However, these data vary in completeness, but have been examined for histories of melanoma in the families of patients with this disease.

No systematic attempt has been made to re-interview all of the 193 patients from whom we have collected questionnaires since 1972. Many of the patients are dead and others live long distances from New Orleans. We have therefore chosen to limit further inquiries to those patients geographically situated near our facility. To date, 12 of the 193 patients have had a second interview at the time of their follow-up visits.

## Results

An analysis of the questionnaires revealed that 14 of 193 patients gave a positive response to the question of a history of melanoma in their families. Two of these patients were husband and wife, and further analysis has not been achieved. One patient with malignant melanoma of the eye gave a history of having a paternal grandfather with a similar lesion. However, ocular melanoma will not be analyzed in this report. Nine families are represented in the remaining 11 patients. Two patients have a brother-sister and 2 patients have a father-daughter relationship. The patients' ages at diagnosis, sites of primaries, and relatives affected with malignant melanoma, are listed in table I. These 11 patients represent 5.7% of the total number of cases studied. Eight of the patients have listed first-degree relatives as the affected family member.

A search of older records revealed an additional 7 patients who in-

*Table I.* Indicating patients with a family history of melanoma with the age at diagnosis, site of primary lesion, and the affected relative

| No. | Patient | Age at diagnosis | Site of primary | Relative with malignant melanoma |
|-----|---------|------------------|-----------------|----------------------------------|
| 1   | K.J.    | 51               | arm             | father of No. 3                  |
| 2   | S.T.    | 18               | arm             | paternal grandfather             |
| 3   | M.J.    | 18               | shoulder        | daughter of No. 1                |
| 4   | L.C.    | 66               | ear             | sister                           |
| 5   | P.E.    | 31               | chest           | brother is No. 10                |
| 6   | F.C.    | 44               | leg             | father                           |
| 7   | J.S.    | 60               | arm             | brother                          |
| 8   | L.F.    | 57               | leg             | nephew                           |
| 9   | J.T.    | 46               | back            | brother                          |
| 10  | D.L.    | 22               | arm             | sister is No. 5                  |
| 11  | T.R.    | 46               | thigh           | uncle                            |

dicated that they had similarly affected relatives. Also, one patient from this group (E. G., age 31 at diagnosis) who previously had no known familial involvement, recently brought her mother (C. G, 70 years old) to be treated for a malignant melanoma of the leg.

Further questioning of the 12 patients studied as they have returned for follow-up has revealed an additional 2 patients with similarly affected relatives. One patient (A. C.) has a great uncle who had melanoma, and the other (P. C.) has a great aunt who had melanoma. Neither patient had known of their affected relative and only after our prompting them to query their family members did these cases become known. The addition of these 2 patients brings the total of patients with affected families to 13 of 193 (6.7%) of the total.

An interesting ancillary finding in the 193 cases studied since 1972 revealed a positive response to family histories of cancer in 4 patients who listed relatives with either bone or soft tissue sarcomas.

## Discussion

It has been accepted that individuals of different ethnic origin have varying predilection for developing malignant melanoma [6, 13]. Preliminary data at our institution seem to substantiate this observation. Death rates from malignant melanoma in Louisiana for Negroes is approximately 0.4/100,000/year. Death rates from malignant melanoma for

Caucasians in Northern Louisiana is approximately 2.4/100,000/year, while that for Caucasians in the parishes along the Mississippi delta is 1.2/100,000/year. These figures are obtained by using the 1970 US Census and the deaths by parish from malignant melanoma for 1960–69. It is our observation that the northern portion of Louisiana has a greater abundance of fair-haired, fair-complexioned people of Northern European, Scottish, or Irish ancestry, while that of Southern Louisiana is more heavily populated with people of Southern European ancestry – particularly French and Spanish.

The extent and mechanisms by which the genetic factors express themselves are unclear. It is anticipated that by studying patients with familial melanoma that additional knowledge can be obtained. Other studies of this ntaure have recognized that these cases with which they were dealing were a minimal number of the total. Our experiences have clearly been the same. The number of patients with similarly affected relatives seems to be proportional to the amount of time spent in obtaining a pedigree history. At any given time, patients have limited knowledge about disease which occurs in their relatives. A full understanding as to the genetics of malignant melanoma will not be known until a relatively large number of patients have been thoroughly investigated as to pedigree information and diseases of family members.

### Conclusion

1. A pedigree of a kindred has been presented indicating the relationship of 4 siblings and a first cousin who have had a total of 9 primary malignant melanomas.

2. The number of patients found to have malignant melanoma with similarly affected family members is proportional to the amount of knowledge obtained about the relatives.

3. A possible familial connection between bone, soft tissue sarcomas, and malignant melanoma is suggested.

### Summary

A series of cases has been analyzed for the occurrence of malignant melanoma in relatives. When routine records are maintained, an incidence of approximately 1% of cases can be found to be familial. When specific questions are asked to all patients, the incidence rises to about 6% of all cases. Information obtained in this manner on secondary cases provides minimal information with regard to the incidence of disease occurring in relatives. Preliminary work suggests that many more patients have malignant melanoma in their families than has previously been recognized.

## References

1  ANDERSON, D. E.: Clinical characteristics of the genetic variety of cutaneous melanoma in man. Cancer 28: 721–725 (1971).

2  ANDERSON, D. E.; SMITH, J. L., and McBRIDE, C. M.: Hereditary aspects of malignant melanoma. J. Am. med. Ass. 200: 741–746 (1967).

3  ANDREWS, J. C.: Malignant melanoma in siblings. Archs Derm. 98: 282–283 (1968).

4  CAWLEY, E. P.: Genetic aspects of malignant melanoma. Archs Derm. 65: 440–450 (1952).

5  KATZENELLENBOGEN, I. and SANDBANK, M.: Malignant melanoma in twins. Archs Derm. 94: 331–332 (1966).

6  LANE BROWN, M. M.; SHARPE, C. A. B.; MacMILLAN, D. S., and McGOVERN, V. J.: Genetic predisposition to melanoma and other skin cancers in Australia. Med. J. Aust. i: 852–853 (1971).

7  LYNCH, H. T. and KRUSH, A. J.: Heredity and malignant melanoma. Can. med. Ass. J. 99: 17–21 (1968).

8  MILLER, T. R. and PACK, G. T.: The familial aspect of malignant melanoma. Archs Derm. 86: 83–89 (1962).

9  SALAMON, T.; SCHNYDER, U. W., and STORCK, H.: A contribution to the question of heredity of malignant melanomas. Dermatologica 126: 65–75 (1963).

10  SCHOCH, E. P.: Familial malignant melanoma. Archs Derm. 88: 445–455 (1963).

11  SMITH, F. E.; HENLY, W. S.; KNOX, J. M., and LANE, M.: Familial melanoma. Archs intern. Med. 117: 820–823 (1966).

12  ST.-ARNEAULT, G.; NAGEL, G.; KIRKPATRICK, D.; KIRKPATRICK, R., and HOLLAND, J. F.: Cutaneous malignant melanoma in identical twins from a set of triplets. Cancer 25: 672–677 (1970).

13  TURKINGTON, R. W.: Familial factor in malignant melanoma. J. Am. med. Ass. 192: 85–90 (1965).

14  WALLACE, D. G. and EXTON, L. A.: Genetic predisposition to development of malignant melanoma. Melanoma and skin cancer. Proc. Cancer Conf. Sydney 1972 (U. C. N. Blight, Sydney 1972).

15  WALLACE, D. C.; EXTON, L. A., and McLEOD, G. R. C.: Genetic factors in malignant melanoma. Cancer 27: 1261–1266 (1971).

Dr. C. M. SUTHERLAND, Tulane University School of Medicine, Department of Surgery, 1430 Tulane Avenue, New Orleans, LA 70112 (USA)

Pigment Cell, vol. 2, pp. 427–432 (Karger, Basel 1976)

# Malignant Melanoma: 'The Red Flag of Oncogenesis'[1]

WILLIAM S. FLETCHER and SALLY PALMER

Department of Surgery, and Tumor Registry, University of Oregon
Health Sciences Center, Portland, Oreg.

## Introduction

In 1971, FRASER *et al.* [3] reported a retrospective series of 154 patients treated for malignant melanoma at the University of California, San
Francisco. The most notable facet of this review was that 20% of the reported patients had other primary malignancies. Of these patients, 46%
had already died because of their disease, making this incidence of other
cancers even more significant.

To determine whether this alarming and important observation was
true in a different population in a different geographical area, the authors
reviewed the experience of the 3 University-affiliated hospitals and the
four private hospitals in the Portland, Oregon, area which serves as the
primary referral source for complicated cancer patients of the Columbia
River Basin. The population encompassed is about 2 million people [2].

The results of this survey indicated a 13% incidence of second primary malignancies at the University of Oregon Medical School, a 12% incidence at the Veterans Administration Hospital, Portland, Oregon, and a
3% incidence at St. Vincent's Hospital, 1 of the 4 private hospitals reviewed. The overall incidence of primary second malignancies when all of
the reported and reviewed hospitals were considered was 11%. This incidence – when compared with the 5.1% incidence of second primary tumors
in a large general tumor clinic population of 37,580, as reported by
MOERTEL *et al.* [5] – is significant at the 0.01 level.

1    Supported in part by Public Health Grants R10 CA 12279 and 1 P01 CA
15065 from the National Cancer Institute, and in part by the American Cancer Society, Oregon Division, and the Oregon Regional Medical Program.

Since that report, the University of Oregon Medical School registry has been completely abstracted and computerized, using the program developed for the Intermountain Regional Medical Program serving the populations of Utah, Montana, Wyoming, Colorado, and Nevada. The registry at St. Vincent's Hospital has also been computerized on the same system making the data from both institutions valid and deleting any duplication of patients.

In the interim, it has been documented that the incidence of other primary tumors in patients with malignant melanoma in the State of Utah alone is 8% [1]. For the whole Intermountain registry, which assesses over 100,000 patients, the incidence is 12.5% [6], essentially about the same as that seen in the University of Oregon Medical School.

The purpose of this communication is to update those data, utilizing only the completely computerized registries, to determine whether the same increased incidence of second primary tumors in patients with malignant melanoma still persists and is indeed valid.

### Method and Materials

Only the data from the University of Oregon Medical School and St. Vincent's Hospital (a private hospital) were considered. All duplications of patients carried on both registries were deleted. Table I indicates the current number of melanoma patients in each hospital, the number of patients with other primary tumors, the number of patients in whom the melanoma was diagnosed first, and the number of patients who had more than one primary melanoma.

Of the 50 patients with other primary tumors seen at the University of Oregon Medical School, 6 patients had 3 or more tumors (6 patients had a total of 20 primary tumors).

Data regarding primary site, age at diagnosis, and sex follow curves which have been presented by many authors [4]. However, all but 6 of the reported patients were Caucasian and these 6 were Negroes. In only one of these did the melanoma arise on a nonpigmented area (sole of the foot). There were no malignant melanomas reported among American Indians, Orientals, or persons of Mexican or other Latin descent which make up the other significant racial groups in the population at risk.

The histology of the second primary tumor in this population is close to that of the previous summary of all Portland hospitals, which was not previously published but may be seen in table II.

Table III indicates the sites of second primary tumors being reported from the University of Oregon Medical School at this time (50 patients, including 4 patients with multiple primary malignant melanoma).

*Table I.* Incidence of multiple primary tumors in patients with malignant melanoma – 1974

|  | University of Oregon Medical School | St. Vincent's Hospital | Total | Percent |
|---|---|---|---|---|
| Total melanoma patients reported | 343 | 151 | 494 | |
| Number of patients with multiple primary tumors | 46 (13.4%) | 17 (11.3%) | 63 | 12.7 |
| Number of patients with multiple melanoma primary tumors | 4 | 3 (1)[1] | 7 (1)[1] | <1 |
| Number of cases in which the melanoma was diagnosed first | 30 (65%) | 12 (70%) | 43 | 66.6 |

1 Seven definite and 1 probable.

## Discussion

It is clear that the increased incidence of second primary malignant tumors in patients with malignant melanoma is statistically valid, at least in the northwestern part of the United States.

It was originally thought that this might represent a peculiarity of patients referred to University hospitals or major medical centers. However, that does not appear to be the case when one considers the fact that the incidence of second primary malignancies changed in a period of 3 years at St. Vincent's Hospital from 3 to 11% with the advent of a modern comprehensive computerized tumor registry. This observation is reinforced by the fact that the overall incidence of second primary cancers in patients with malignant melanoma in the Intermountain Regional Medical Program's registry is on the order of 12.5%. This registry encompasses all of the hospitals and patients in a 5-state area. Therefore, it becomes increasingly important to document not only the incidence of a particular cancer, but what happens to that patient thereafter.

The possibility that the population at risk might be a major factor in the data presented was considered. The population at risk in the Colum-

*Table II.* Melanoma study, 6 Portland hospitals – 1971 [2]

| | |
|---|---|
| Total number of melanoma patients | 699 |
| Number of double primary tumors | 63 |
| Number of patients with 3 or more tumors | 11 |
| Number of patients with multiple primary melanomas | 4 |
| | |
| *Histology of second primary tumors* | |
| Malignant melanoma | 4 |
| Multiple skin | 24 |
| Leukemia | 1 |
| Hodgkin's disease | 1 |
| Sarcoma of 4 types | 5 |
| Cervix | 5 |
| Ovary | 2 |
| Vagina | 1 |
| Vulva | 2 |
| Prostate | 5 |
| Testis | 1 |
| Penis | 1 |
| Colon | 3 |
| Rectum | 5 |
| Kidney | 1 |
| Bladder | 2 |
| Lip | 3 |
| Lung | 2 |
| Breast | 2 |
| Endometrium | 1 |
| Primary unknown | 2 |

bia River Basin is primarily fair-skinned people of Western European origin, i.e. Nordic, Teutonic, Anglo-Saxon, and persons of Gaelic descent. This still appears to be a major factor. It is particularly noteworthy that non-Caucasians at risk to the same environmental exposures such as sunlight, urban living, and agricultural carcinogens did not develop the disease. These are primarily Indians, Orientals, and Latins, none of whom, in this series, developed a malignant melanoma.

Thus, it can be seen that there are multiple factors that work to develop a malignant melanoma or other cancer. Probably the most important of these in the genesis of malignant melanoma is the genetic factor. The second most important is whatever carcinogenic stimulus may be applied to that genetic predisposition, be the carcinogenic stimulus exposure

*Table III.* Histology of second primary tumors, University of Oregon Medical School – 1974

| | |
|---|---|
| Malignant melanoma | 4 |
| Breast | 2 |
| Colon/rectum | 4 |
| Parotid gland | 2 |
| Prostate | 1 |
| Thyroid | 1 |
| Lung | 1 |
| Lymphoma | 2 |
| Leukemia | 2 |
| Endometrium | 1 |
| Cervix | 5 |
| Ovary | 2 |
| Vagina | 1 |
| Sarcoma | 3 |
| Mesothelioma | 1 |
| Undetermined | 2 |
| Multiple skin | 16 |
| Total | 50 |

to sunlight, viruses, hydrocarbons, or other known carcinogenic stimuli. The possibility of an immunologic deficit has not yet been studied.

It is of interest that most of the second primary tumors arose in squamous epithelium while the bulk of the remainder were of histologic types currently thought to be of possible viral etiology. These include sarcomas, Hodgkin's disease, leukemia, and carcinoma of the cervix.

In the earlier publication [2], the incidence of a previous malignancy was roughly 50% while 3 years later, the incidence of the previous malignancy has dropped to about 30% and the melanoma was diagnosed first in about 70% of the cases. This indicates that the medical and lay population are more aware of the risk of malignant melanoma and that persons with melanoma are being treated earlier and more effectively. More than half of the patients described earlier are already dead because of their malignant melanoma; many of these were people in the 20- to 50-year age group. In short, patients with malignant melanoma are being diagnosed earlier and are being treated more effectively. Therefore, the survivors appear to be at a greatly increased risk of developing another primary cancer and must be followed not only for their malignant melanoma but with great attention to the possible development of a second primary cancer.

## Summary

The incidence of second primary malignancies in a population of 494 malignant melanoma patients was reviewed and found to be 63 or 12.7%. This is more than double the incidence of second primary tumors in a general tumor clinic population. Over half of these generally young patients are dead and no longer at risk. The diagnosis of a malignant melanoma should be thought of as 'the red flag of oncogenesis' with the patient not only being at high risk of recurrence, but also at risk of developing one or more other primary cancers. In short, the diagnosis of malignant melanoma is virtually tantamount to an expectation of death from cancer.

## References

1   COWAN, L. B.; SMART, C. R., and MOSLANDER, V.: Melanoma in Utah. Rocky Mt. med. J. 68: 29–32 (1971).
2   FLETCHER, W. S.: The incidence of other primary tumors in patients with malignant melanoma. Pigment Cell, vol. 1, pp. 255–260 (Karger, Basel 1973).
3   FRASER, D. G.; BULL, J. G., jr., and DUNPHY, J. E.: Malignant melanoma and coexisting malignant neoplasms. Am. J. Surg. 122: 169–174 (1971).
4   McCARTHY, W. H. (ed.): Melanoma and skin cancer. Proc. Int. Cancer Conf., Sydney 1972.
5   MOERTEL, C. G.; DOCKERTY, M. B., and BAGGENSTOSS, A. H.: Multiple primary neoplasms. I. Introduction and presentation of data. Cancer 14: 221–230 (1961).
6   SMART, C.: Personal commun. (1972).

Dr. WILLIAM S. FLETCHER, University of Oregon Health Sciences Center, 3181 S.W. Sam Jackson Park Road, Portland, OR 97201 (USA)

# Glossary

ACTH. See Adrenocorticotrophic hormone.

Adenosine triphosphate (ATP). A nucleotide synthesized mainly in mitochondria, through the Embden-Meyerhof pathway; principal means of cellular energy transfer; present in cytoplasm and nucleus of the cell. Cyclic AMP is formed from ATP by adenyl cyclase. See Adenyl cyclase, Cyclic AMP, Embden-Meyerhof pathway, and Mitochondria.

Adenyl cyclases. A group of enzymes which catalyze the formation of cyclic AMP from ATP in response to specific hormones such as MSH, ACTH, epinephrine, glucagon, luteinizing hormone, antidiuretic hormone, and others. Normal melanocytes, and at least some melanoma cells, have adenyl cyclase systems which respond specifically to MSH. Non-MSH-responsive adenyl cyclases are found in other tissues. See Adenosine triphosphate, Cyclic AMP, ACTH, Ephinephrine, and MSH.

Adrenaline. See Epinephrine.

Adrenergic nerves. Postganglionic sympathetic nerves, activated by, or liberating norepinephrine (noradrenaline). The melanophores of teleost fishes are adrenergically innervated; their $\alpha$-adrenergic receptors mediate melanosome aggregation, while their $\beta$-adrenergic receptors are involved in pigment dispersion. See Norepinephrine.

Adrenochrome. A red oxidation product of adrenaline.

Adrenocorticotrophic hormone (ACTH). Polypeptide hormone produced by the anterior lobe of the pituitary, in response to stressful stimuli, resulting in the production of corticosteroids by the adrenal cortex. The action of ACTH in stimulating the nutrition, growth, and function of the adrenal cortex is mediated by cyclic AMP. The first 13 amino acids in the ACTH polypeptide chain are identical with those of the $\alpha$-melanocyte-stimulating hormone (MSH). See Corticosterone, MSH, and Cyclic AMP.

Albinism. Congenital absence or reduction of pigment. An inborn error of metabolism, inherited as an autosomal recessive trait, characterized by the partial or total absence of melanin in the skin, hair, and eyes. The melanocytes are structurally normal; however, there is probably a block of deficiency in the pathway between tyrosine and melanin. Albinos are rarely afflicted with melanoma, but have a high incidence of squamous cell carcinoma.

*Allogeneic.* Pertaining to genetically dissimilar individuals of the same species.

*Allogeneic inhibition.* The growth inhibitory effects on cells, due to an antigenic dissimilarity, which allogeneic cells exert on each other when in contact, both *in vitro* and *in vivo*.

*Allograft.* A graft derived from an allogeneic donor.

*Amelanotic melanoma.* Malignant neoplasm, derived from melanocytes, but not forming melanin. See Melanoma.

*Aminophylline.* One of the family of methylxanthines which inhibit phosphodiesterase; it is used in the measurements of adenyl cyclase activity to prevent hydrolysis of accumulating cyclic AMP. See Adenyl cyclases, Cyclic AMP.

*Antibody-mediated immunity.* Humoral immunity depending directly or indirectly on the capacity of circulating protective antibodies to intercept antigens, which are then neutralized or opsonized.

*ATP.* See Adenosine triphosphate.

*Autochthonous.* Found in the part of the body in which it originates, as in the case of an autochthonous tumor; a spontaneous tumor borne by the host of origin.

*Autologous.* Derived from the subject itself.

*B-16 mouse melanoma.* A spontaneous, metastasizing pigmented melanoma, which arose in the skin, at the base of the ear, in a C57BL/6J strain mouse in 1954. It is transplantable in the strain of origin. Most lines carry the LDH-elevating virus. See Melanoma, LDH-virus.

*Basal cells.* Cells forming the basal layer of the stratum germinativum of the epidermis. Basal cells are the principle dividing cell population, and are especially subject to actinic neoplastic transformation. Since melanocytes frequently accompany basal cell tumors, the pigment they produce may lead to an erroneous clinical diagnosis of melanoma. This is of prognostic importance since basal cell carcinomas are relatively benign compared with melano-carcinoma.

*Birthmark.* A circumscribed benign growth in the skin which is evident at birth and frequently pigmented. A congenital nevus of any type. See Nevus.

*Bloch reaction.* Development of melanin *in vitro*; observed in melanocytes following the addition of dopa, described by the Swiss dermatologist, B. BLOCH, 1878–1933.

*Blue nevus.* A nevus, covered by smooth skin, which appears to be blue, or blue-black. The lesion is composed of pigmented spindle cells in the lower dermis; the unusual color is due to the quantity of melanin and its location in the dermis. Clinically, there are several varieties; the Jadassohn-Tieche and the cellular blue nevus are the most common. The latter is sometimes misdiagnosed as melanosarcoma. Malignant blue nevi are extremely rare. See Nevus.

*Carotenoids.* Lipid soluble, yellow to orange-red pigments universally present in photosynthetic tissues of plants; also found in marine invertebrates, fish, amphibians and in feathers.

*Catecholamine.* Generic term for compounds containing a catechol group and an amine group, generally considered to be derivatives of $\beta$-phenylethylamine. The catecholamines, dopamine, epinephrine, and norepinephrine, are of importance in the sympathetic nervous system, and are melanin-aggregating agents when applied to adrenergically innervated fish melanophores.

*Cell line M40.* Derived from a human melanoma; has separate and distinct sites for fetal-associated and tumor-specific antigens.

*Cell-mediated immunity.* See Thymus-derived lymphocytes.

*Chediak-Higashi syndrome.* Pleiotrophic syndrome in man, characterized by autosomal recessive inheritance, dilution of pigmentation in eye, skin, and hair, giant granules in the melanocytes and leukocytes, photophobia, susceptibility to infection and early death.

*Chloasma (mask of pregnancy).* Abnormal collections of pigment covering a relatively large and diffuse skin area. Hyperpigmentation may occur as a result of the action of hormones, friction, heat, light, application of various irritant substances to the skin. Melasma is specifically associated with pregnancy, or systemic diseases such as tuberculosis, cancer, and endocrine diseases.

*Cholinergic nerves.* Postganglionic, parasympathetic nerves which secrete acetylcholine at their axon terminals. Adrenergic, rather than cholinergic nerves, are apparently involved in the innervated melanophores of fish. See Adrenergic nerves.

*Chromatophores.* Pigment-bearing cells of invertebrates and lower vertebrates, which are derived from the embryonic neural crest and are capable of effecting color changes by concentrating or dispersing their pigment granules. Specific examples are: erythrophores, iridophores, xanthophores, and melanophores.

*Chromatotrophic hormone (CTH).* Synonymous with MSH or intermedin; refers to actions on iridophores, as well as melanophores. See MSH.

*Cloudman S-91 mouse melanoma.* A classical, transplantable, metastasizing mouse melanoma discovered by A. M. CLOUDMAN in 1937. The original tumor arose in the skin at the base of the tail of a DBA strain female mouse. Melanotic and amelanotic variants are available. Most lines carry the LDH-elevating virus. See Melanoma.

*Corticosterone.* Steroid hormone produced by the adrenal cortex in response to ACTH production by the pituitary. Corticosterone is the major steroid produced in mice, rats, and other rodents; whereas cortisol is the major glucocorticoid in human beings. When elevated, these hormones have adverse effects upon the immunological system, including involution of lymph nodes, spleen, thymus, and a lymphocytopenia, with a resultant impairment of cell-mediated immunity. See Adrenocorticotropic hormone, Thymus-derived lymphocytes, and LDH-virus.

*Cross syndrome.* Oculocerebral syndrome encompassing hypopigmentation of hair and skin, gingival fibromatosis, microphthalmia, oligophrenia, spasticity, and athetoid movements.

*Cyclic AMP (3',5'-cyclic adenosine monophosphate).* Nucleotide formed from ATP by adenyl cyclases. Cyclic AMP mediates the effects of MSH upon melanocytes and melanophores, and is also the biochemical mediator of various other hormone-induced cellular responses. See Adenyl cyclase, Adenosine trophosphate, Adrenocorticotropic hormone, Cyclic nucleotide phosphodiesterase and MSH.

*Cyclic nucleotide phosphodiesterase.* Enzyme found in tissues containing adenyl cyclase, which catalyzes the conversion of cyclic 3',5'-AMP to

5'-AMP. This enzyme is inhibited by methylxanthines, such as caffeine, aminophylline and theophylline. See Adenyl cyclase, Cyclic AMP.

*Dendrites.* Elongated, branched protoplasmic processes characteristic of cells derived from the neural crest, including melanocytes, chromatophores and nerve cells. In the latter they conduct nerve impulses toward the cell body.

*Deoxyribonucleic acid (DNA).* Helical molecule constructed of a sequence of paired nucleotides on a deoxyribose backbone. DNA bears the genetic code, which is transcribed to messenger RNA, and carried to the ribosomes where it is translated into proteins. Substitution of synthetic nucleotides for naturally occurring ones has resulted in a lessening of tumorigenicity in some tumor cell lines. In melanoma cell lines, melanogenesis has also been suppressed by such substitution.

*Dermal chromatophore unit.* A compound functional unit which brings about color changes in fish and amphibians, consisting of the integrated response of melanophores, xanthophores, and iridophores, that provides the mechanism for integumental color change in response to hormonal stimulation either in the intact animal or *in vitro.*

*Dermis (corium).* The subepithelial connective tissue component of the skin, which is derived from the embryonic mesoderm. See Epidermis.

*DNA.* See Deoxyribonucleic acid.

*Dopa (3,4-dihydroxyphenylalanine).* Amino acid, intermediate product in the oxidation of tyrosine by oxidases (tyrosinase, dopa oxidase, peroxidase) to melanin. The naturally occurring amino acid is in the L-form. L-Dopa is

also involved in the synthesis of catecholamines.

*Dopa oxidase.* The mammalian enzyme which converts dopa to dopaquinone in the process of melanin synthesis. Although the terms dopa oxidase and tyrosinase are used interchangeably, it has not been unequivocally established that mammalian dopa oxidase can use tyrosine as a substrate. See Raper theory, Tyrosinase, and Peroxidase.

*Dopamine.* A catecholamine intermediate in the formation of norepinephrine and epinephrine (adrenaline) from dopa. See Dopa, Epinephrine, and Norepinephrine.

*DTIC (dimethyltriazeno imidazole carboxamide).* Inhibits L-dopa oxidation *in vitro,* and has been used as a chemotherapeutic agent against melanoma.

*Ectoderm.* Outermost of the three primary embryonic germ layers, and source of neural tissue, the neural crest, sense organs, epidermis, melanocytes, and chromatophores. See Neural crest.

*Embden-Meyerhof pathway.* Metabolic, glycolytic pathway by which glucose is converted to alcohol or to lactic acid, yielding ATP, in the cell. See Adenosine triphosphate.

*Endoplasmic reticulum (ER).* A system of subcellular structures consisting of interconnected tubules and vesicles (cisternae) that occupy the cytoplasm of metabolically active cells. The microsome fraction obtained from disrupted cells is derived from the endoplasmic reticulum and has a high RNA content. The ER is postulated to be involved in the transfer of enzymes, including tyrosinase and dopa oxidase, from ribosomes to Golgi vesicles, in the formation of premelanosomes.

*Ephelid.* See Freckle.

*Epidermal melanin unit.* Melanocyte

plus an associated pool of keratinocytes (Malpighian cells) the number of which may vary. The melanocyte and the Malpighian cells appear to operate closely together, with the melanocyte synthesizing the pigment and donating it to the Malpighian cells. They can be considered to comprise a structural, as well as a functional unit that is analogous in some respects to other compound cellular functional units such as the nephron. See Melanocyte, Keratinocyte.

*Epidermis.* Outer stratified squamous keratinizing epithelium of the skin, which is derived from the embryonic ectoderm. In addition to being a protective covering for the entire body, the epidermis gives rise to hair, feathers, scales, nails, hoofs, and several types of glands. It is composed of five layers. See Dermis.

*Epinephrine (adrenaline).* A catecholamine having hormone action, produced by the adrenal medulla; it inhibits the release of MSH and ACTH from the pituitary, and causes melanin aggregation in teleost and amphibian melanophores. See Catecholamines.

*Erythrophore.* Chromatophore containing a red (pteridine or carotenoid) pigment that occurs in some fishes and crustaceans. See Carotenoid and Pteridine pigment.

*Eumelanin.* The dark brown variety of melanins, widely distributed in the tissues of animals and birds. The pigment is usually formed from tyrosine or dopa under the catalytic influence of tyrosinase (dopa oxidase). See Phaeomelanin.

*Eyestalk.* Site of chromatophorotrophin production in crustaceans.

*Familial melanoma.* Melanoma which occurs in more than one member of the same human family. Initial data suggests that an autosomal dominant gene with incomplete penetrance may be involved.

*Fortner hamster melanomas.* A series of 'spontaneous' pigmented tumors which arose over a period of time in a colony of hamsters maintained in the laboratory of J. G. FORTNER. Various melanotic and amelanotic lines are maintained by transplantation in Syrian golden hamsters.

*Freckle (ephelid).* A tan to brown macule found on areas of skin exposed to sunlight. Freckles are not present at birth, and do not appear until after infancy, despite exposure to sunlight. However, the role of sunlight in the development of freckles is indisputable. There is an heritable tendency. See Lentigo.

*Gallophaeomelanins.* Group of phaeomelanic pigments of high molecular weight (2,000–50,000) which occur in hair, fur, and feathers. They are insoluble in dilute acids, but dissolve in alkalies giving yellow-brown solutions which display no defined absorption maxima in the ultraviolet and visible region. See Phaeomelanins and Trichosiderins.

*Genes for melanogenesis.* Genes which control the various synthetic steps, including enzymes, involved in melanogenesis. Abnormalities in any of these genes can result in various pigmentation disorders. See Familial melanoma, Albinism, Cross, and Chediak-Higashi syndromes.

*Gloger's rule.* 'Darkest-colored animals are generally found in the warm, humid tropics; grading to the lightest-colored animals in the cold, dry arctic regions.'

*Golgi apparatus.* Intracellular complex of vesicles and fine tubules, adjacent to the nucleus. Its function may include coating the products of exocrine secretion with a protein envelope, and the secretion of complex carbohydrates. The Golgi apparatus is postulated to be the site of origin of the enzymic components of the premelanosomes.

Guanophore. Chromatophore containing reflecting platelets which are partially composed of guanine. See Iridophore.

Halo nevus. A pigmented nevus surrounded by a halo of acquired leukoderma. Ultrastructural investigations indicate that the early inflammatory reaction consists of active stimulated lymphocytes and monocytes migrating from blood vessels to form close association with nevus cell nests. Nevus cell destruction is associated with macrophages involved in phagocytosis of cytoplasmic remnants and pigment granules. Antibodies against the cytoplasm of melanoma cells have been found in the sera of patients with regressing halo nevi.

Harding-Passey mouse melanoma. A classical, transplantable pigmented mouse tumor discovered in the laboratory of R. A. PASSEY in 1925. The original tumor arose spontaneously in the ear of a non-inbred mouse, and will grow in a variety of mouse strains. This tumor exhibits a high population of pigment-containing macrophages, and a low capacity for metastasizing. Most lines carry the LDH-elevating virus. See Melanoma.

Hermansky-Pudlak syndrome. Albinism associated with hemorrhagic diathesis, due to a platelet storage pool deficiency.

Hogben and Slome melanophore index. Measure of the degree of pigment dispersal in melanophores.

Humoral immunity. See Antibody-mediated immunity.

Hypothalamus. A region at the base of the brain, situated in close proximity to the pituitary. The hypothalamus produces a number of neuro-hormones which regulate the release of various pituitary hormones, including MSH. See MIF, MRF, and MSH.

Iglesias rat melanomas. Several spontaneous, transplantable pigmented tumors discovered by R. IGLESIAS, Santiago, Chile, in A×C strain rats. The first tumor was transplanted successfully in 1957. See Melanoma.

Intermedin. The same as MSH, a term used by some authors working with melanophores. The term was originally used to indicate that the hormone is produced by the pars intermedia of the hypophysis. See MSH.

Iridophore. Chromatophore containing iridescent guanine-containing granules, which occurs in the skin of cephalopods, fishes, and reptiles. See Guanophore.

Iridosomes (reflecting platelets). Granules containing guanine, found primarily in iridophores.

Keratinocyte (Malpighian cell). The epidermal cell which synthesizes keratin, stores melanin, and together with the melanocyte forms the binary cell system of the epidermis. The keratinocyte develops through successive stages of basal cell, prickle cell, and granular cell, eventually producing the noncellular, fibrillar material, keratin. See Epidermal melanin unit.

Langerhans' cell (suprabasal clear cell). Dendritic, star-shaped, nonpigmented cell situated in the epidermis. The Langerhans' cell contains nonmelanized disc-shaped organelles bearing some resemblance to melanosomes; however, it is tyrosinase and dopa-negative. It is considered by some to be a phagocytic cell which engulfs degenerate melanocytes in piebald and vitiligenous skin.

LDH-virus (lactate dehydrogenase-elevating virus). Benign RNA-virus ubiquitously distributed in materials routinely transplanted in mice, including transplantable melanomas. The virus infection causes an elevation in several plasma enzymes, including lactate dehydrogenase, from which its name is derived. Of greater experimental concern, this virus causes modifications of the immunological system which may compromise experimental results.

*Lentigo.* A well circumscribed, round, pigmented macular lesion ranging in color from light tan to dark brown or even black. Lentigos, in contrast to senile lentigo, are not dependent upon sunlight; they may appear on any part of the body and are often found at birth, which distinguishes them from freckles. They differ from junctional nevi in that they are not potentially malignant. See Freckle, Nevus.

*Lipofuscin.* Golden brown pigment, considered to be a derivative of lysosomes, and found in certain tissues of older animals, especially in neurones and the cells of the myocardium. Lipofuscin is considered to be a component of neuromelanin, but is also postulated to be a degenerate 'wear and tear' pigment. See Lysosome, Neuromelanin.

*Lipophore.* Older collective term for erythrophores and xanthophores, used because of the solubility of their pigments in lipid solvents.

*Lymphotoxin.* Factor obtained from tissues of tumor-bearing mice; has the ability to kill tumor cells *in vitro,* similar to the action of living spleen cells.

*Malignant melanoma.* The term 'malignant melanoma' is a redundancy, and should not be used since melanomas are assumed to be malignant, unless specifically designated as juvenile melanomas, or 'benign', as in some ocular varieties. See Melanoma.

*Malpighian cells.* Keratinocytes which are closely associated with melanocytes in the epidermal melanin unit. Melanosomes produced by melanocytes are transferred to the Malpighian cells, which were named after the Italian anatomist, histologist, and embryologist, M. Malpighi, 1628–1694. See Epidermal melanin unit, and Keratinocytes.

*Melanin.* A generic term for a wide variety of natural pigments responsible for shades of black and brown found in plants and animals. Melanin is an insoluble, high molecular weight polymer derived from the enzymic oxidation of phenols, starting with tyrosine. In the case of vertebrates, melanin is synthesized in melanosomes, a cellular organelle within melanocytes or melanophores. See Eumelanin and Phaeomelanin.

*Melanin as semiconductor.* Melanins have been demonstrated to be amorphous semiconductors; some melanin-binding drugs alter this conductivity, as well as the threshold switching properties of melanins.

*Melanoblast.* An immature pigment cell; a precursor of the melanocyte and melanophore. See Melanocyte, Melanophore.

*Melanocyte.* A pigment synthesizing cell. A secretory cell, derived from the neural crest, that produces a specialized organelle, the melanosome, containing enzymes (dopa oxidase, tyrosinase, peroxidase) which catalyze the oxidation of the natural precursor tyrosine to an insoluble, dense polymer, melanin.

*Melanocyte-stimulating hormone.* See MSH.

*Melanogenesis.* Formation of melanin is probably initiated in the premelanosome and continued in the melanosome of the melanocyte or melanophore. In the presence of tyrosinase, dopa oxidase, or peroxidase, tyrosine is first oxidized to dopa; the dopa is then oxidized to dopa-quinone, which in turn is converted through several intermediates into a pigmented polymer, melanin.

*Melanoma.* Malignant neoplasm, derived from melanocytes. Malignant amelanotic varieties occur, also originating from melanocytes but not forming melanin.

*Melanoma-associated antigens.* Isolated from melanoma cells grown *in vitro*; appear to be glycoproteins. The melanoma antigens are distinct from known murine transplantation antigens.

*Melanophage.* Macrophage which has ingested or phagocytized melanin. A confusing term which should be abandoned.

*Melanophore.* A dermal melanocyte of cold-blooded vertebrates, constituting the pigmentary effector system (aggregation and dispersion of melanosomes within these melanophores).

*Melanosome.* An organelle that is surrounded by a membrane and contains a highly organized internal structure of longitudinally oriented strands or concentric lamellae that have a regular pattern of dense particles with a characteristic periodicity. The organelle may be spherical or elipsoid and may be from 0.5 to 1.0 $\mu$m in length, and from 0.2 to 0.3 $\mu$m in diameter. Melanosomes contain the melanin-synthesizing enzyme dopa oxidase (tyrosinase). See Melanocyte.

*Melanotrophin.* Synonymous with MSH, intermedin, and chromatophorotrophin.

*Melatonin (5-methoxy-N-acetyltryptamine).* Hormone produced by the pineal gland which lightens MSH-darkened skin; effects are specific for melanophores, having no effect on iridophores. Melatonin is responsible for dark-adaptation in larval amphibians. See MSH.

*Messenger RNA.* A ribonucleic acid that carries the code for a particular protein from nuclear deoxyribonucleic acid (DNA), and acts as a template for the formation of that protein. See Nuclear acidic proteins.

*Methylxanthines.* A family of compounds which competitively inhibit the hydrolysis of cyclic AMP by phosphodiesterase. See Aminophylline, Cyclic AMP, Phosphodiesterases.

*Microtubules.* Cellular organelles which, in melanocytes, appear to be involved in melanin aggregation in *Fundulus* melanophores, and possibly also in frog and other melanophores.

*MIF.* See MSH-release-inhibiting factor.

*Mitochondria.* Subcellular organelles of various size and shape, limited by an outer smooth membrane and an inner membrane showing infoldings (cristae mitochondriales). Mitochondria are the major sites of energy transduction and ATP synthesis in the cell. They possess cytochrome oxidase and other Krebs' cycle enzymes. See Adenosine triphosphate, and Embden-Meyerhof pathway.

*Mole (lay term for intradermal nevus).* A pigmented lesion in the skin, usually benign, resulting from the proliferation of melanocytes. See Nevus.

*MRF.* See MSH-releasing factor.

*MSH (melanocyte-stimulating hormone, also known as intermedin).* A polypeptide hormone of 13–22 amino acid residues, produced by the pars intermedia of the pituitary. MSH stimulates melanocytes and melanophores to produce pigment. In lower vertebrates, MSH effects melanin dispersion in melanophores, and is the only hormone of major importance in regulating iridophore responses. These effects are mediated by cyclic AMP. There are two types of MSH, $\alpha$ and $\beta$. MSH is related chemically to ACTH. See ACTH, Cyclic AMP.

*MSH-releasing factor (MRF)*. Postulated hypothalamic hormone which may release MSH from the pars intermedia of the pituitary. See MSH.

*MSH-release-inhibiting factor (MIF)*. Hypothalamic hormone which inhibits the release of MSH from the pituitary. See MSH.

*Neural crest*. Ectodermal embryonic site, lateral to the neural tube, from which cells of the adrenal medulla, nerve cells, and other dendritic cell arise.

*Neural pigments*. See Neuromelanin, and Lipofuscin.

*Neuromelanin*. Intraneuronal pigment; considered to be melanized lipofuscin. See Lipofuscin.

*Nevus*. A general term applied to discolored patches in the skin. Pigmented nevi may be either congenital or acquired lesions, and are due to benign melanocyte proliferation; pigmented nevi may become wholly or partially amelanotic. Certain pigmented nevi have malignant potential. Epithelial nevi are congenital hyperplastic lesions of epidermal cells which may appear to be pigmented as a consequence of the activity of associated melanocytes. Connective tissue nevi are congenital lesions in which there is a localized thickening of the dermis. Vascular nevi are those due to malformations of cutaneous blood vessels. Junctional, intradermal, and compound nevi are important clinical classifications.

*Norepinephrine (noradrenaline)*. A catecholamine; precursor of epinephrine produced by the adrenal medulla; also principal transmitter substance in sympathetic adrenergic neuro-effector junctions; a vasoconstrictor; reverses the effects of MSH upon teleost melanophores.

*Nuclear acidic proteins (NAP)*. Proteins associated with chromatin which are believed to be associated with genetic expression. MSH treatment of Cloudman mouse melanoma cells *in vitro* results in differences in the NAP as well as increased melanin content.

*Oncorna viruses*. Oncogenic RNA viruses with 70S RNA, RNA-directed DNA polymerase, and a particle density of 1.16–1.19 g/ml. These viruses have been found in various animal melanomas, and similar particles have been detected in human melanomas. Their etiological relationship to human tumors is uncertain. See RNA, RNA viruses.

*Parkinson's disease*. Paralysis agitans, a disease of the central nervous system which is associated with loss of pigment by the cells of the substantia nigra of the brain. This disease responds in some cases to the therapeutic administration of L-dopa.

*Peroxidase*. Enzyme catalyzing the oxidation of various substances, such as diphenols, aromatic amines, and peroxides. Peroxidase may be involved in the oxidation of tyrosine to dopa during melanin and/or catecholamine synthesis in mammals. Peroxidase has been detected in some melanoma preparations.

*Phaeomelanins*. The term includes all red, yellow, orange and brown pigments which are formed by a deviation of the eumelanin pathway involving interreaction of cysteine with dopa quinones produced by the enzymatic oxidation of tyrosine. See Gallophaeomelanins and Trichosiderins.

*Phenylalanine ammonia-lyase*. Enzyme which degrades the amino acid phenylalanine, and inhibits the growth of B-16 melanoma *in vivo*.

*Phosphodiesterases.* Enzymes found in tissues containing adenyl cyclase; these enzymes are involved in the biochemical mechanisms for converting cyclic AMP to 5'-AMP. They are also found in snake venom. See Cyclic AMP, Cyclic nucleotide phosphodiesterase, MSH.

*Piebaldism.* Localized hypomelanosis of skin and hair, which may be inherited either as an autosomal dominant or recessive trait, and histologically characterized by the complete absence of melanocytes, or by the presence of abnormal melanocytes, in contrast to the morphologically normal melanocytes found in albinism.

*Pineal gland (epiphysis).* Endocrine gland rising from the roof of the third ventricle of the brain, which produces serotonin and melatonin. See Melatonin.

*Pituitary (hypophysis).* An endocrine gland attached to the infundibulum of the brain, which is under the general control of the hypothalamus. The anterior portion of the pituitary secretes ACTH and other hormones, while the closely related MSH is produced by the pars intermedia. See MSH, ACTH.

*Pleiotrophic syndrome.* See Chediak-Higashi syndrome.

*Premelanosome.* An immature melanosome. A cytoplasmic granule in melanocytes which is the site of melanin formation. See Melanosome.

*Primordial organelle.* Postulated chromatophore organelle of lower vertebrates which may develop into a melanosome, pterinosome, or iridosome, depending upon specific developmental cues.

*Prosencephalon.* The anterior division of the embryonic brain, which forms the cerebral hemispheres.

*Pteridine pigments.* Yellow crystalline bicyclic bases found in pterinosomes; for example, xanthopterin (2 amino, 4',6'-dihydro pteridine). Pteridine pigments were first discovered in the wings of butterflies (Greek *pteron*, wing). See Pterinosomes, Erythrophores, and Xanthophores.

*Pterinosomes.* Granules containing pteridine pigments, found in lower vertebrate erythrophores.

*Purine pigments.* Principal pigments of iridophores (guanine, hypoxanthine and adenine). See Iridophores, Iridosomes.

*Quinones.* Intermediates in the formation of melanin from tyrosine.

*Raper theory.* The biochemical scheme proposed by H. S. RAPER in 1927, to account for the metabolic pathway leading from tyrosine to melanin.

*Reflecting platelet.* See Iridosome.

*Retinal pigment epithelium.* Innermost layer of the eye, which synthesizes melanosomes in embryonic life. The cells of the retinal pigment epithelium are interdigitated with the rods and cones of the neural retina.

*Retinal pigment hormones.* Crustacean hormones that regulate pigment movements in the retina.

*Ribonucleic acid (RNA).* Single or double stranded chains of ribonucleotides. The three major types of ribonucleic acid in cells are messenger RNA, ribosomal RNA, and transfer RNA. RNA is concerned with the transfer of the genetic code, carried in DNA, to the cellular site of protein synthesis. Certain viruses possess the only known double stranded RNA. See Deoxyribonucleic acid.

*Ribosomes.* RNA-rich, cytoplasmic granules that function in protein and enzyme synthesis; site of tyrosinase/dopa oxidase synthesis.

*RNA.* See Ribonucleic acid.

*RNA C-type viruses.* RNA viruses which have been detected in many animal tumor cell lines, including Greene hamster melanoma cells.

*RNA viruses.* See RNA C-type viruses, Oncorna viruses, LDH-virus.

*Serotonin (5-hydroxytryptamine).* Pineal indole, which acts to disperse melanin in *Xenopus* melanophores. See Melatonin.

*Substantia nigra.* See Parkinson's disease.

*Syngeneic (isogenic, isologous).* Implies a degree of genetic identity between mammals of the same species, enabling acceptance of homografts. Occurs naturally in identical twins and may be achieved experimentally in mice by about 20 successive generations of brother-sister mating.

*Tanning.* Uniform darkening of the skin following exposure to sunlight or other effective radiation. Following irradiation, there appear to be two effects: (1) an immediate oxidation of existing melanin in the skin, making it darker; (2) after a few days an increase in tyrosinase/dopa oxidase activity, resulting in the formation of more melanin. Increased proliferation of latent epidermal melanocytes or stem cells may also occur.

*Thymus-derived lymphocytes (T cells).* Effector lymphocytes of cell-mediated immunity. T cells act against malignant cells, including melanoma cells. T cells can be separated from other leukocytes on the basis of their receptors for sheep RBCs. These small lymphocytes are usually long-lived, and recirculate through the blood stream and the cortical areas of the lymphoid tissues, returning to the blood via lymphatic vessels.

*Trichosiderins.* Group of phaeomelanic pigments, originally considered to contain iron (hence the name), which occur in hair, fur and feathers. Most trichosiderins have characteristic pH-dependent colors and display well-defined absorption maxima in the visible and ultraviolet region. In contrast to gallophaeomelanins, they are soluble in both dilute acids and alkalies. See Phaeomelanins and Gallophaeomelanins.

*Tyrosinase (dopa oxidase).* Aerobic oxidase; copper-protein complex found in plants and insects which catalyzes the oxidation of both tyrosine and dopa. Although the term 'tyrosinase' has been used interchangeably with dopa oxidase in reference to mammalian melanogenesis, the role and characterization of mammalian 'tyrosinase' is also called catechol oxidase, polyphenol oxidase, and phenolase. The systematic name and number is 1.10.3.1 $o$-diphenol:oxygen oxidoreductase. The recommended trivial name is $o$-diphenol oxidase. See Dopa oxidase, Peroxidase.

*Tyrosine phenol-lyase.* An enzyme which degrades the amino acid tyrosine, and has inhibitory effects on the growth of B-16 melanoma *in vivo*.

*Vitiligo (leukoderma).* Condition in which there are patches of depigmentation of the skin. Postulated to be due to replacement of melanocytes in the basal layer of the epidermis by Langerhans' cells. Vitiligo is noncongenital. See Langerhans' cells.

*Xanthophore.* Chromatophore occurring in fishes, amphibians, and certain reptiles, containing yellow pigment, composed of pteridines, flavines and carotenoids.

# Author Index

# Subject Index